Mad Skills Exercise Mixtape

Volume 2

100+ Illustrated Garage Gym Workouts

Ben Musholt

First edition published in 2020 by BPM Rx, Inc.

ISBN: 9798673889824

BPM Rx and Strength Mob are registered trademarks of BPM Rx, Inc.

www.BPMRx.com
www.BenMusholt.com

This book is dedicated to my Father.
Thank you for sharing your love of books, martial arts, and creativity.

www.EdMusholt.com

DISCLAIMER

The material contained in this book is for informational purposes only. BPM Rx Inc. and Ben Musholt advise that the exercises and workouts described in this book can be strenuous, and may not be suitable for all individuals. The author makes no claim to the safety of the movements or techniques in this book, and advises consultation with a qualified professional to determine if they are appropriate for you. It is strongly recommended that the reader consult with a physician before engaging in any of the physical activities described in this book, or any other exercise routine. The publisher and author disclaim any and all liability for any injury or conditioned sustained via performance of the exercises in this book, and may NOT be held liable for any damages from the practice of said exercises.

Your health and safety are most important.

Be smart: Consult with professionals, train with caution, and use appropriate exercise progressions.

Intro

Welcome to the Mad Skills Exercise Mixtape – Volume Two. In this installment, we will be exploring 100+ workouts that can be done in your garage gym. This book is a companion to the *Mad Skills Exercise Encyclopedia* and is a follow-up to the first mixtape. The front half of the book (Side A) explores routines that can be performed with common garage gym items, like your barbell, kettlebells, dumbbells, and a pull-up bar. The second half of the book (Side B), introduces a steel mace for additional variety in your training. The purpose of this mixtape is to provide exposure to numerous exercise combinations that fit together into effective garage gym workouts.

If you've already worked through volume one, then the following intro pages will be a repeat for you. I would encourage you to reread them, however, as a reminder about the workout structure and general movement advice.

Workout Structure

The workouts that you'll encounter all stick to a common training structure. The format is a three-tiered system of the warm-up, circuit training, and cool-down. The warm-up generally entails two bodyweight or light-weight exercises to get your heart rate up and prepare you for more intense exercise. Use the warm-up[1] as a time to prime your nervous system and get your joints ready for action.

The circuit training portion of each workout is the heart and soul of mixtape. In this middle section, you'll find three to four exercises that address *leg strength*, *upper body pulling strength*, and *upper body pushing strength*. By hitting these three categories, and varying the type of leg strengthening between sessions, circuit training like this provides a powerful whole-body workout.

---

[1] By the way, don't feel limited to only perform the two movements listed in the warm-up section. Add enough movement until you feel your body is sufficiently prepared for heavier exercise.

Intro

The last section of each workout adds another two bodyweight movements to the session. These final exercises are often different calisthenics, like push-up variations or core strengthening movements. Think of these as the finishing touches to each workout. They will help you cool down after the more intense exercises of the circuit. They may also help address any body regions that might not have been targeted by the previous three to four exercises.

2-3-2 Method

2 Warm-up Exercises

3 (or 4) Circuit Exercises

2 Cool-down Exercises

Use What You've Got

Don't be discouraged if you don't have every piece equipment displayed in the book. It can take years to build out your garage gym—there's no reason to go broke purchasing all of the gear at once! The best recommendation is to be flexible and creative in your use of what exercise tools you *do* have.

Intro

For many movements, a dumbbell can be a great substitute for a kettlebell. If you don't have a weight bench or a plyo box, a stairwell can work well for jumps and split squats. If you don't have a pull-up bar, many of the hanging movements can be imitated from gymnastics rings. Likewise, if you don't have a sandbag, load up a duffle bag or a backpack.

The one sticking point here is that you are probably going to want to purchase a barbell sooner than later. Garage gym training centers around the barbell for numerous skills. Once you add a barbell to your at-home arsenal, you won't ever look back.

Why You Won't See Specific Reps, Sets, or Weight Recommendations

As you dive into the workouts, you'll notice that they don't have associated reps and sets, or prescribe a certain weight to lift. Why have these been omitted? It's because each reader is starting from a different point and has access to a different set of equipment. Perhaps you don't have a 50 lb kettlebell, or your dumbbells don't go up to 25 lbs. It could be that you are just starting to build your garage gym and don't have a full array of weight plates yet. More importantly, maybe you are new to the fitness journey and aren't ready for the intensity that someone else can tolerate.

Prescribing a workload at a specific resistance level is bound to be too much for some, and not enough for others. The diagrams are meant to illustrate the variety of ways that movements can be pieced together for an effective garage gym workout. If you want a personalized approach to fitness, you'll need to meet one-on-one with a coach.

Intro

However, that doesn't mean that you are totally on your own here. By sticking to a few simple parameters, you can adjust each workout into a productive session. In terms of general guidelines, here is a basic framework to follow:

Warm-up

The initial phase of your workout should last between *5 to 10 minutes*. You want it to be long enough to prepare you for action, but not so long that it wears you out for the bulk of the session. In general, a good target is to perform **50 to 100 reps of each motion**. An example could be 100 jumping jacks, and 50 prisoner lunges. It could also be 50 mountain climbers, and 100 twisting jumps. If the movement is locomotive, like a bear crawl or a crab walk, set a target distance of 15 to 30 feet and run it for a few lengths.

There is always the exception though, so be mindful and adjust as necessary. Burpees are a good example. You might find them in the warm-up, but trying to do 50 to 100 would be overkill. It might make more sense to do 10 to 20 burpees. Similarly, beginners might be toasted after 25 air squats, so doing more would only limit their abilities in the circuit training portion. Use your head, and understand that this part of the workout is only meant to get you ready for the next portion of the session.

Additionally, don't think you have to perform each exercise distinct from the other one. The two warm-up movements can be done sequentially, or you can alternate back and forth until you are sufficiently prepped.

Prior to heavy lifting with the barbell, it's smart idea to do a warm-up set or two at a lighter weight. Jumping directly to your target load might be too strenuous right off the bat. Stay vigilant so you can have a long and injury-free training career.

INTRO

Circuit Training

Recall that each circuit is going to consist of three to four movements. To turn these exercises into an effective circuit, you want to **cycle through the movements for three to five "sets"**. If you are a beginner, or are pressed for time, cycle through the movements three times. If you want a heavier-duty workout, push yourself to complete five or more cycles. Four rounds through seems to be a sweet spot. When a four-round circuit is combined with the warm-up and cool-down, you should be able to complete the workout in about 30 minutes.

Now, how many repetitions of each exercise should you perform? As a rule of thumb, **5 to 12 repetitions of an exercise are a good target**. Bodybuilders might use higher rep ranges, and power lifters might use lower ones, but they have specific training goals in mind. For the purposes of an at-home fitness regimen, 5 to 12 reps are a safe target. Of course, the caveat is that you have to be using enough resistance for the movement to be effective.[2] The idea is that you should be fatigued at the end of the target rep range, but still have enough gas to complete the motion with good form. Danger happens when you are too spent to safely lift the weight anymore.

What about bodyweight or static exercises? Once you are strong enough to crank more than a dozen pull-ups or other bodyweight movements, you should start thinking about adding external weight. Wearing a weight vest or holding a dumbbell can provide the additional stimulus for continued strength development. In terms of static exercises like L-sits, planches, and levers, aim to hold the position for 5 to 10 seconds. Exercises that specifically target the core, like planks, can be held for 10 to 30 seconds.

---

2 Some resisted exercises like kettlebell swings naturally lend themselves higher rep ranges. A 15, 20, or even 30- rep set of kettlebell swings is fine in some scenarios.

V

Intro

Movement Advice

Don't be sloppy.

You've only got one body, so don't go thrashing it about! As you perform an exercise, imagine yourself as a dancer with exquisite poise from the top of your head all the way to your tiptoes. If you were to record yourself on video, how would your body look? Would it appear centered, symmetric, and balanced? If not, focus on the quality of your movement and posture before adding resistance or difficulty.

Listen to your body.

As you work your way through the workouts in this book, you are going to encounter a wide variety of new movements. As you try them out, pay attention to how your body feels. If a skill seems seriously awkward, it could be that your alignment is way off, or you aren't strong enough for it yet.

If you have pain with a movement, then something isn't right. Try to adjust your stance, positioning, or movement pattern. If little tweaks don't help, get it checked out. Maybe a physio needs to address some underlying injury. A visit with a fitness coach could help adjust your form or provide a substitute movement.

Trust your gut. If a movement doesn't jibe with your body, swap it for an alternative.

Be smart about loading.

Injuries related to fitness are often the result of doing too much too soon. Jump into a workout routine after months off, and BOOM an injury flares up. Increase the resistance or the difficulty of a movement too fast, and you are setting yourself up for disaster. Being cautious about how you introduce and increase load is a crucial characteristic for the garage gym athlete.

For example, if you can't perform a movement through its target range of motion without resistance, then don't go adding extra load. Master the bodyweight version before adding more challenge. Master air squats before dumbbell front squats. Master split jumps before resisted split jumps. You get the picture.

In a similar way, don't advance to single limbed skills until you have sufficient strength with the double limbed version.[3] Only attempt single arm hangs after you can perform a double arm hang for a healthy amount of time. Only attempt pistol squats versions once you can move through the array of split squats with confidence.

Another common-sense recommendation is that if you can't support yourself in the beginning position of the movement, don't attempt the rest of the motion. Inverted skills are the best reference point. If you can't safely support your torso through your shoulders at the top of a pike or jackknife push-up position, don't think about trying the full movement. Your head and neck are too valuable.

---

3 *Open chain* exercises like dumbbell shoulder presses or bicep curls are an exception to the "double before single limb" rule.

Intro

Understand how to use exercise progressions.

As someone who wants to train at home, it will be helpful to know how to adjust the exercises in this book to fit your ability level. Some movements may be way too easy. Some may be way too hard. Rather than skip those sections of each workout, figure out how you could make the movement easier or harder to match your ability level.

Common progressions include:

- **Unloaded » Loaded**
- **Less resistance » More resistance**
- **Assisted » Unassisted**
- **Slow » Fast**
- **Kipping » Strict**
- **Small range of motion » Full range of motion**
- **Symmetric double limb » Asymmetric double limb » Single limb**
- **Short levers » Long levers**
- **Simple » Complex**
- **Single plane » Multi-plane movements**

Appendix B at the end of the book has a number of common progressions to get you started.

Effort = Outcomes.

When your goal is to build strength and muscle, then your body needs the stimulus to add muscle mass and connective tissue capacity. Training at an intensity that is below this threshold is fine, but it won't lead to the gains you seek. That means that when you settle in for the circuit training portion of each session, you need to put in the work. Go hard, but be safe about it.

This idea is summarized by the principle of *progressive overload*. By gradually increasing the total workload between training sessions, your body will adapt through improved strength.

Note how this cycles back to why you won't find specific reps/sets or weight prescriptions in this book. It's up to YOU to continually push the needle on your training. It's up to you to gradually add more weight to each exercise. In the absence of more resistance—maybe your home gym isn't fully complete yet—increase your overall workload via more reps or sets of the movements.

If you don't put in the effort, don't expect the outcomes.

Are you someone who needs more accountability
on your fitness journey?
Head over to **benmusholt.com/coaching** to learn about virtual
coaching options.

Get After It

I hope you enjoy exploring the workouts in the following pages. Don't worry about doing them in order. In fact, skip around if you want. When you perform a workout that felt amazing, mark it so that you can repeat it again.

Garage gym circuit training is convenient, low cost, and effective. As you challenge yourself with the sequences illustrated in this book, take pride in how you are crafting yourself into a more well-rounded athlete

Good luck on your journey. Whatever your fitness goals are, know that these workouts are helping to build a more capable version of yourself. Now go and get after it!

3

Side A

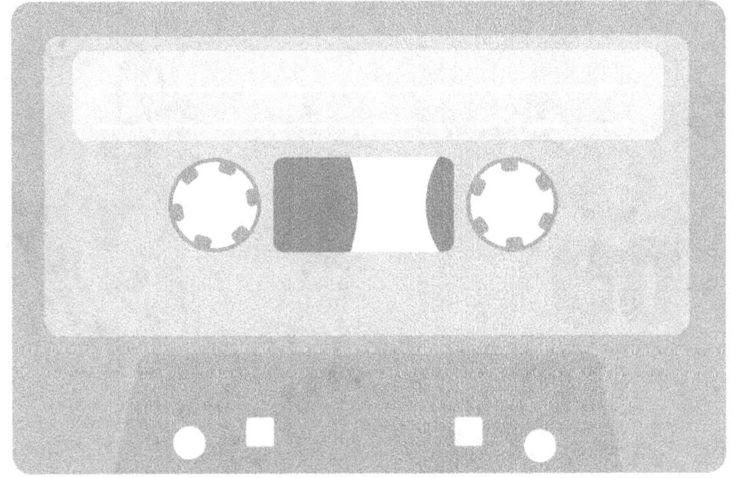

SIDE A

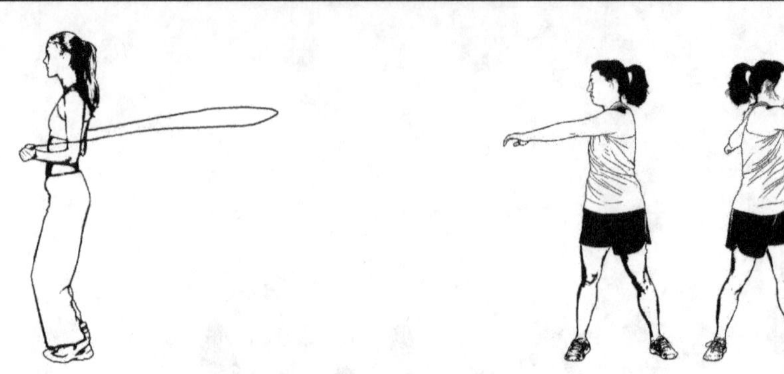

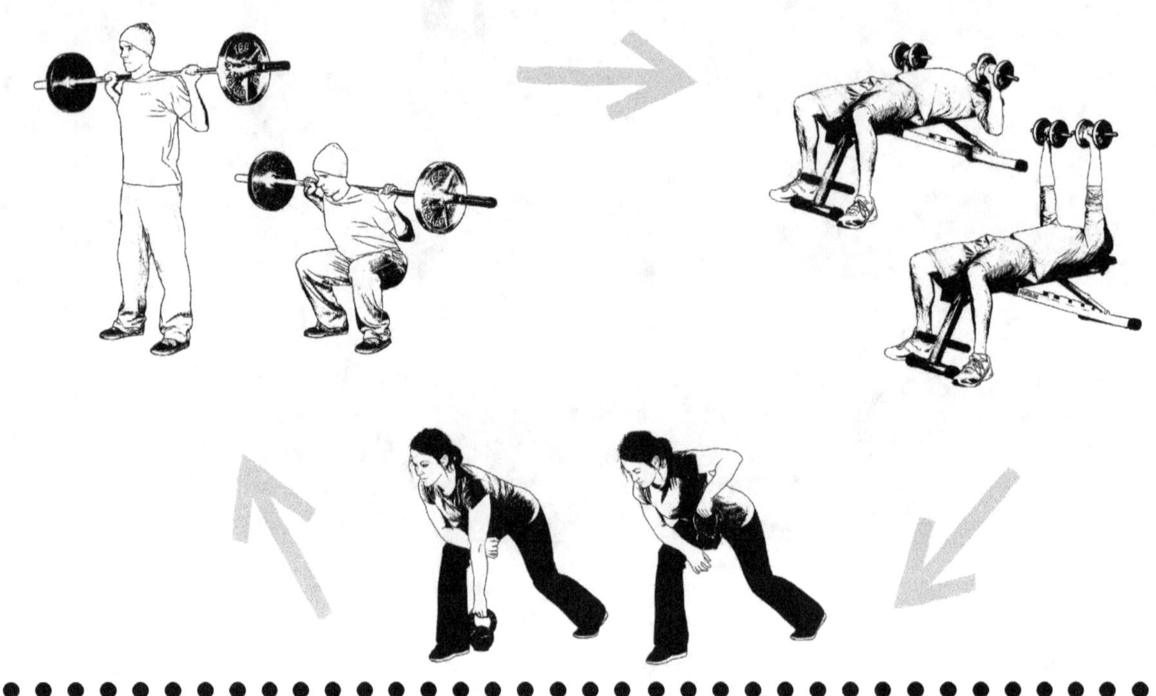

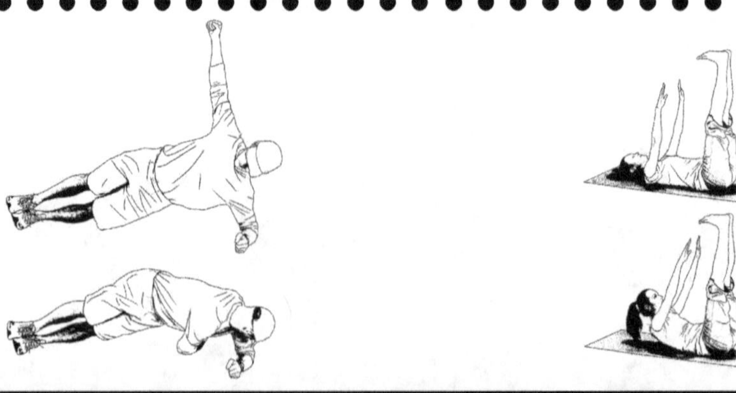

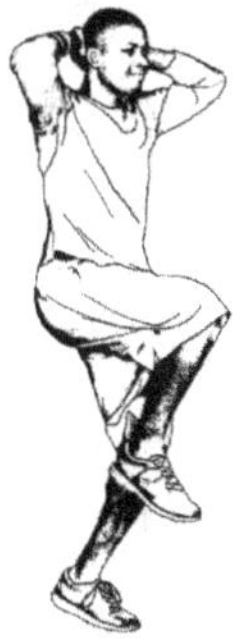

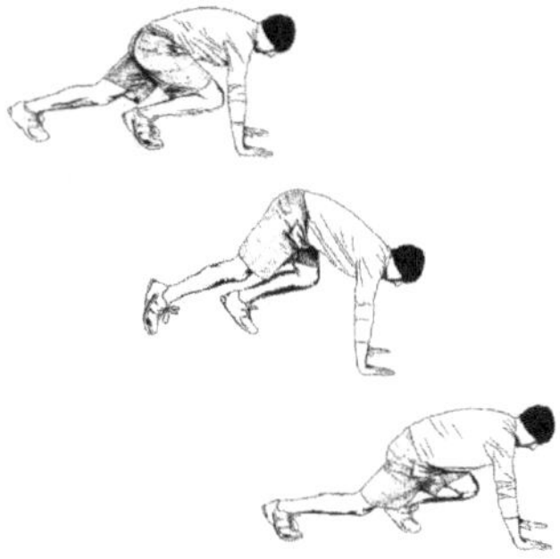

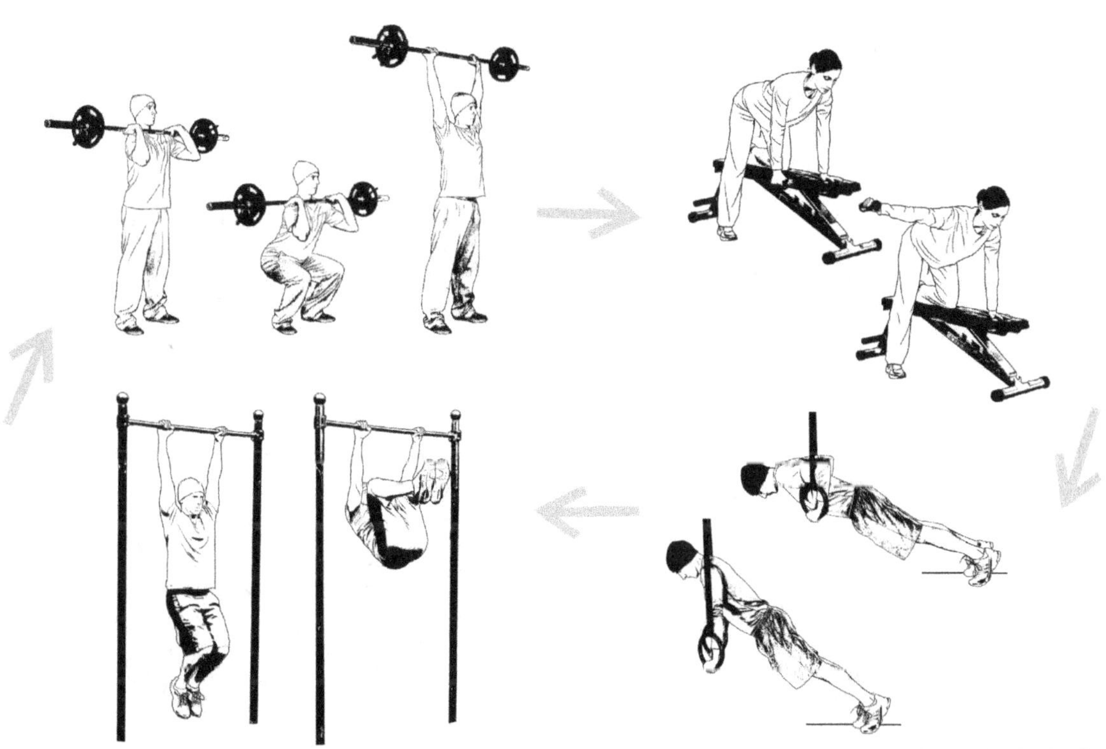

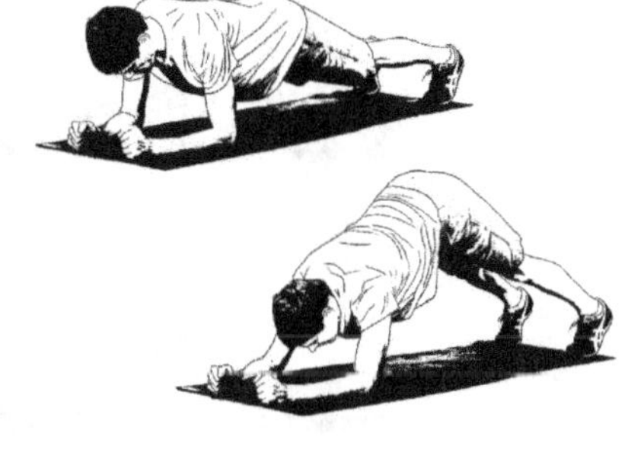
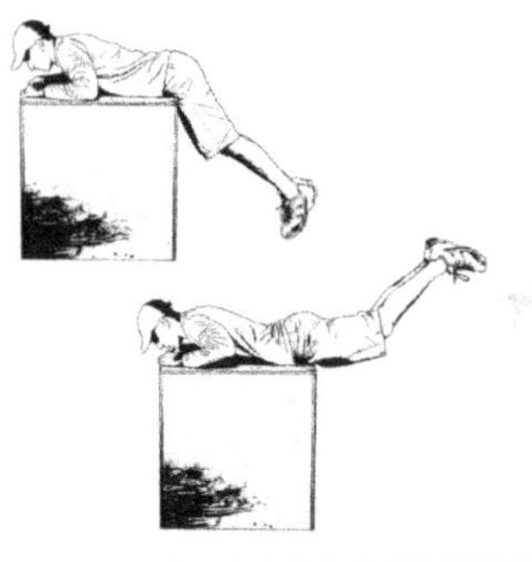

SIDE A

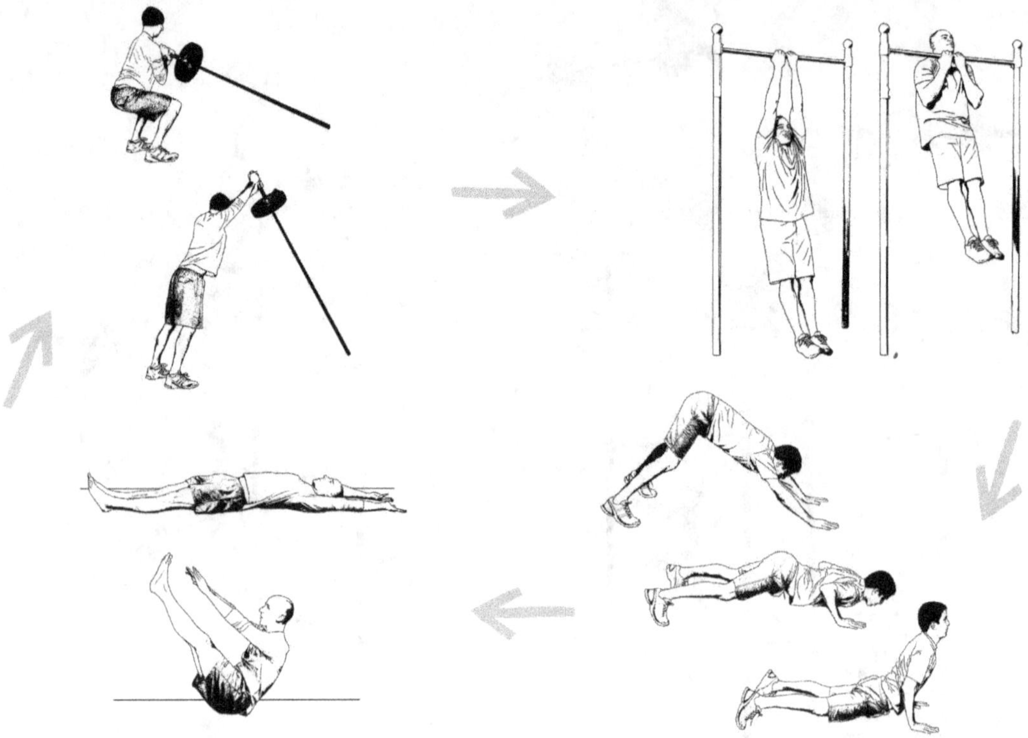

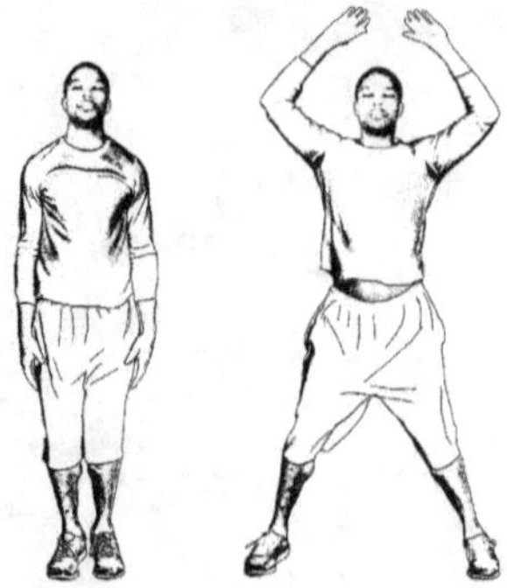

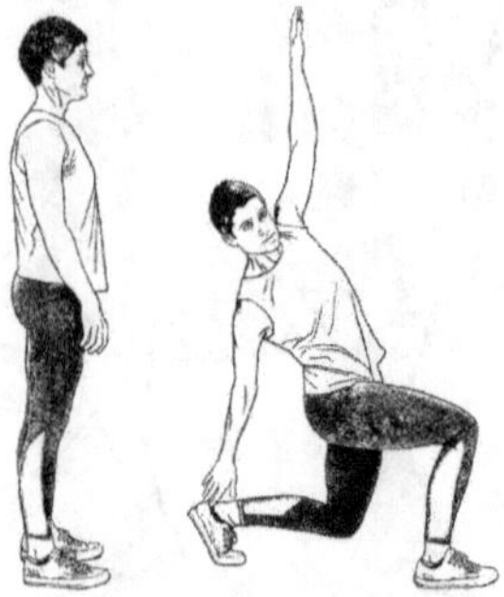

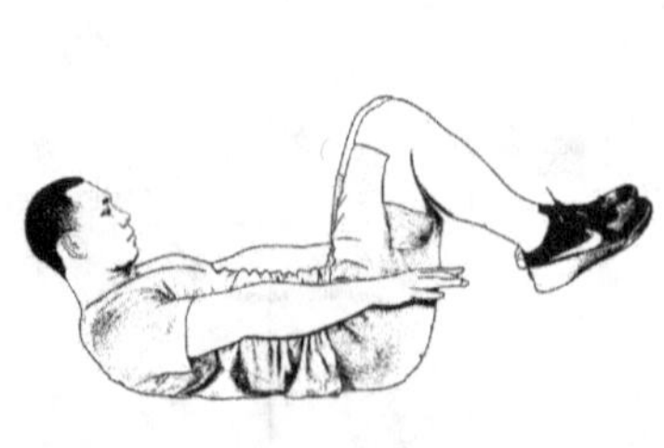

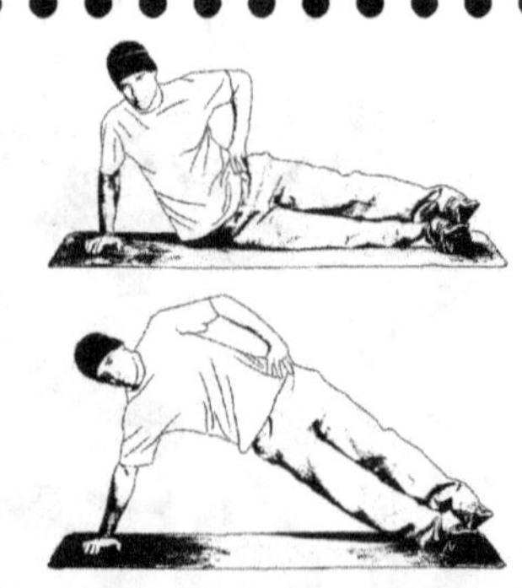

SIDE A

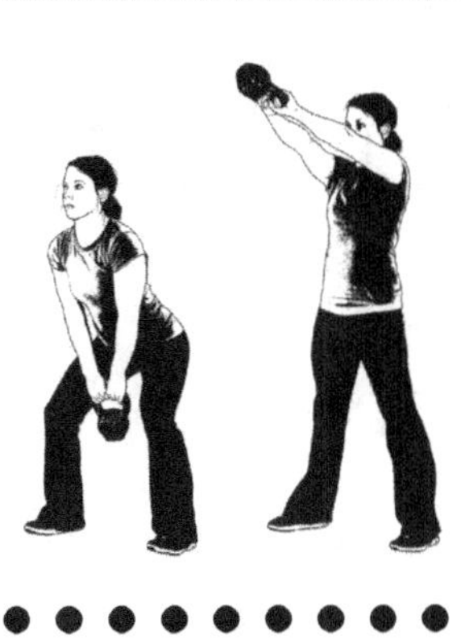

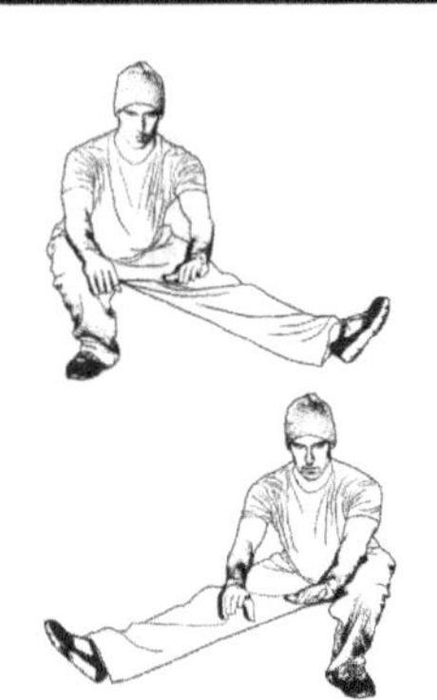

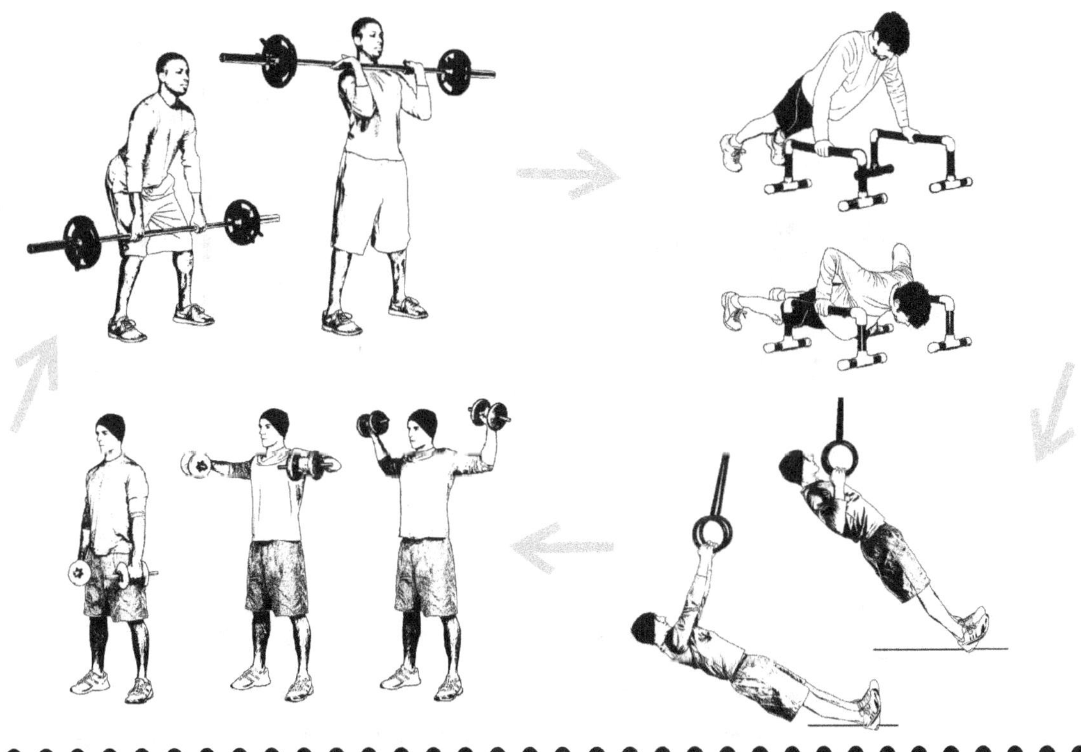

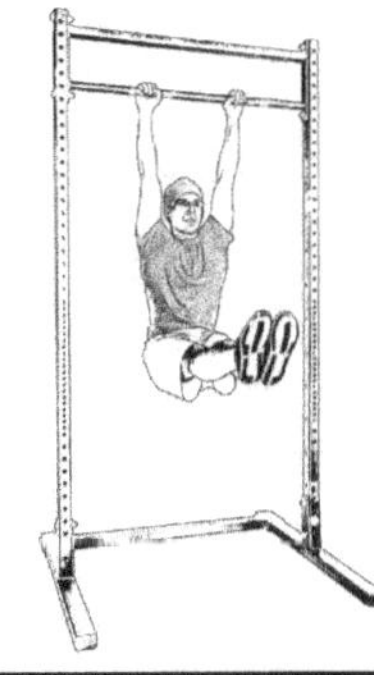

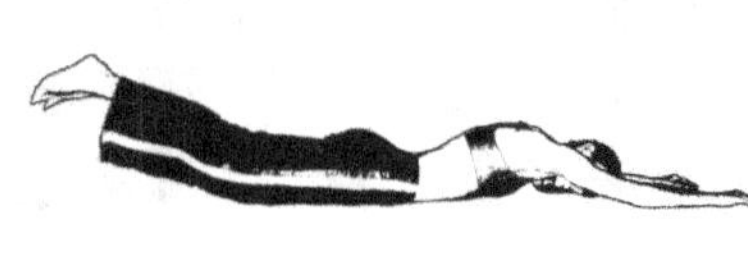

SIDE A

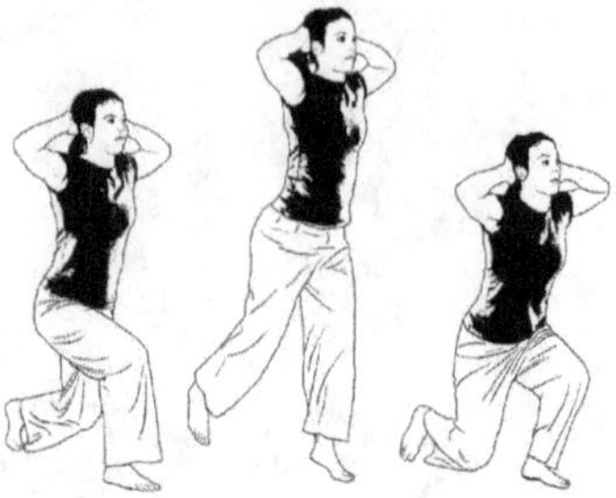

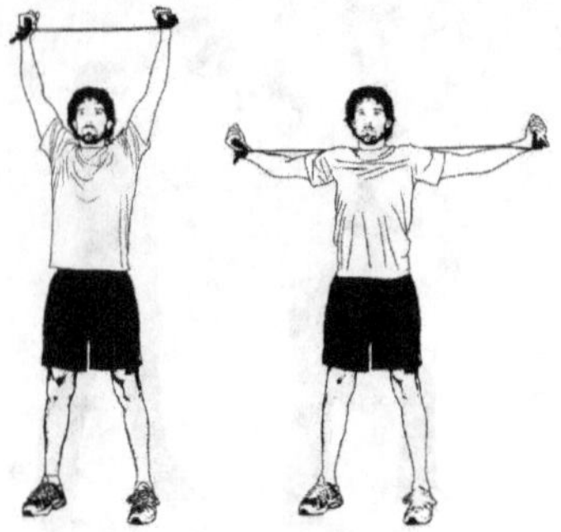

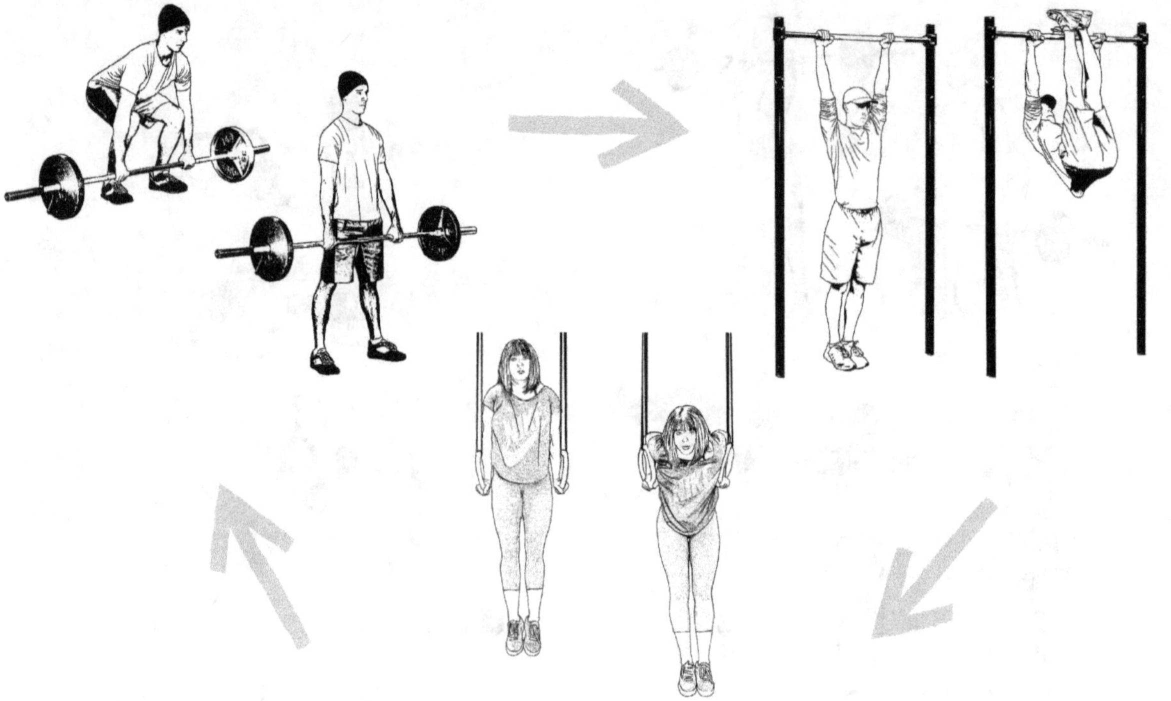

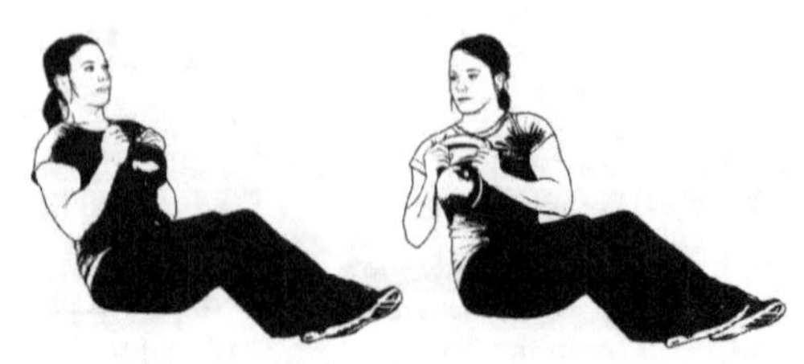

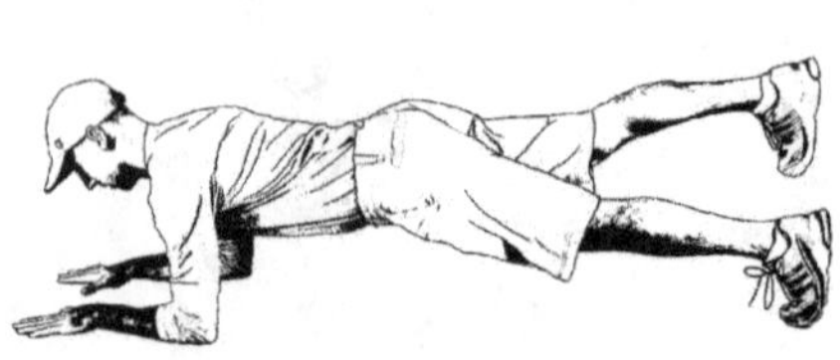

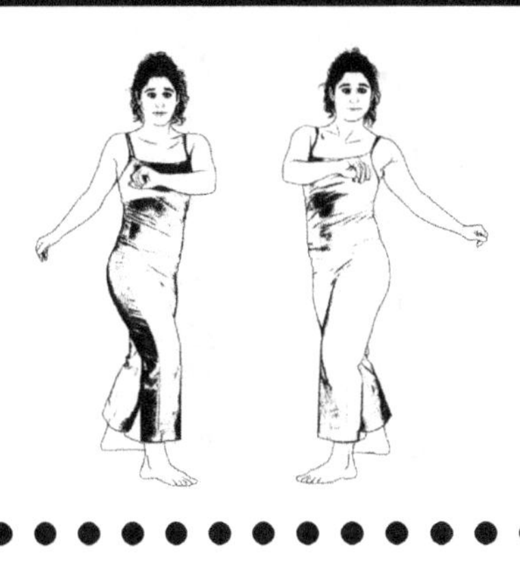
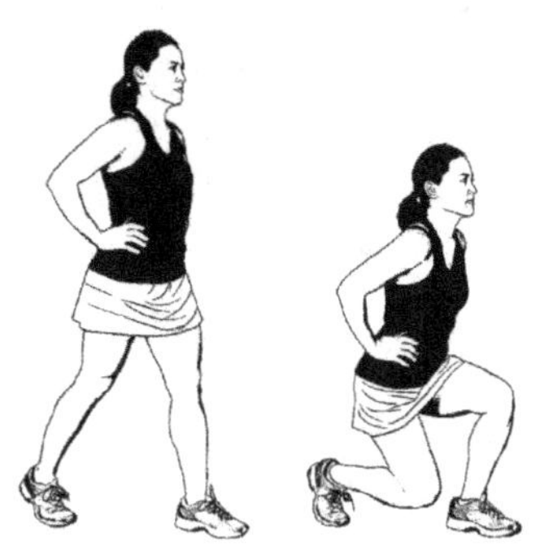
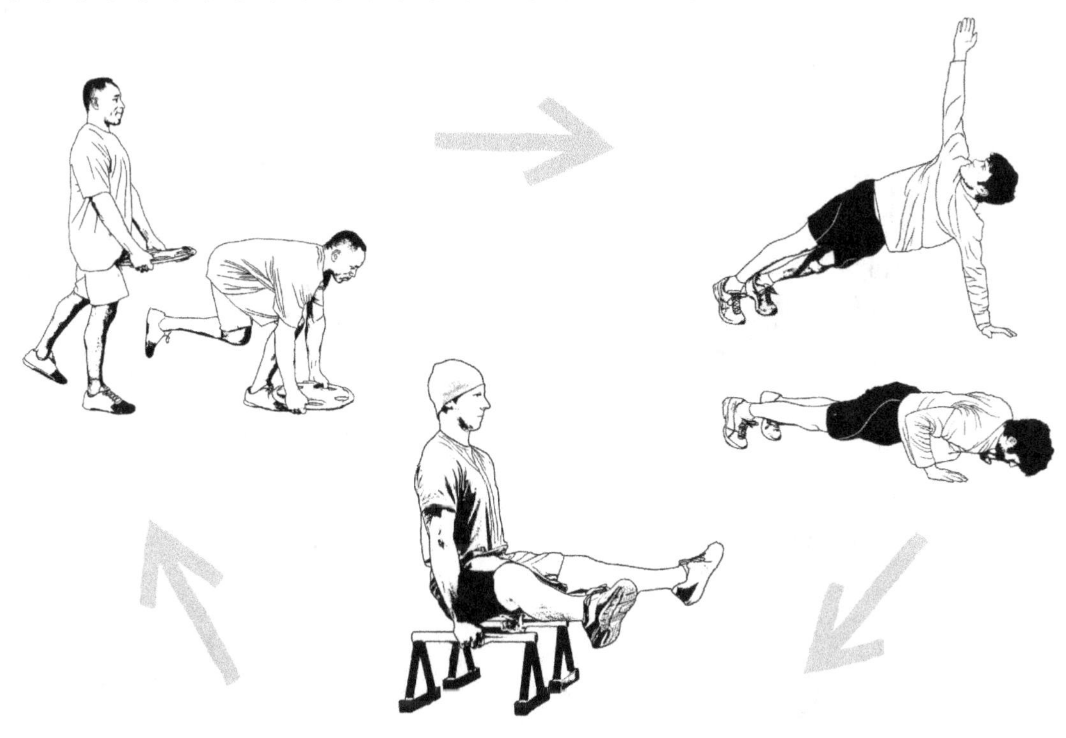
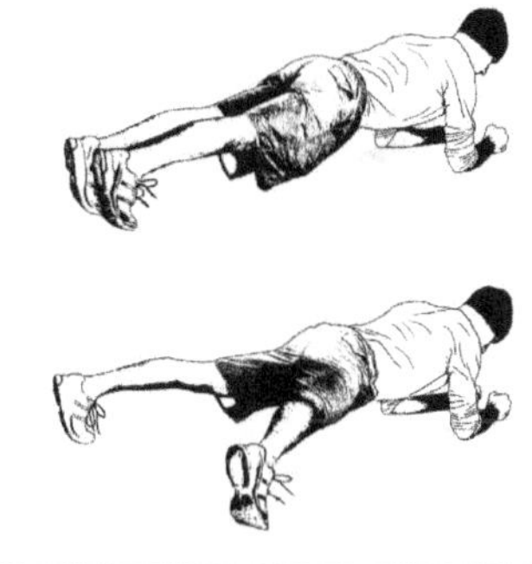
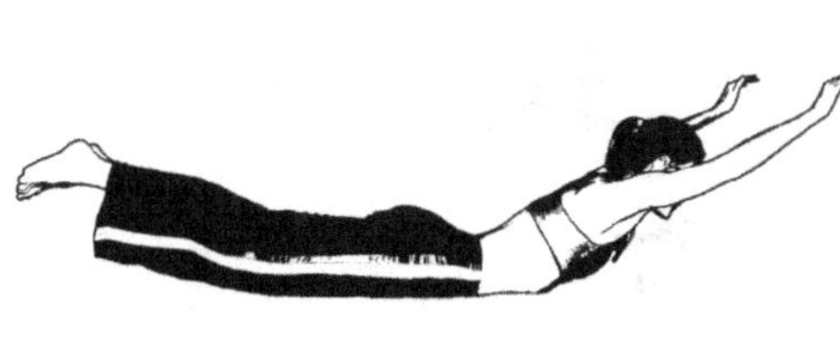

SIDE A

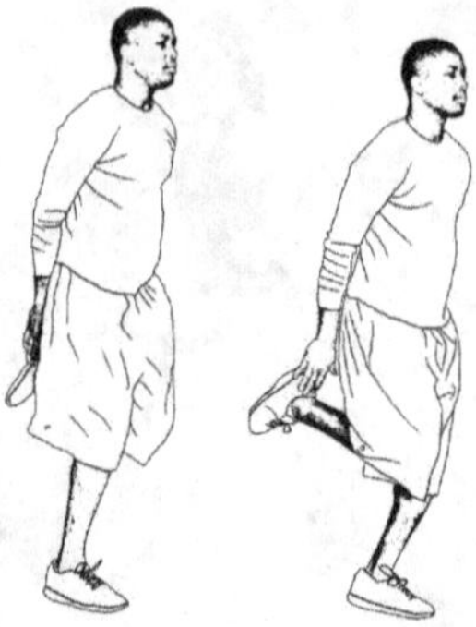

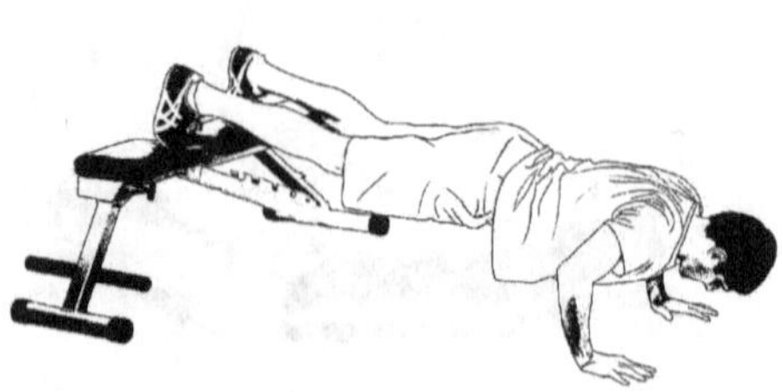

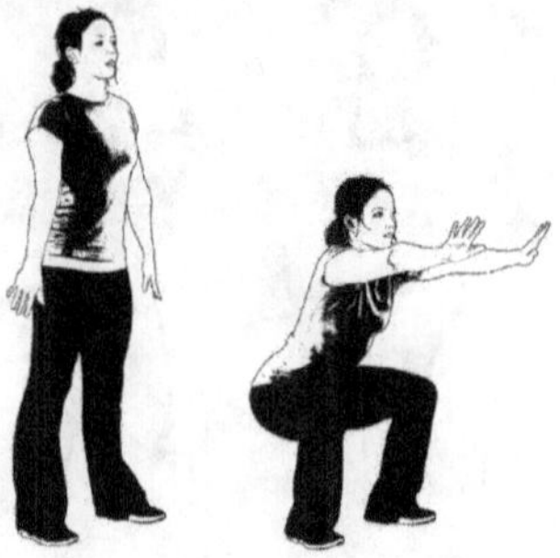

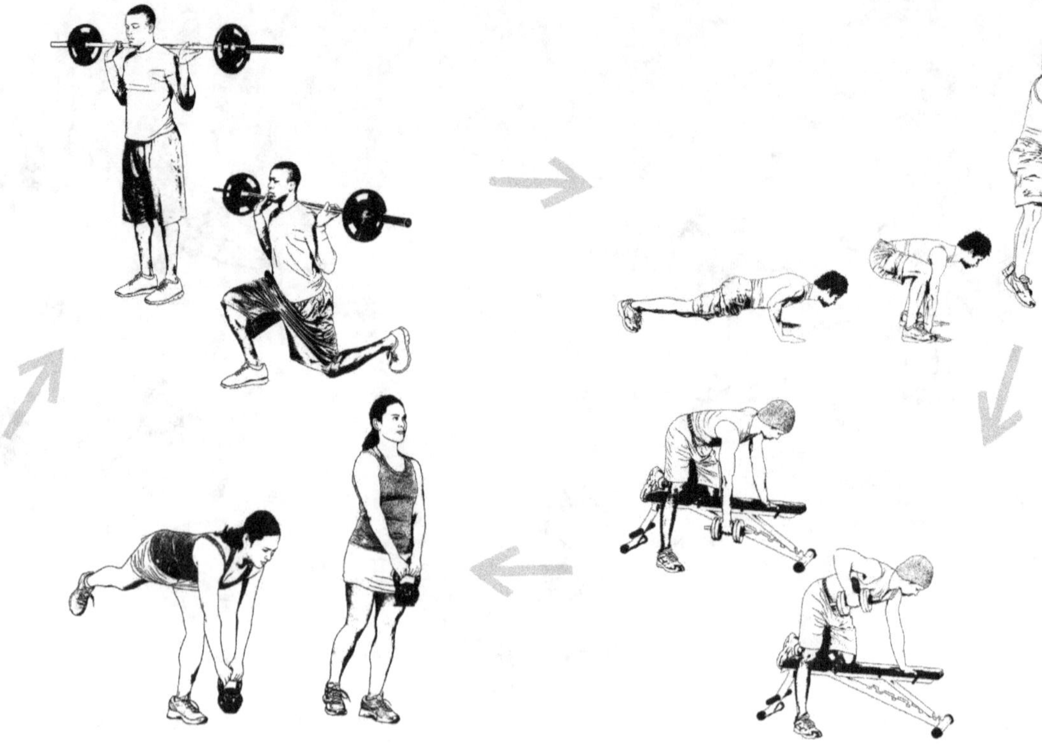

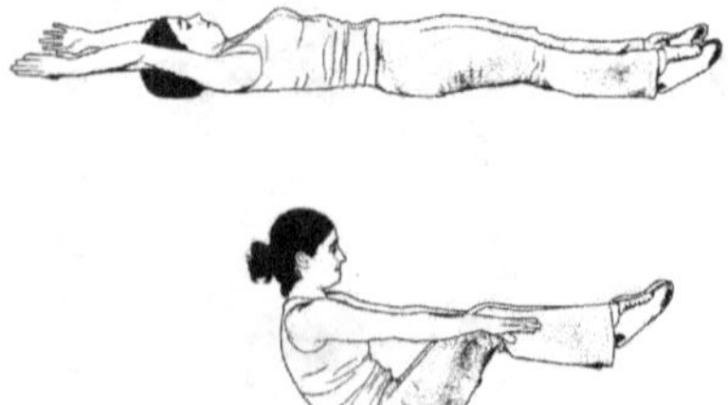

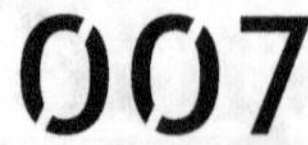

SIDE A

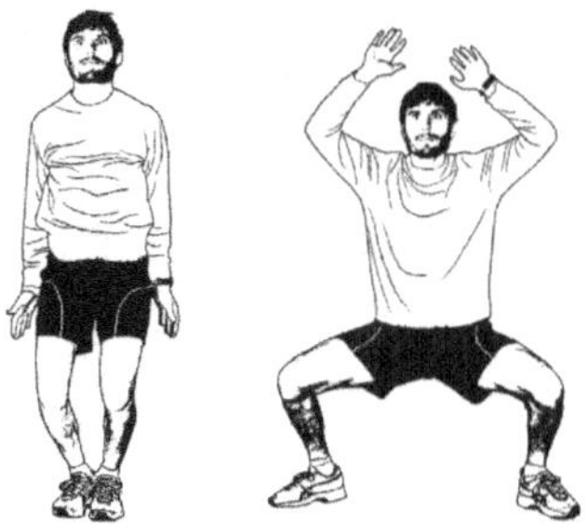

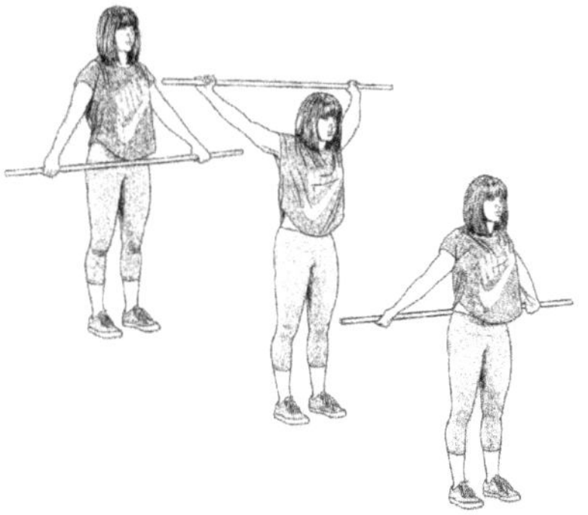

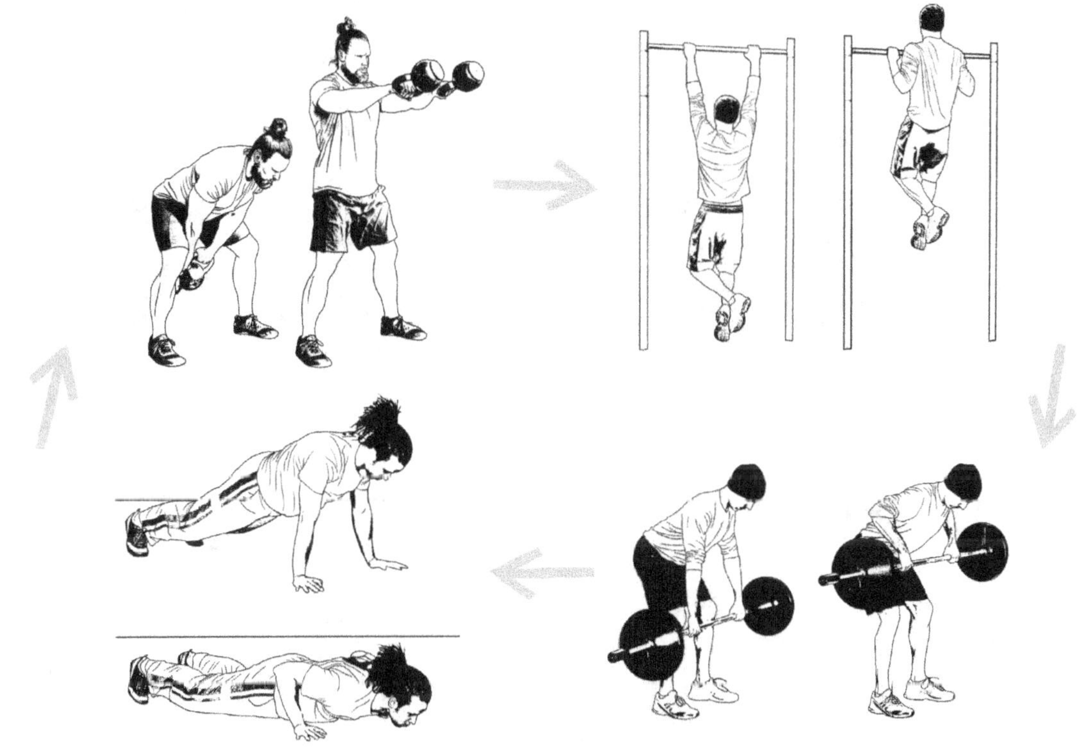

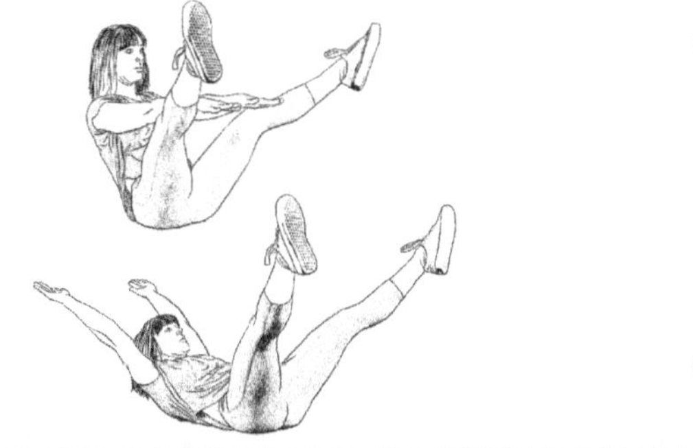

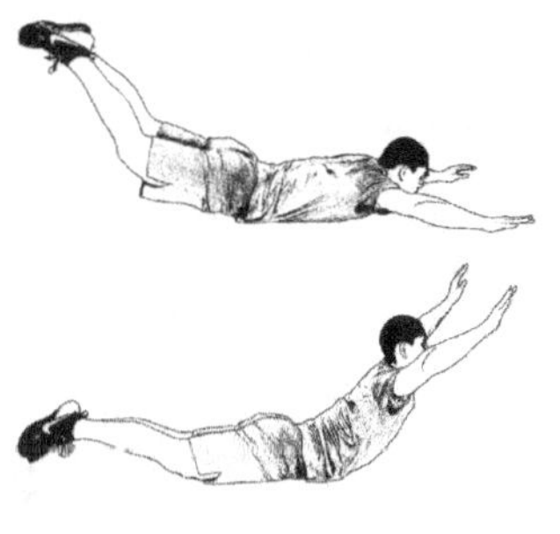

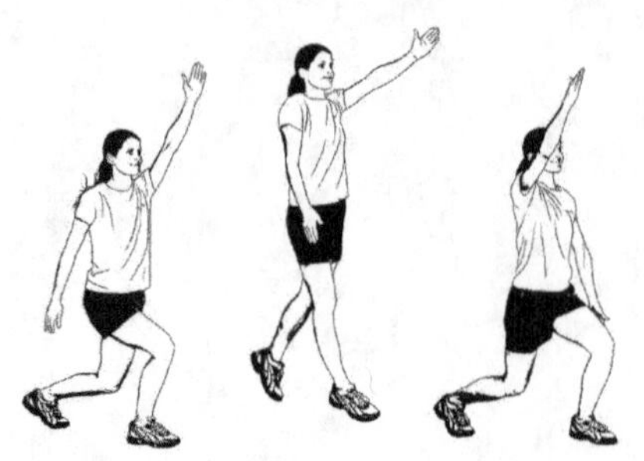

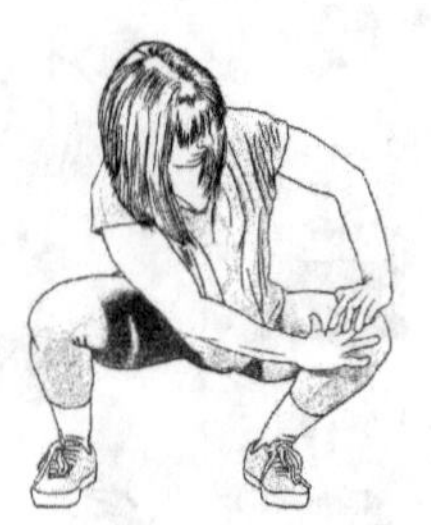

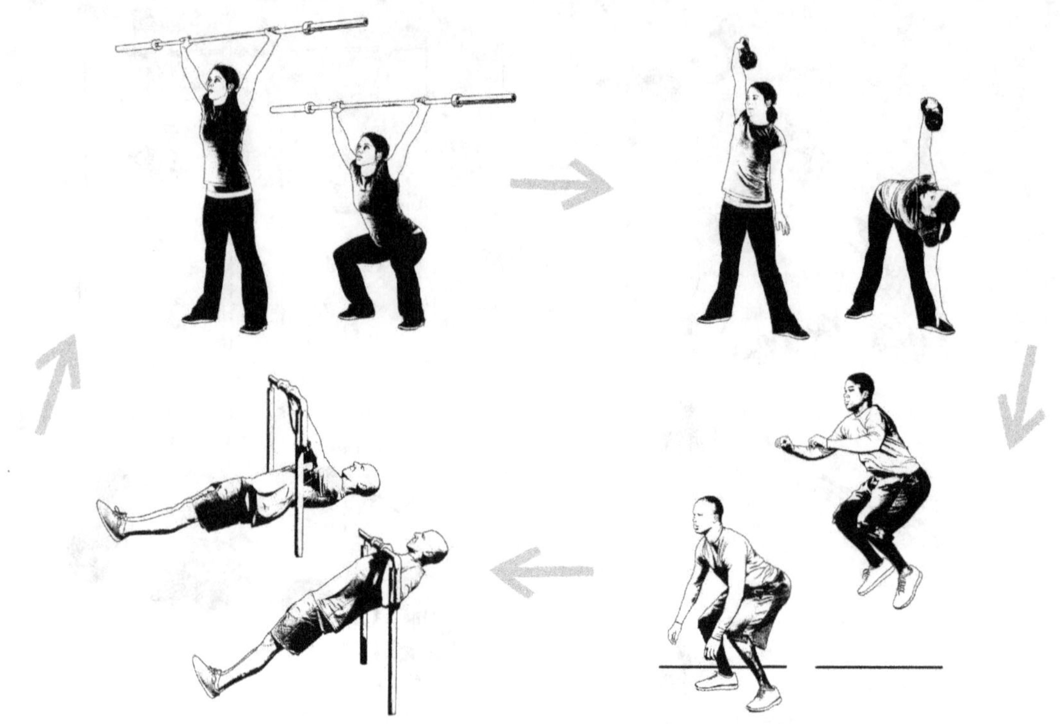

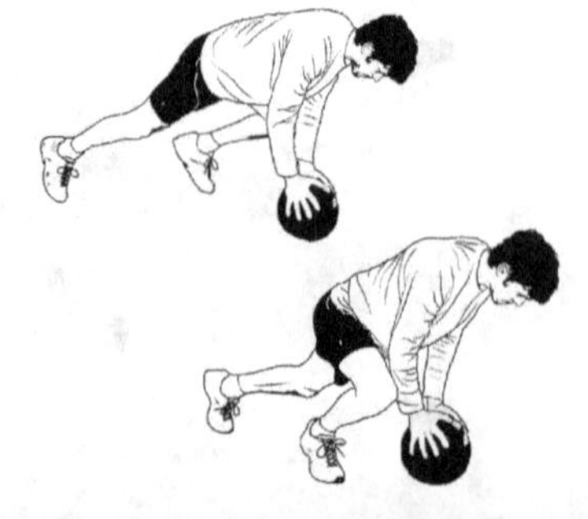

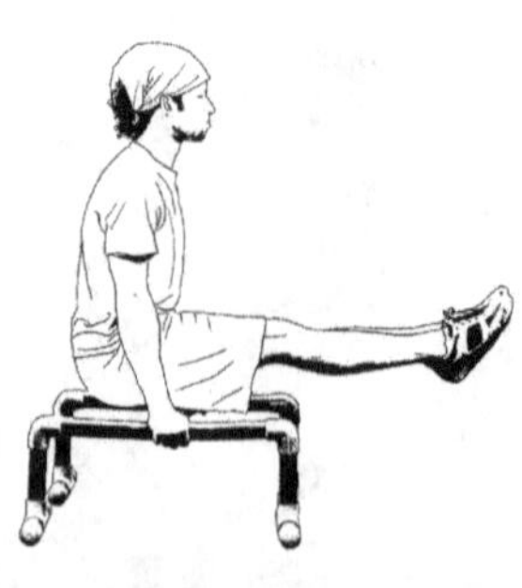

SIDE A

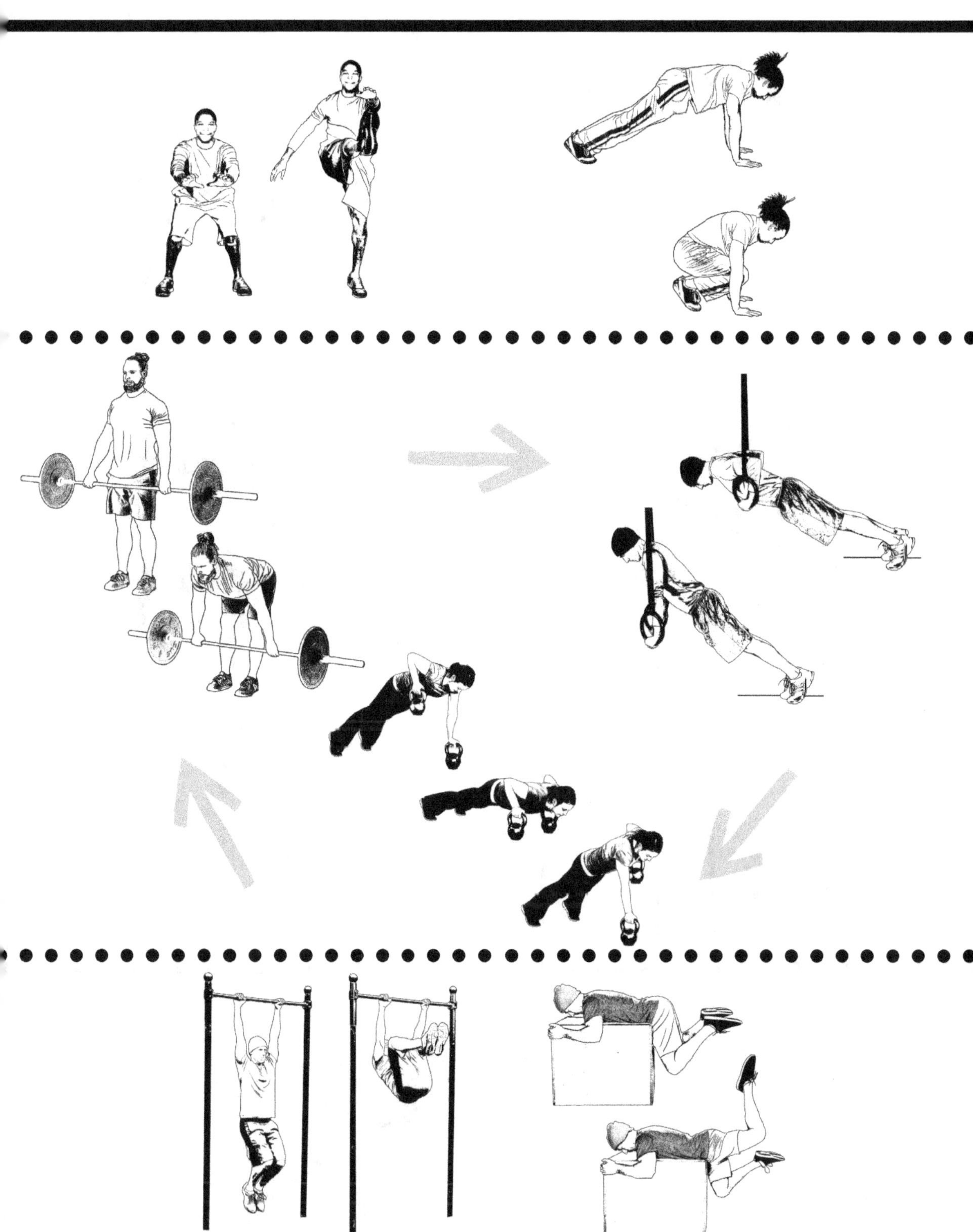

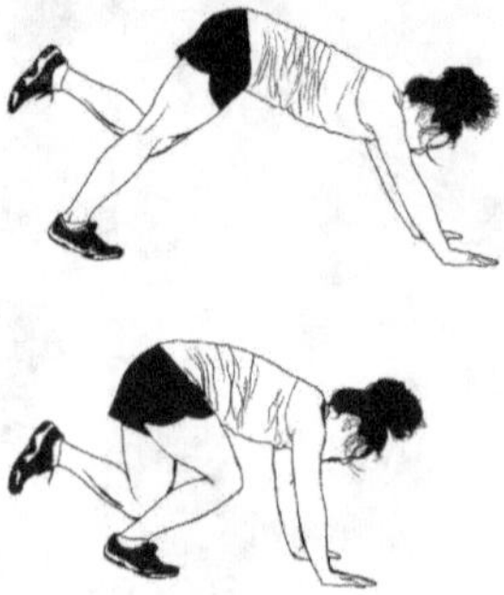

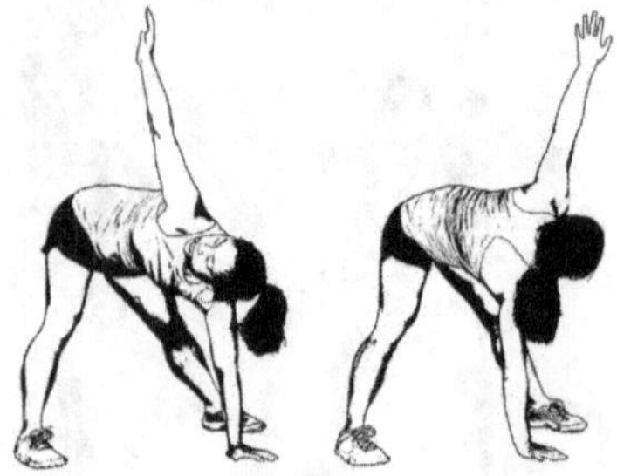

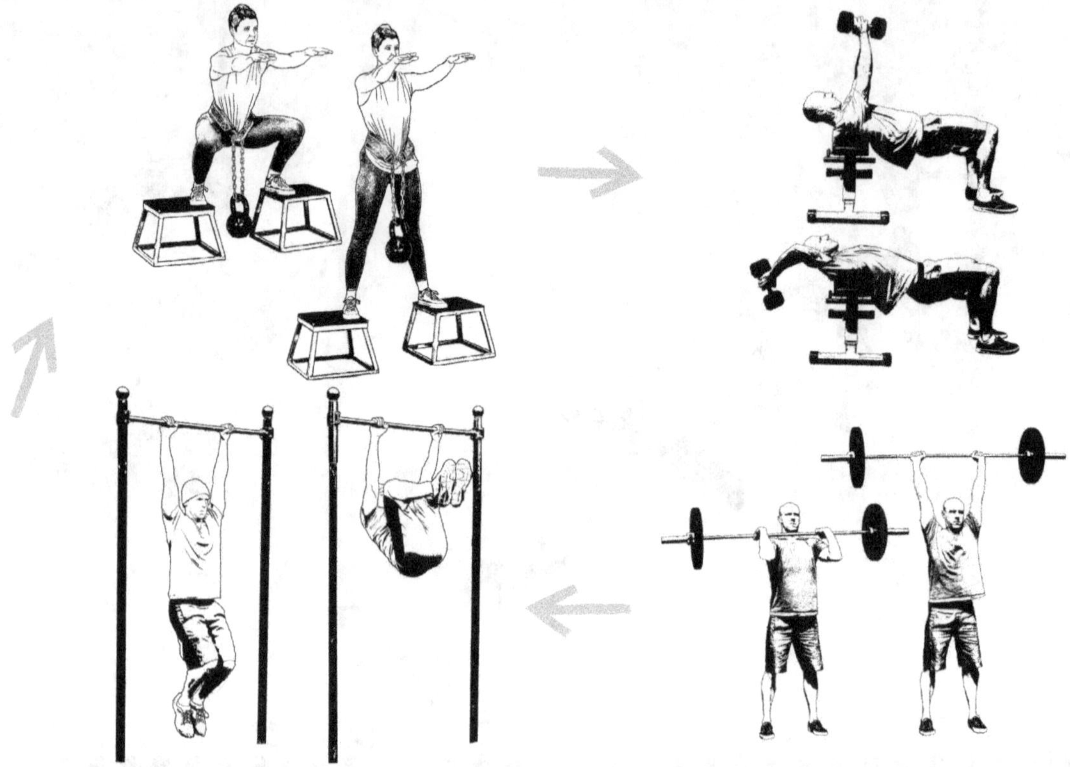

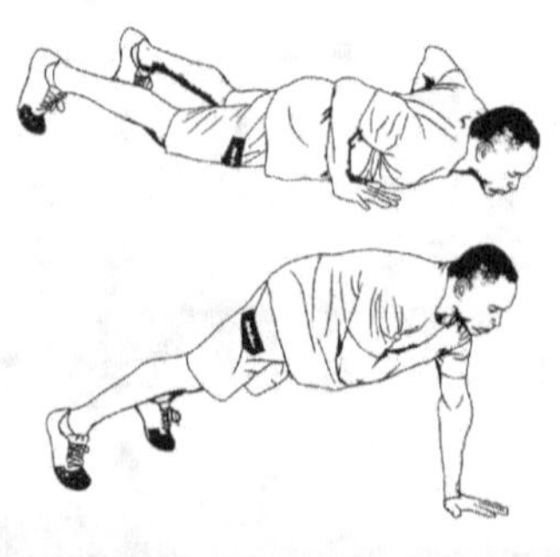

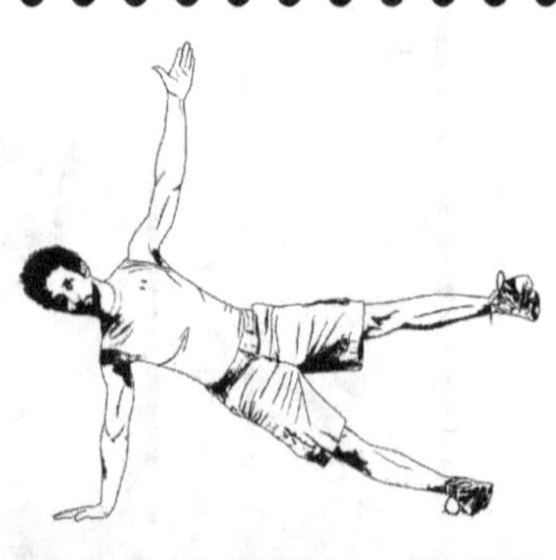

SIDE A

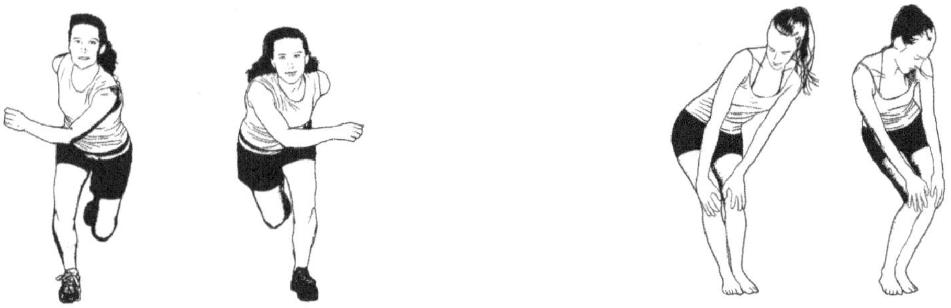

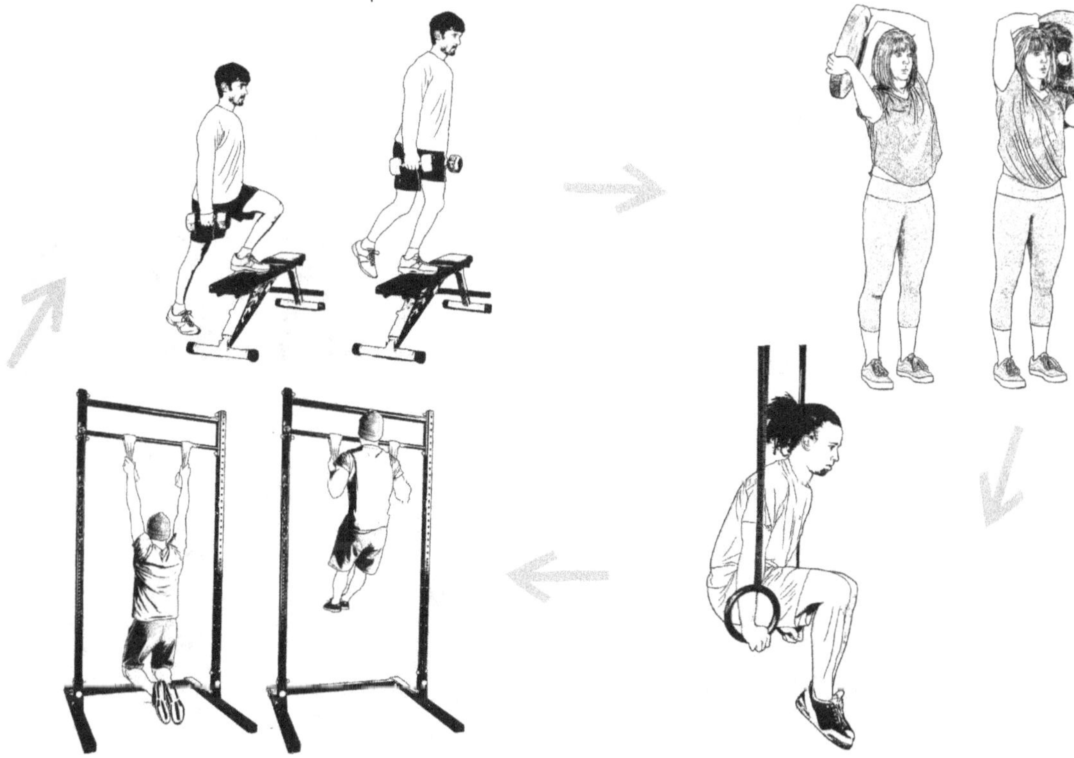

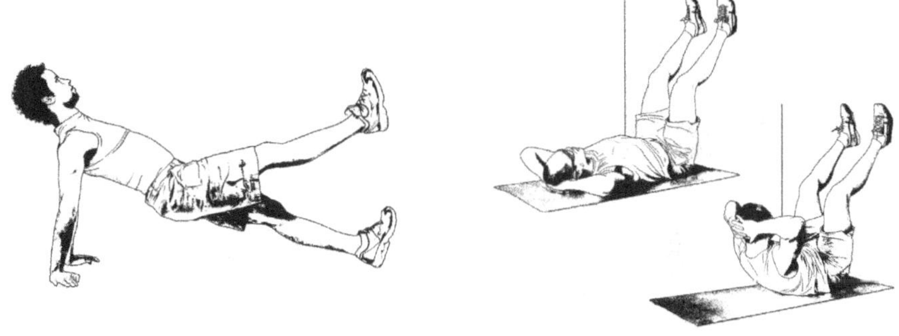

SIDE A

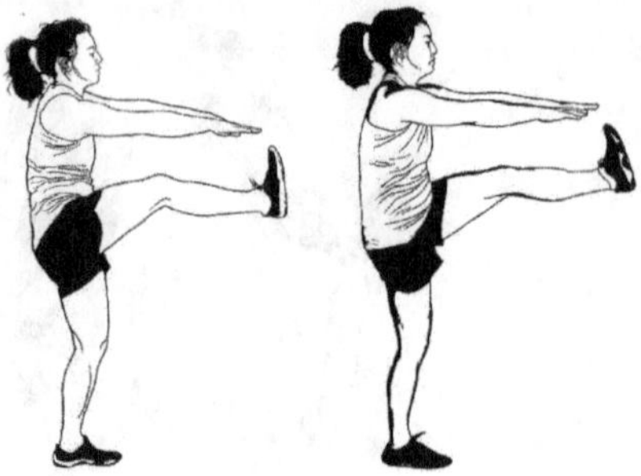

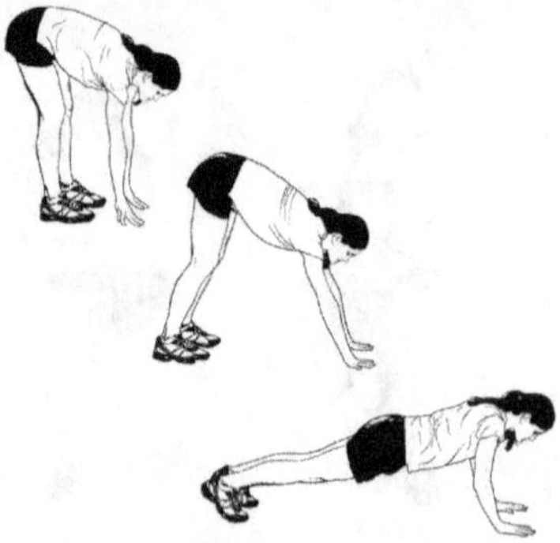

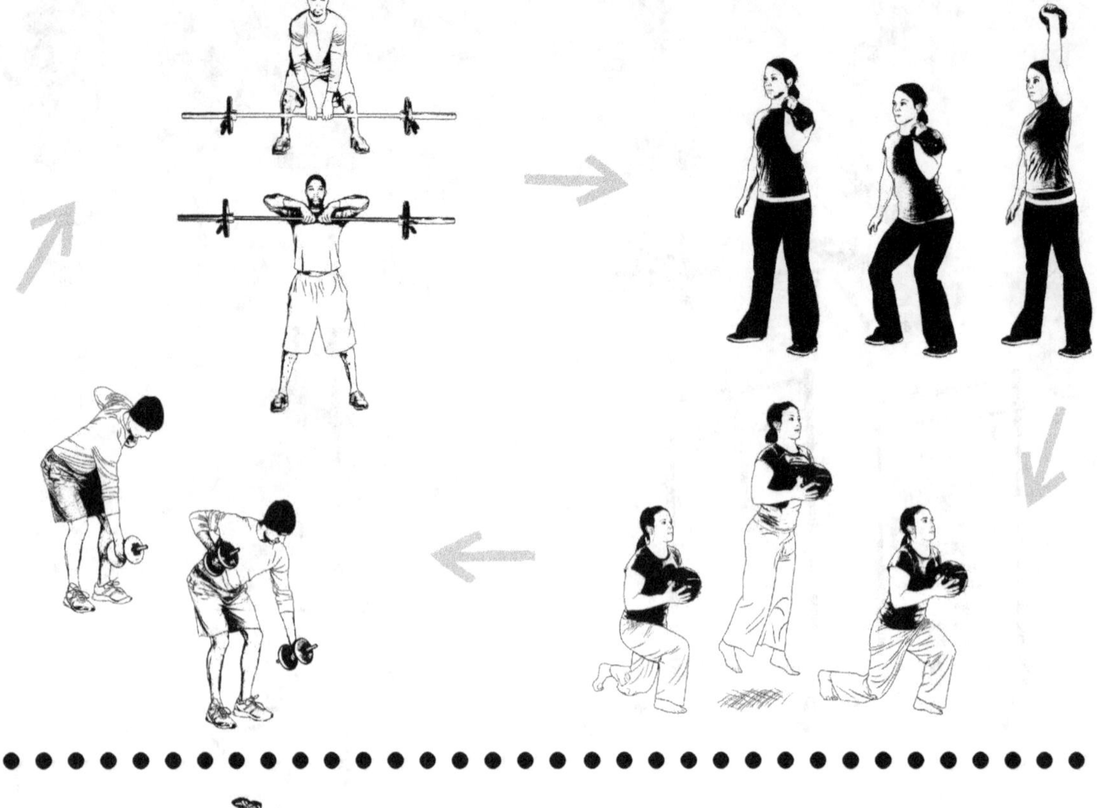

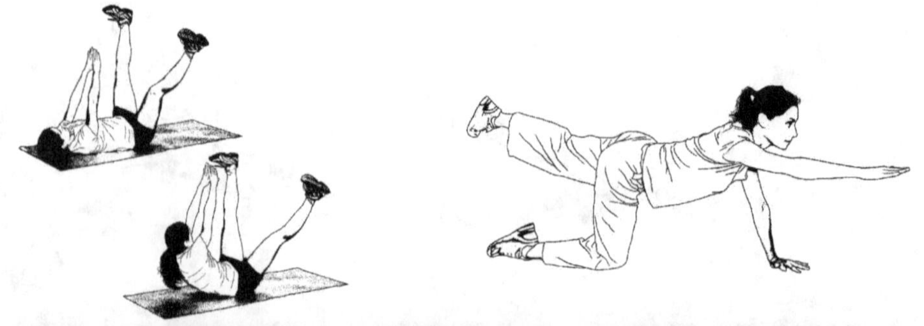

SIDE A

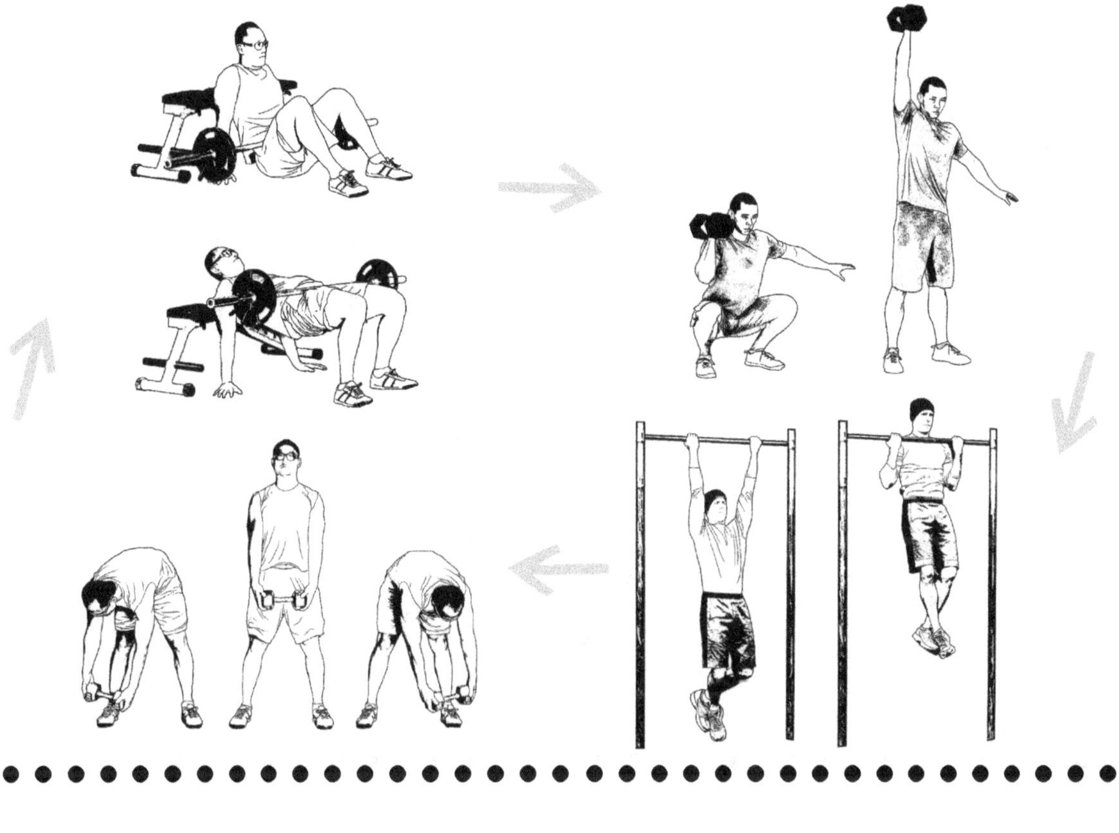

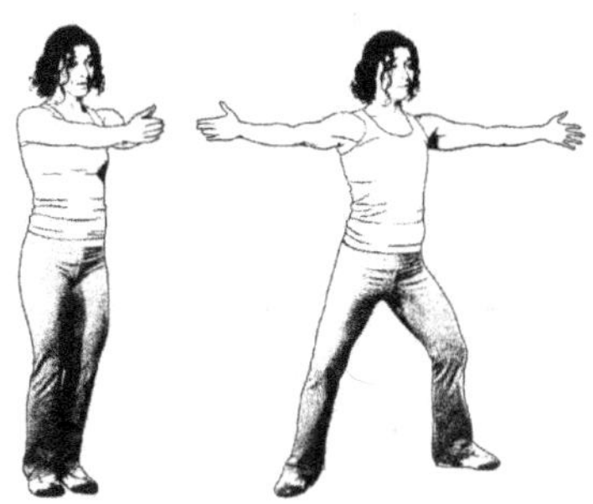

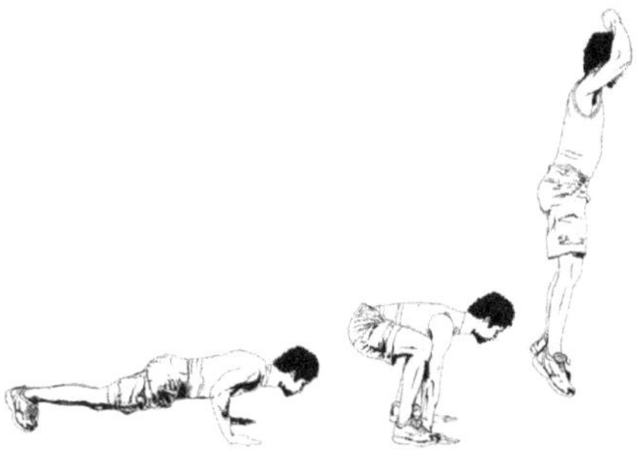

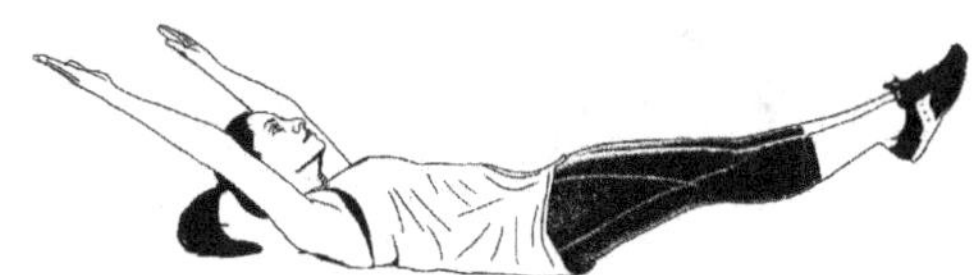

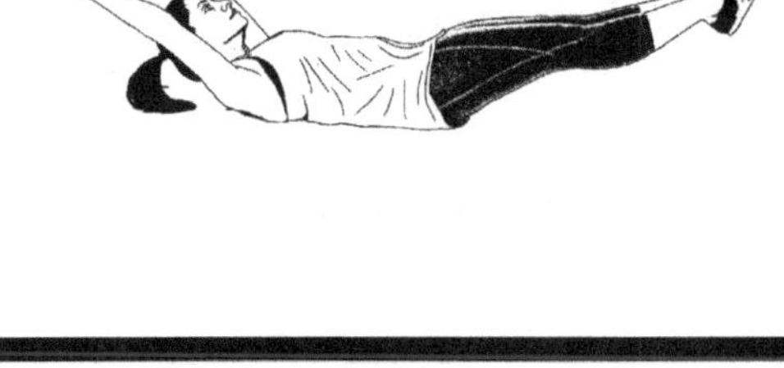

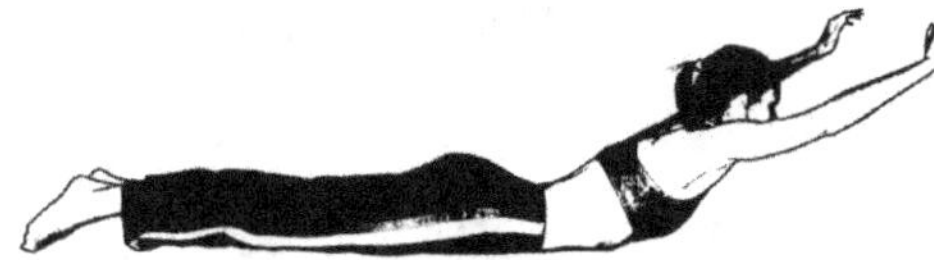

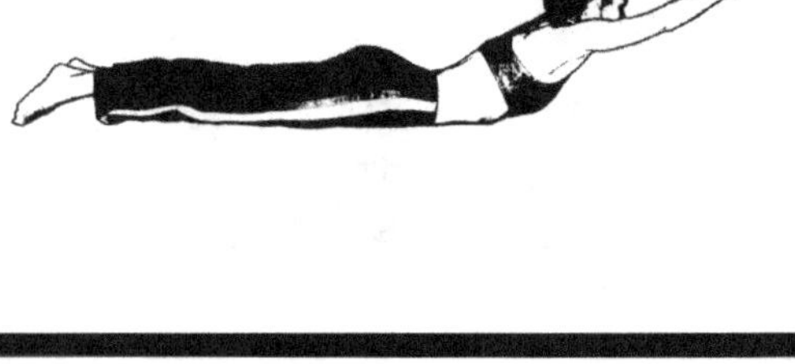

SIDE A

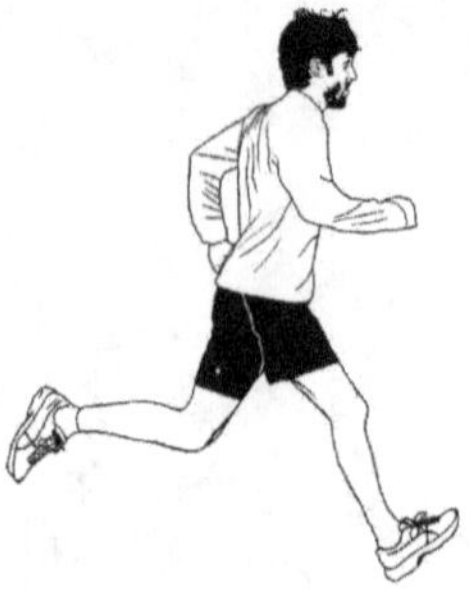

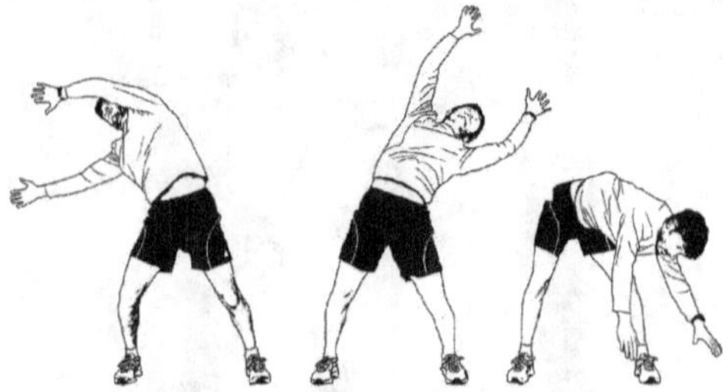

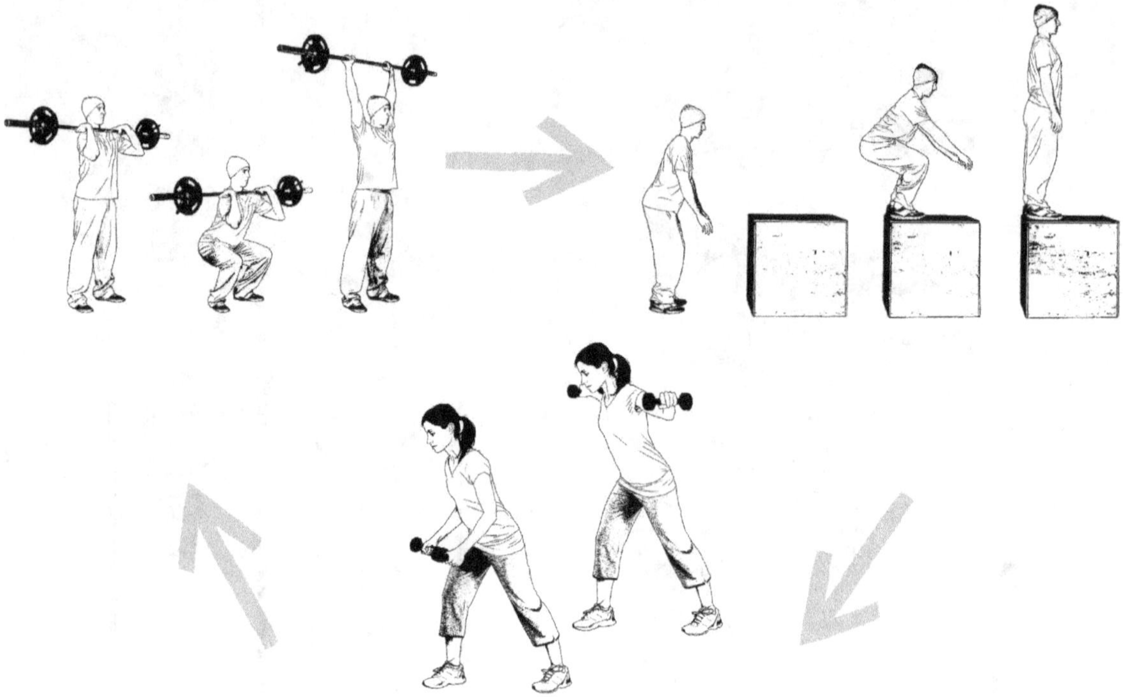

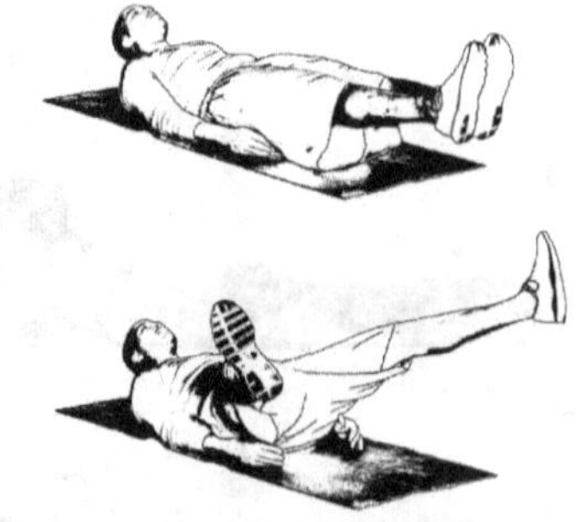

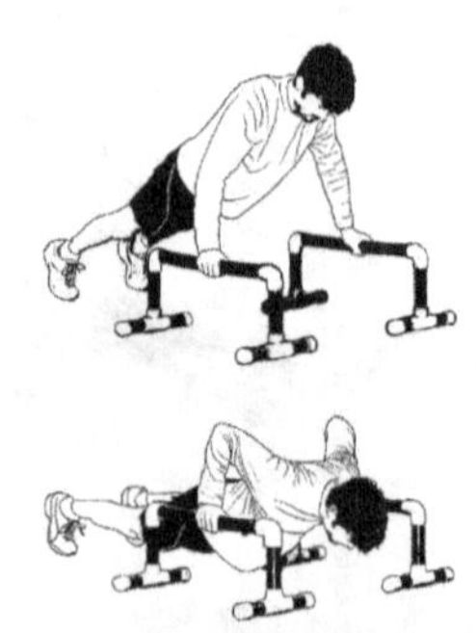

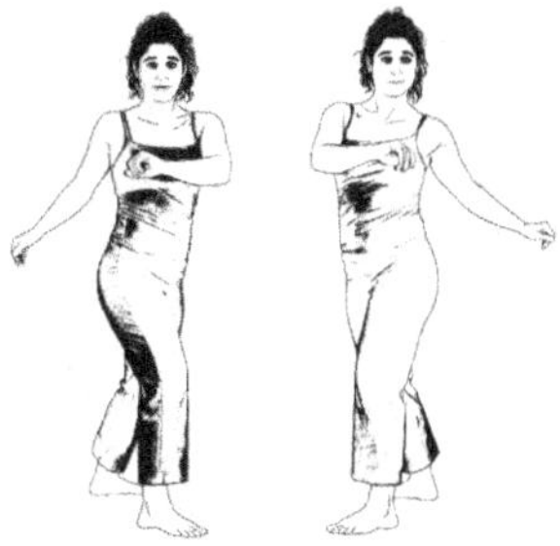

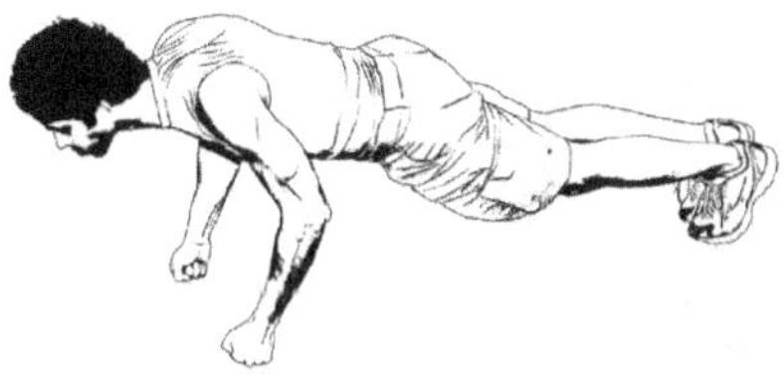

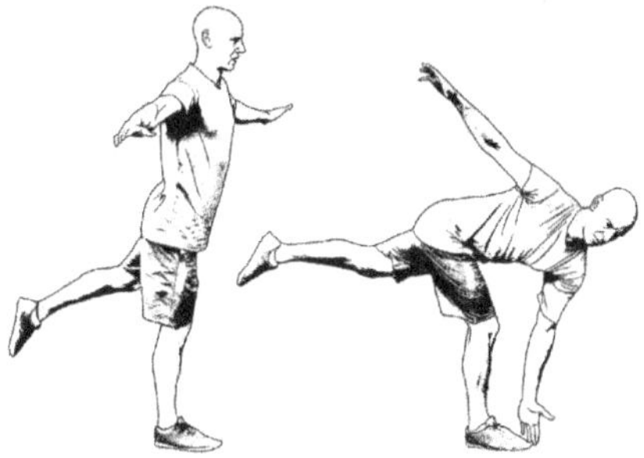

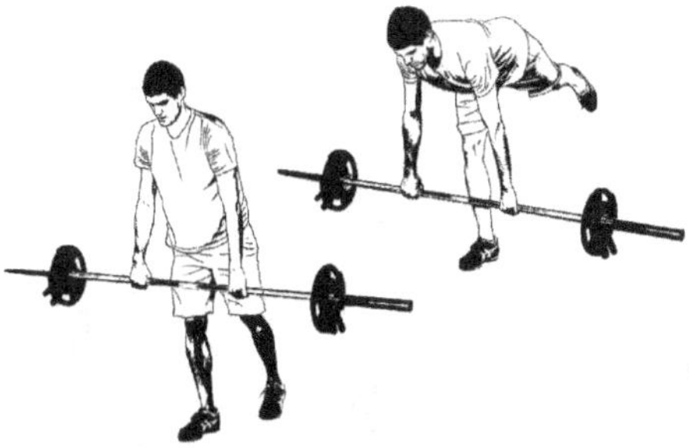

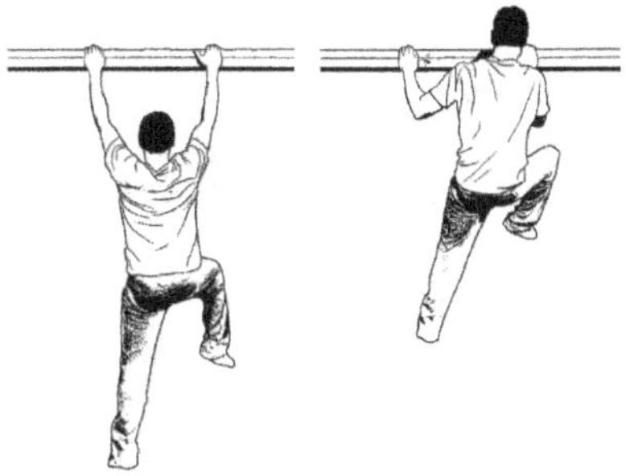

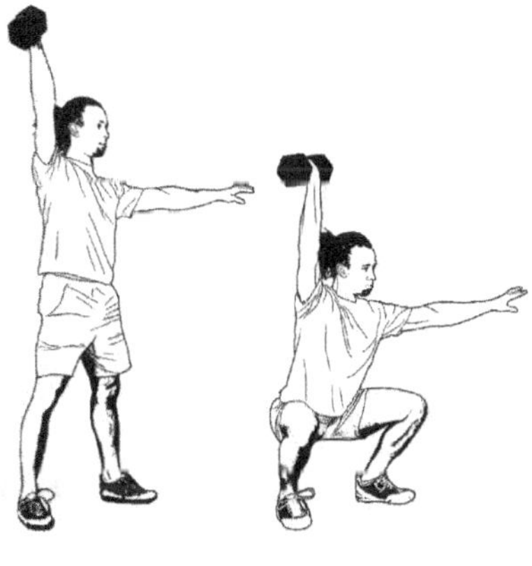

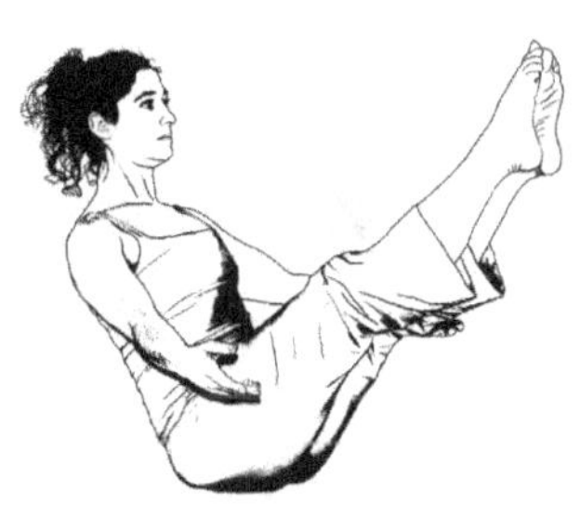

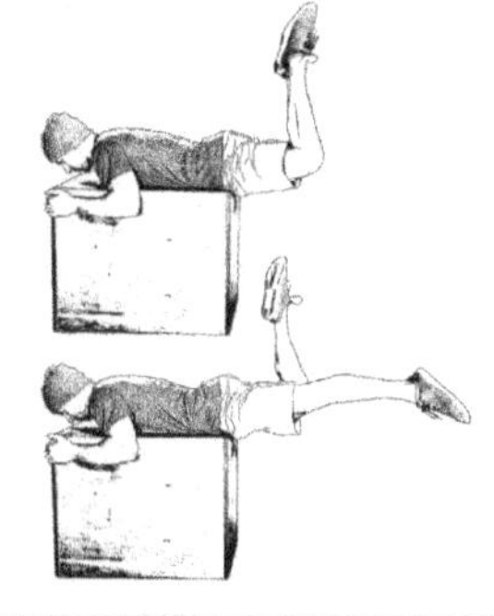

SIDE A

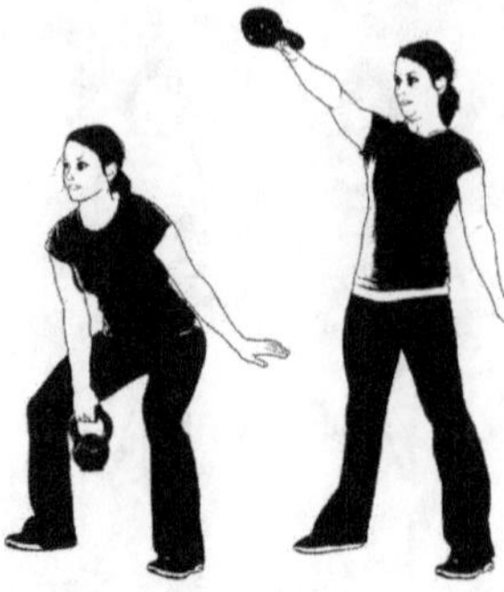

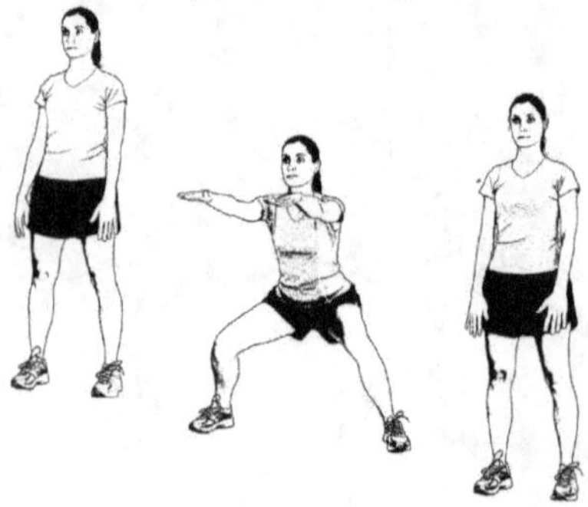

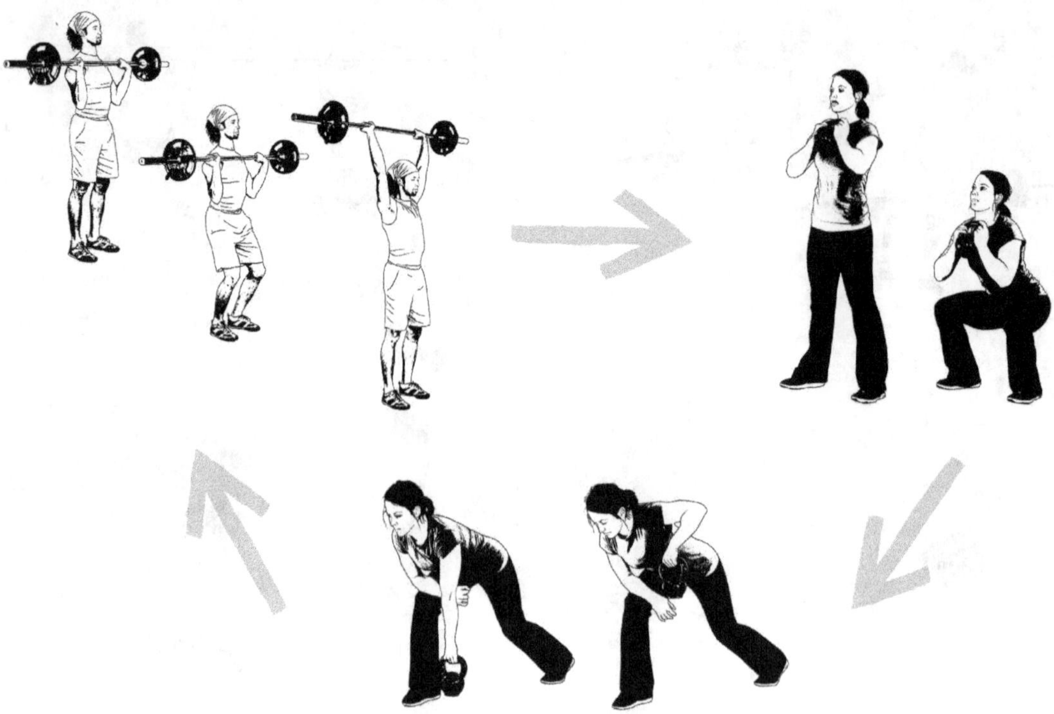

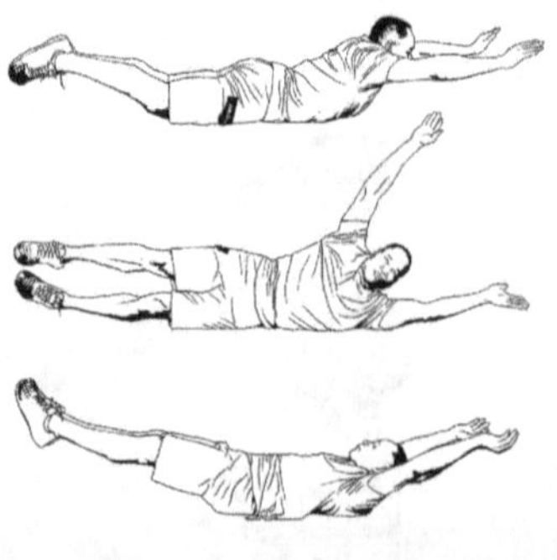

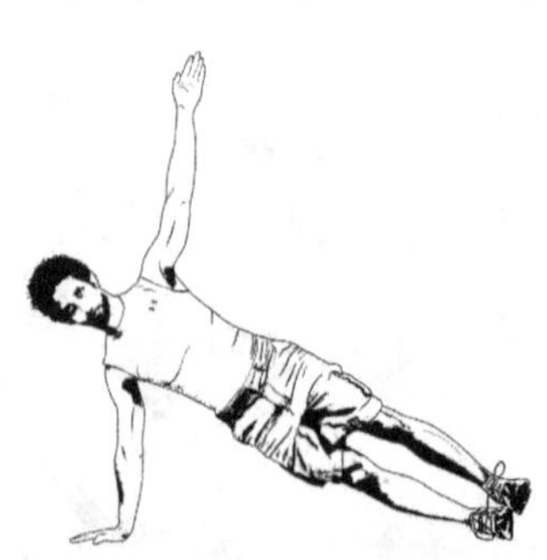

SIDE A

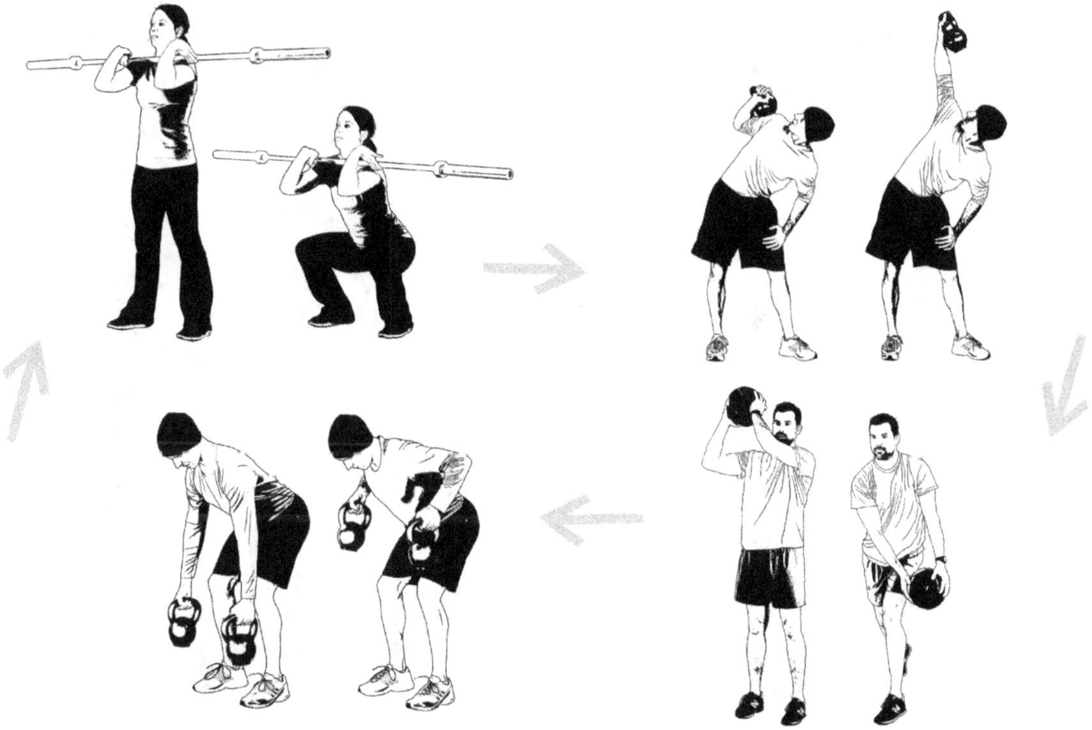

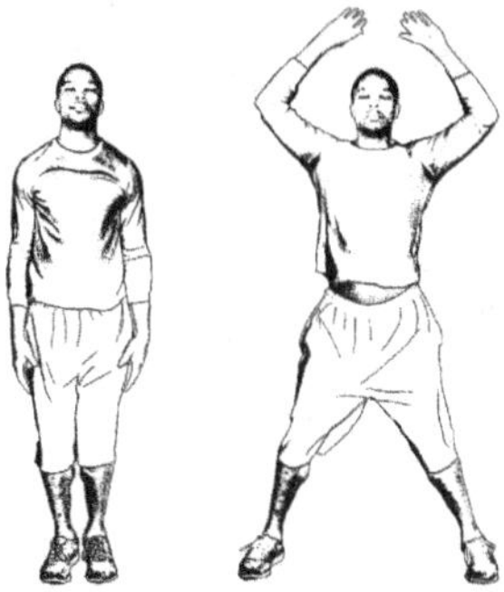

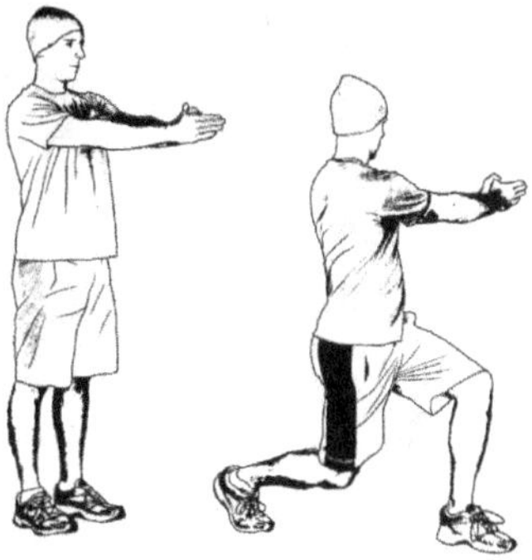

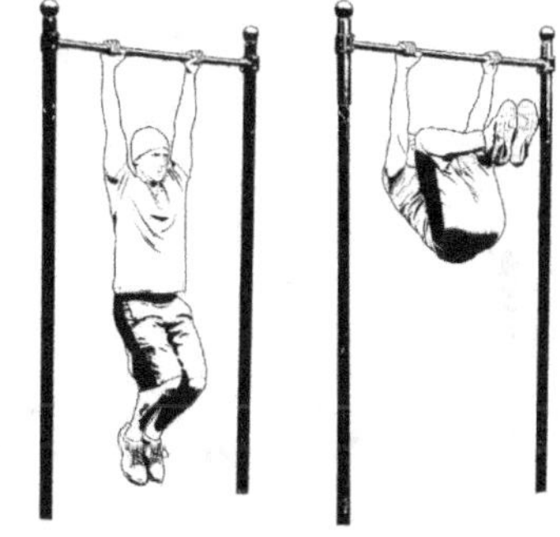

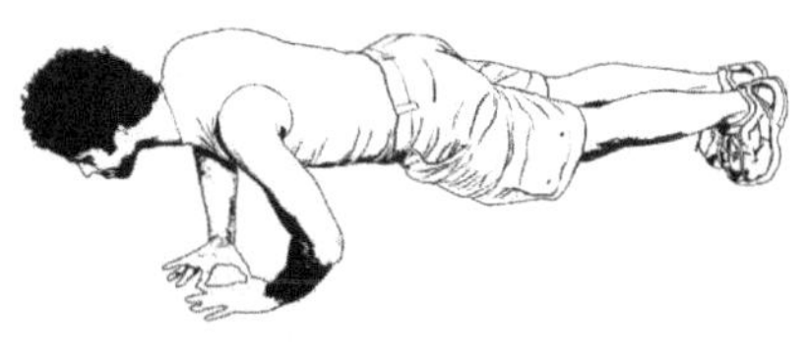

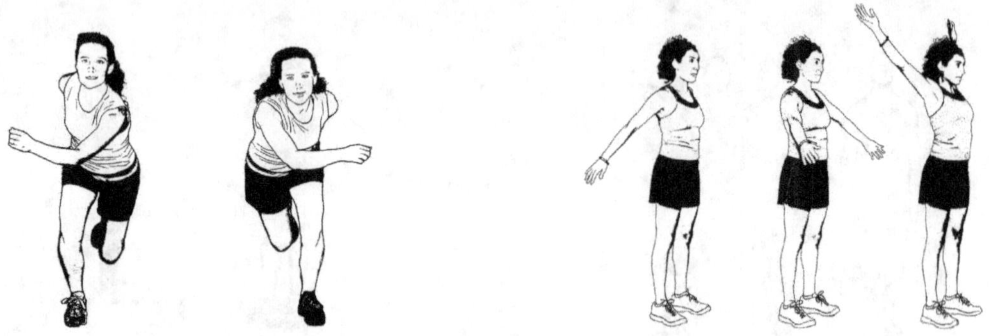

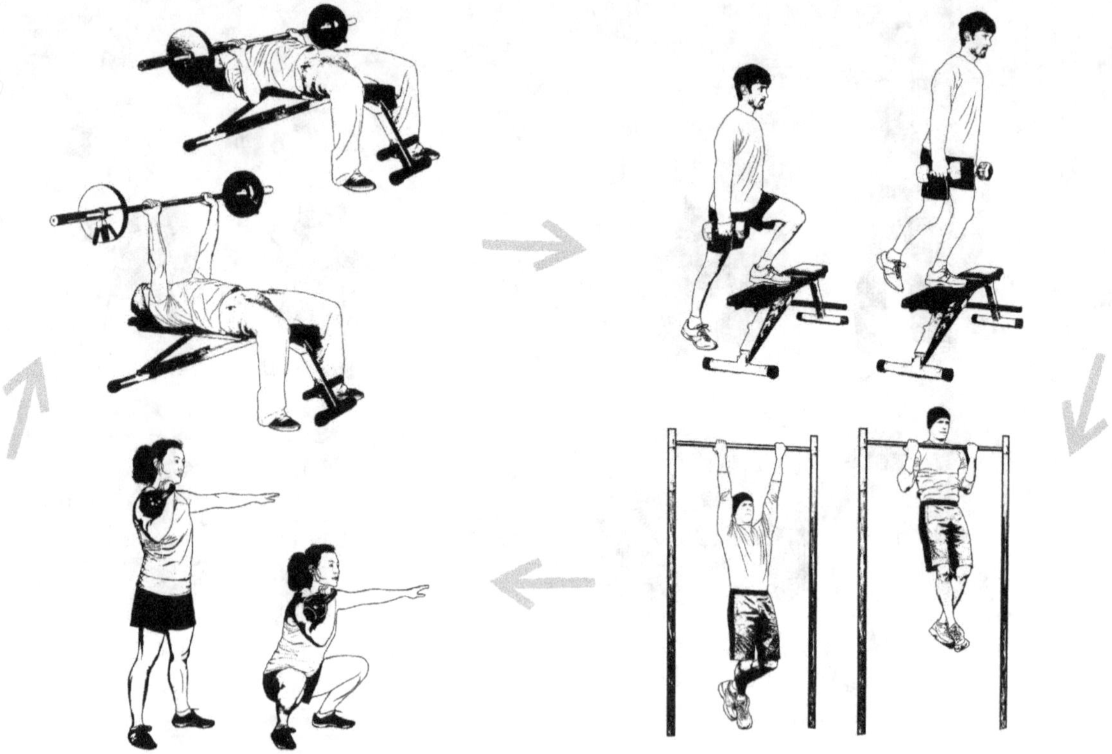

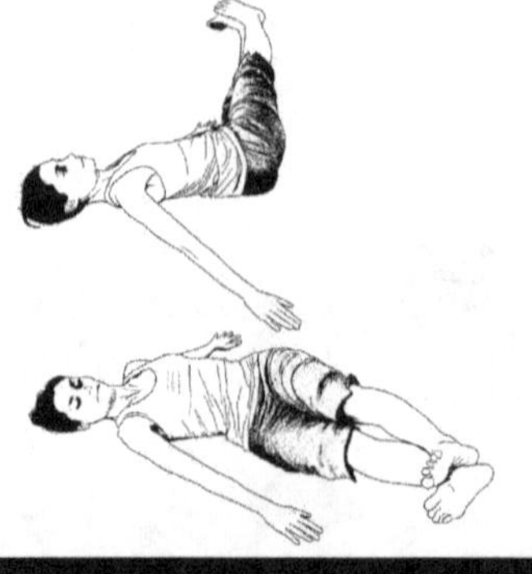

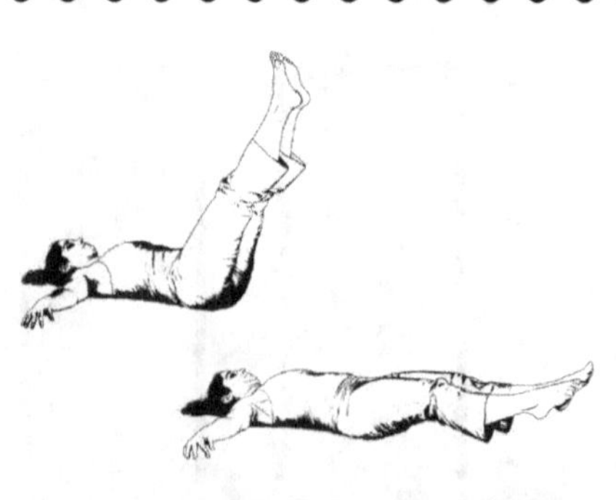

SIDE A

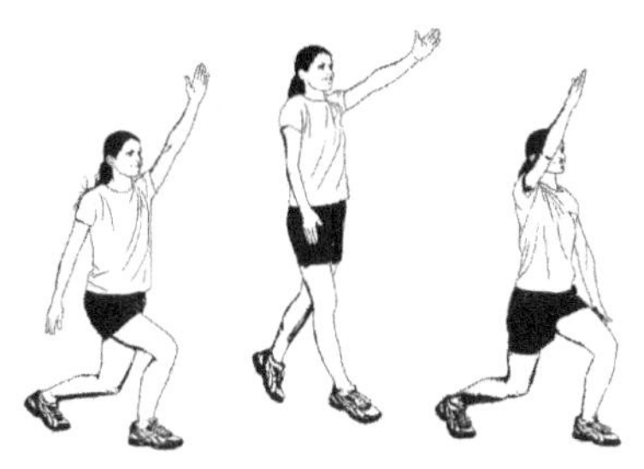

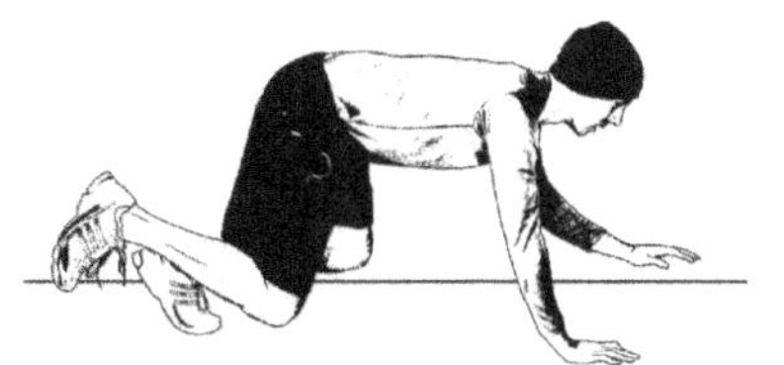

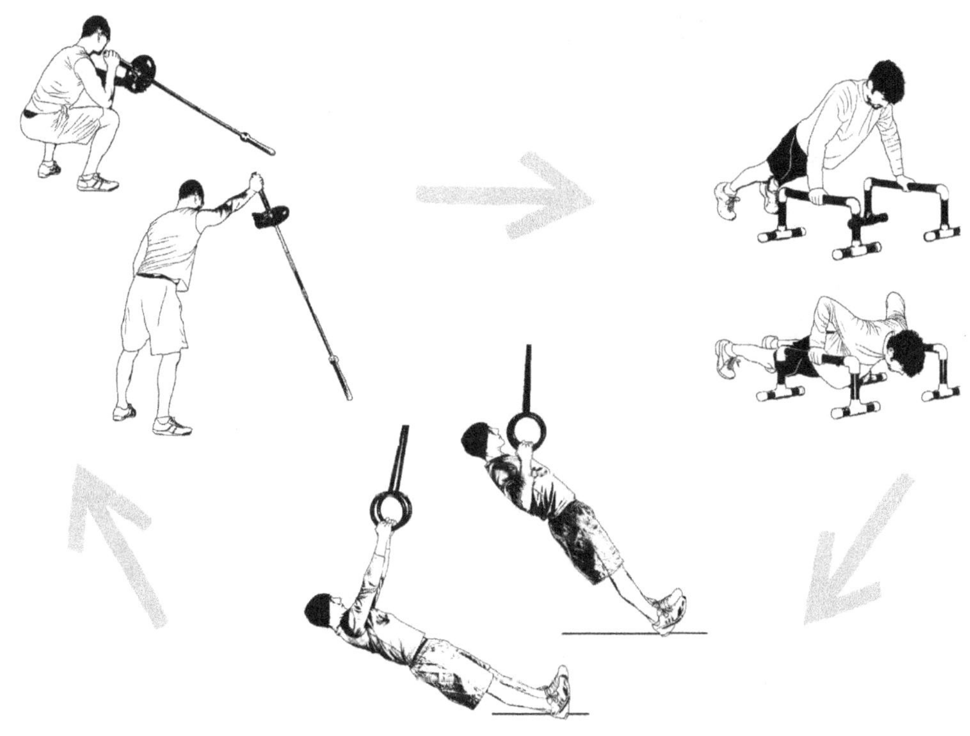

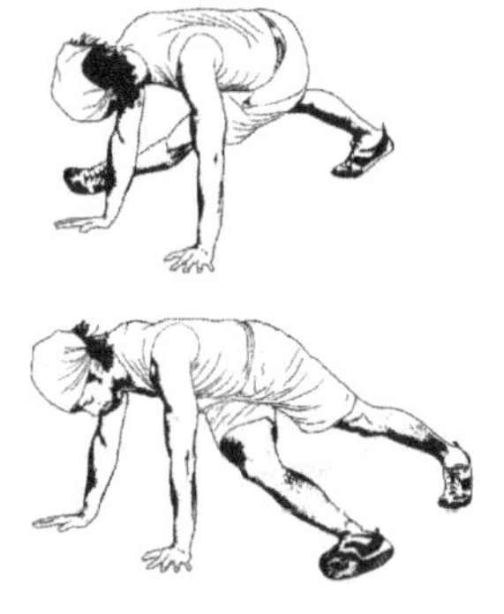

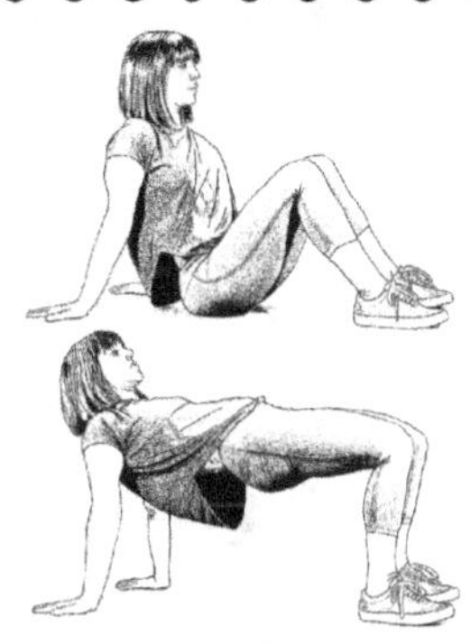

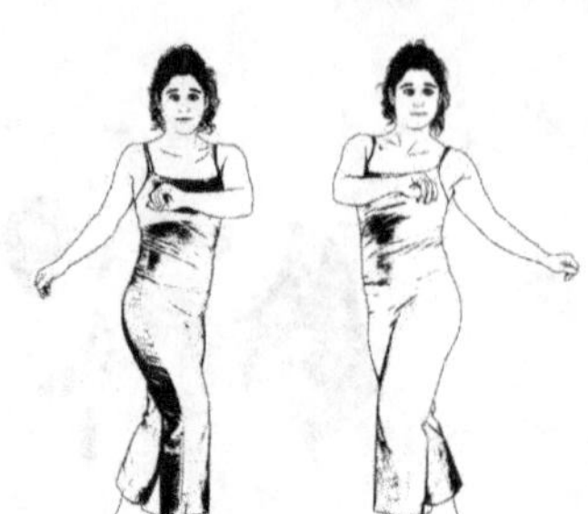

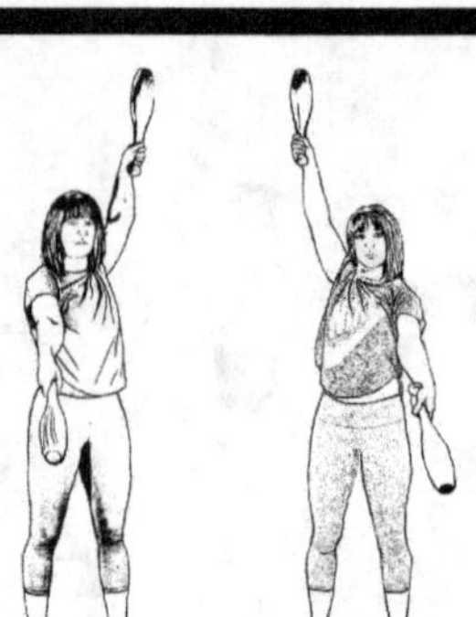

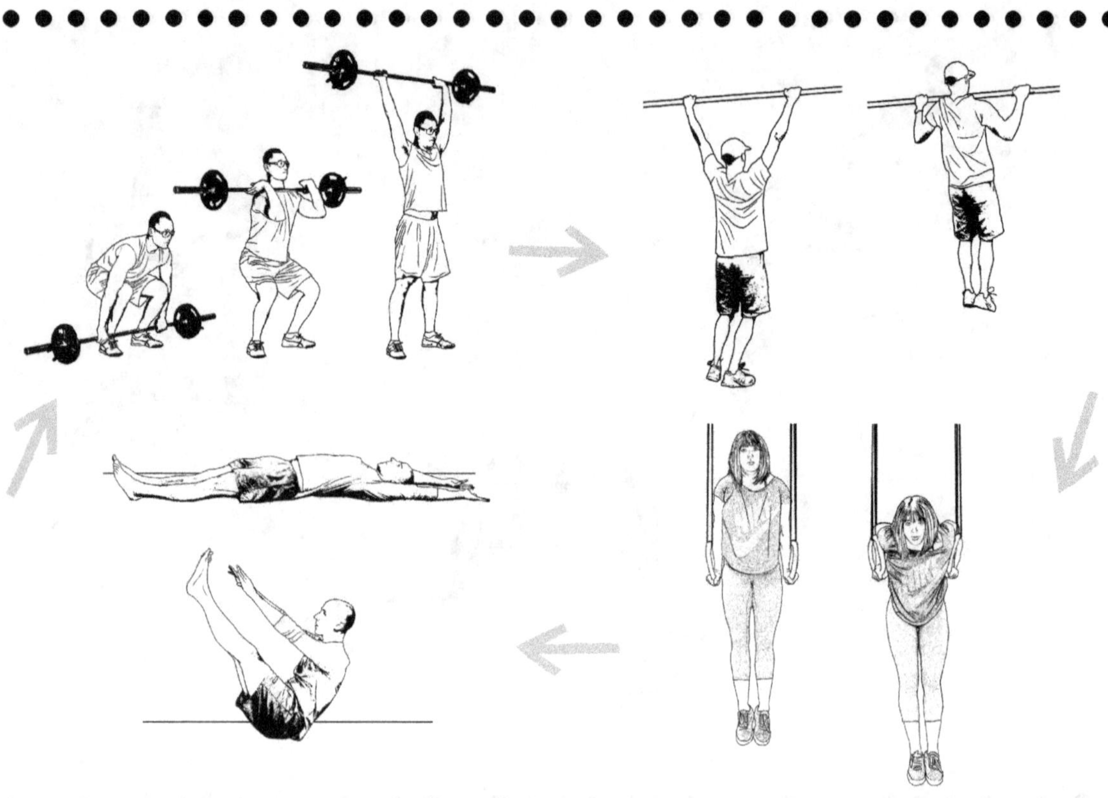

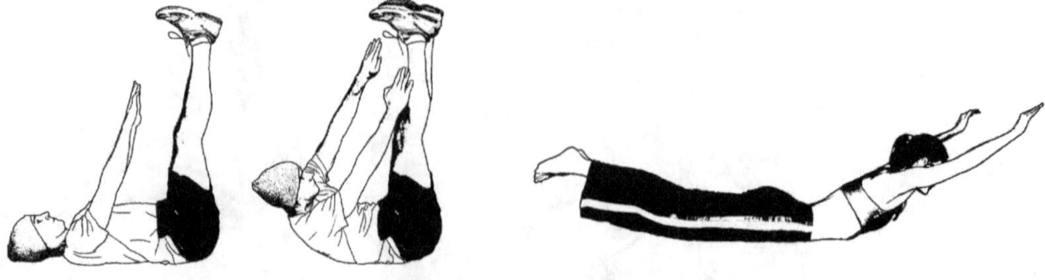

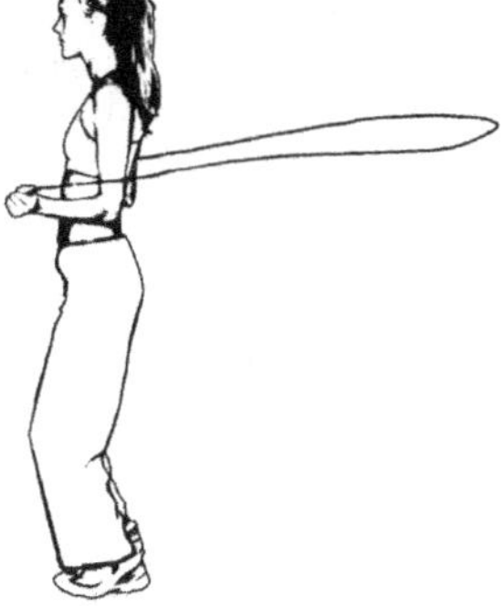

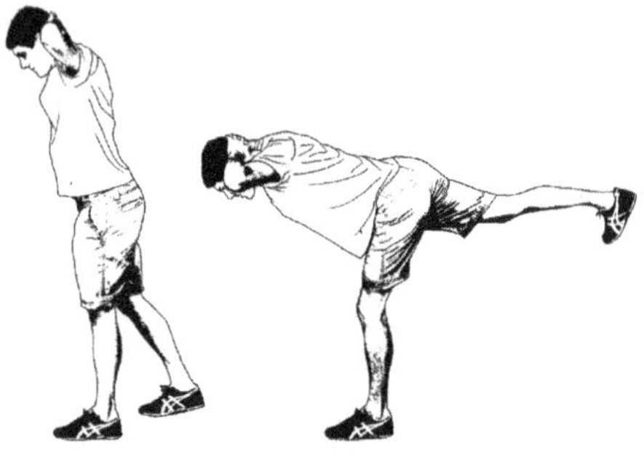

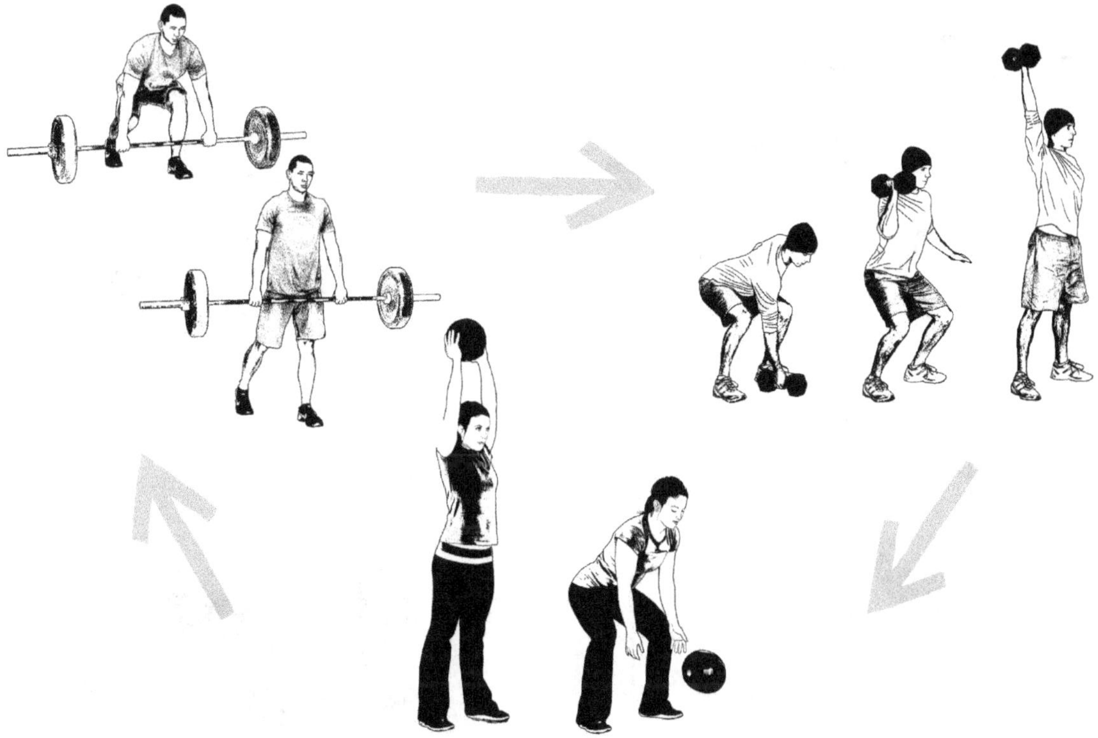

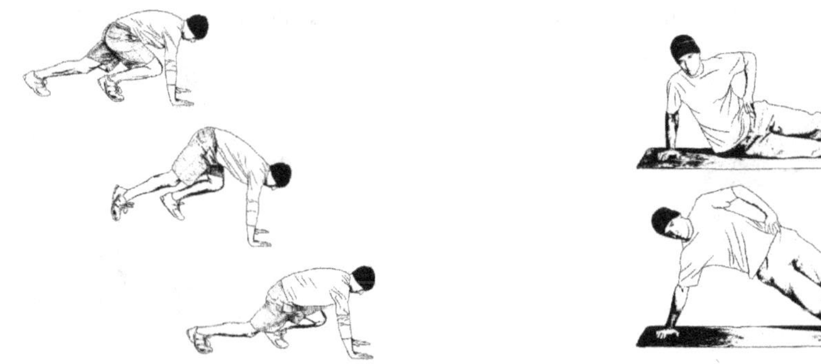

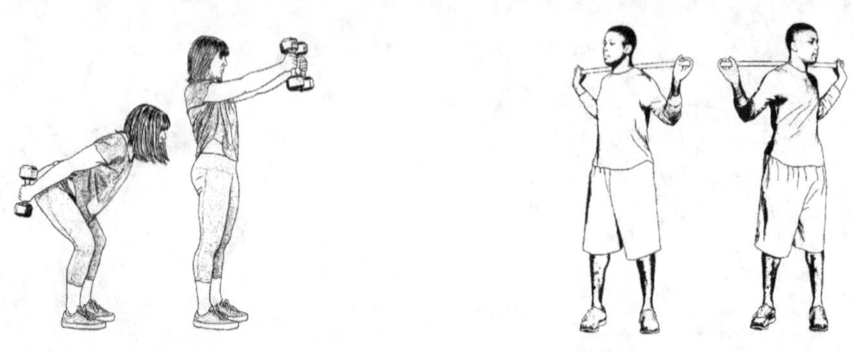

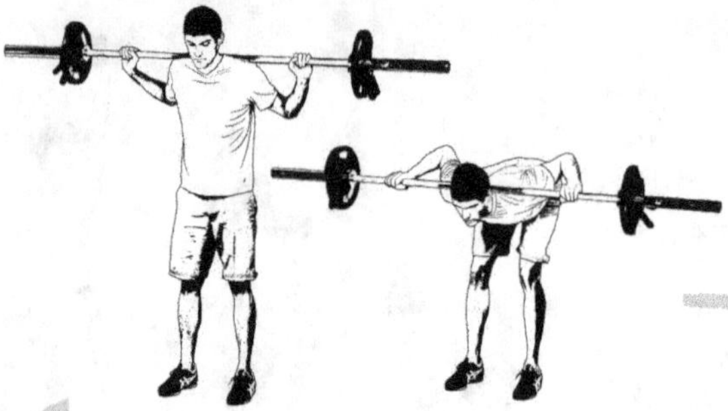

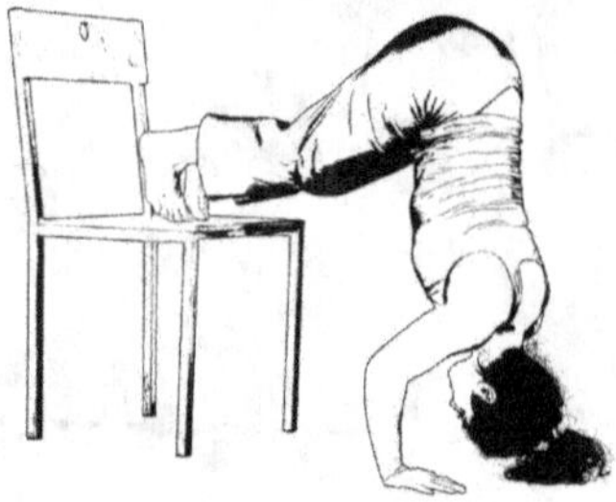

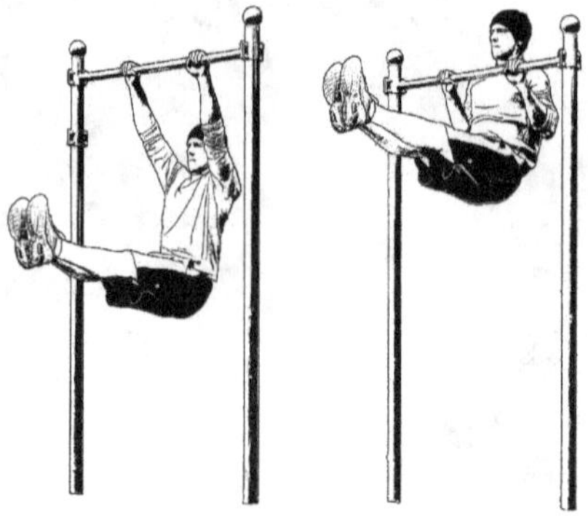

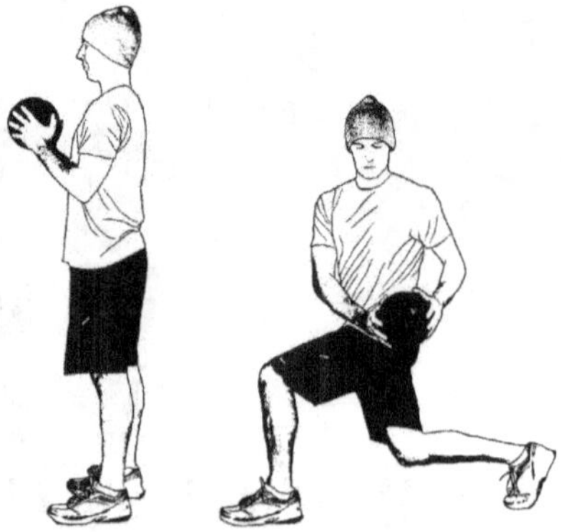

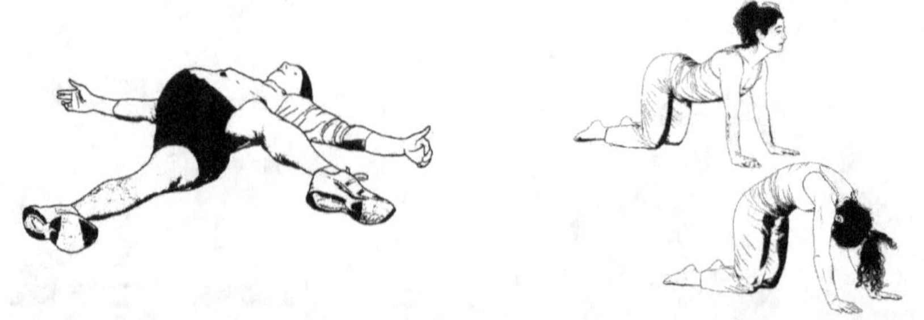

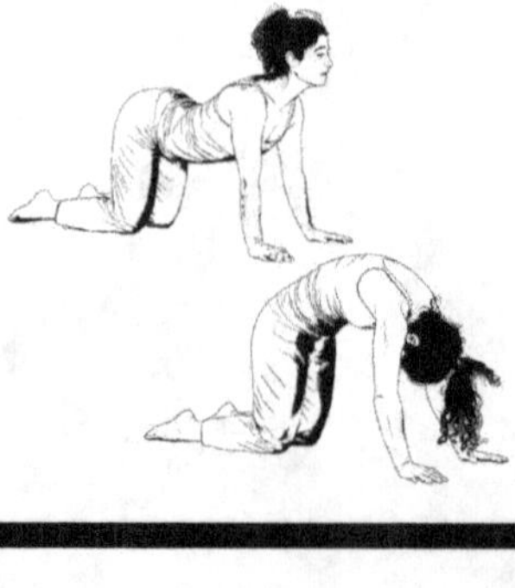

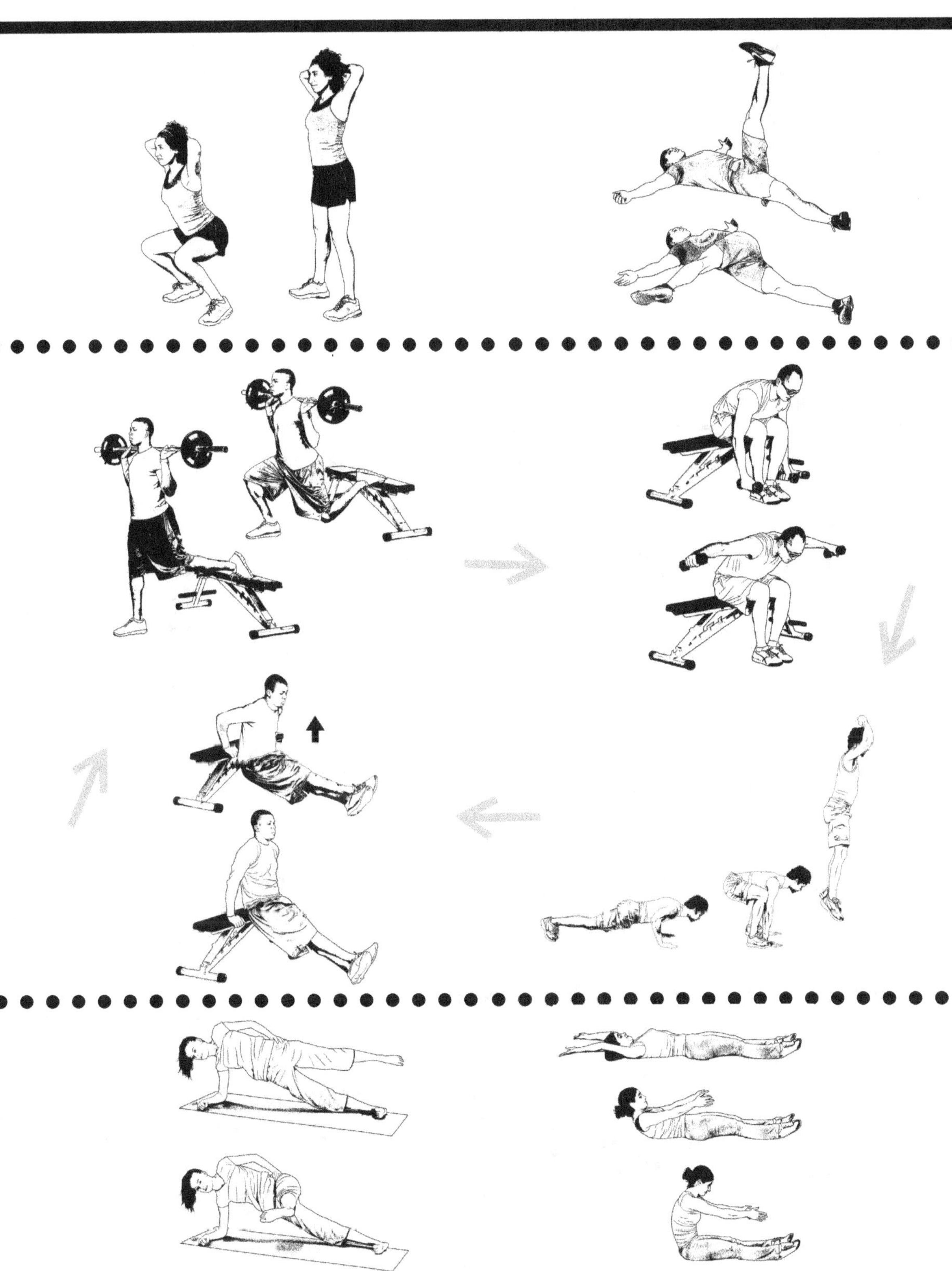

SIDE A

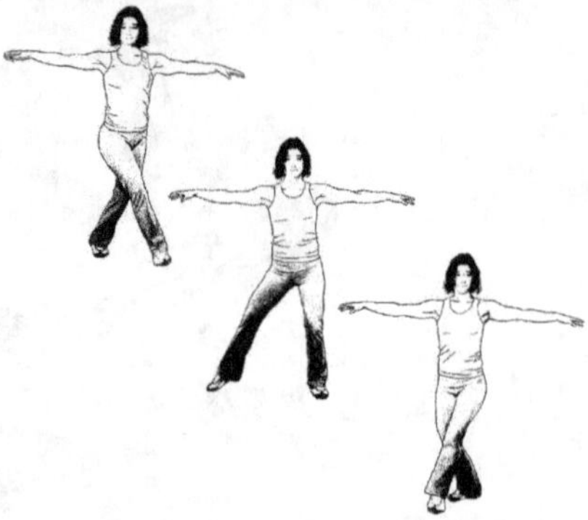

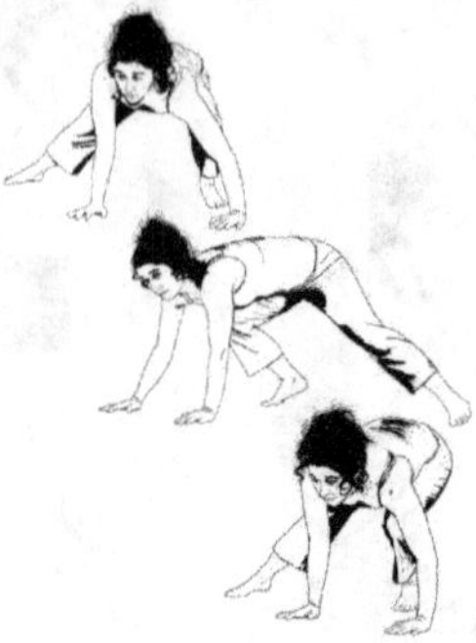

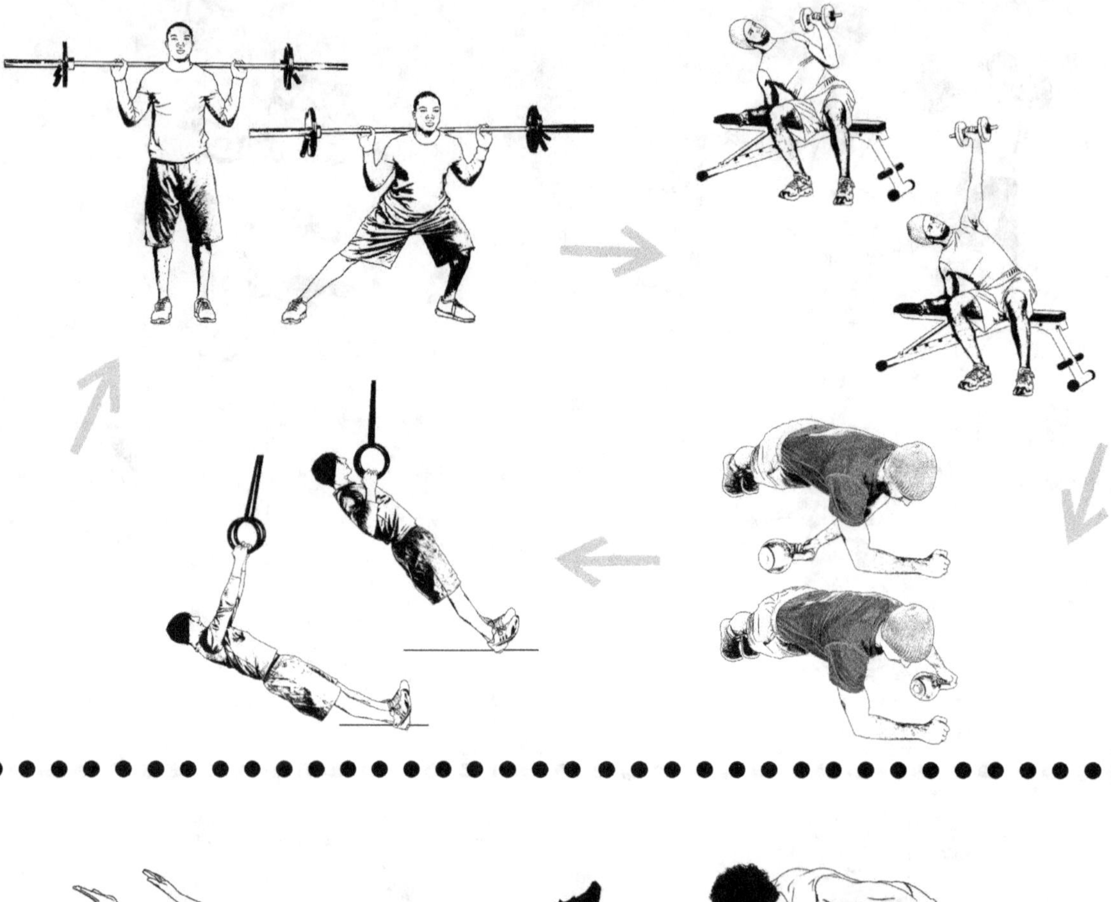

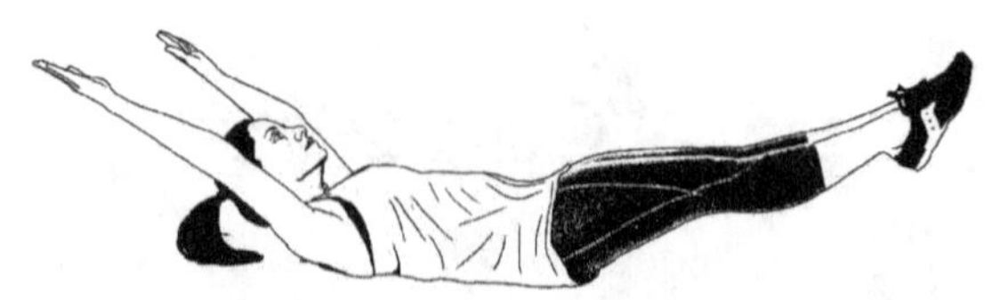

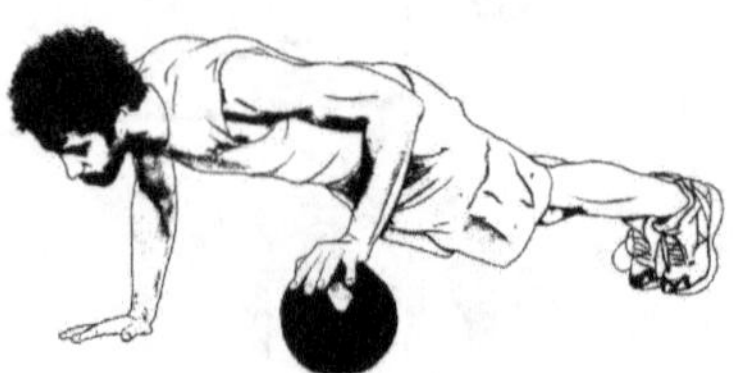

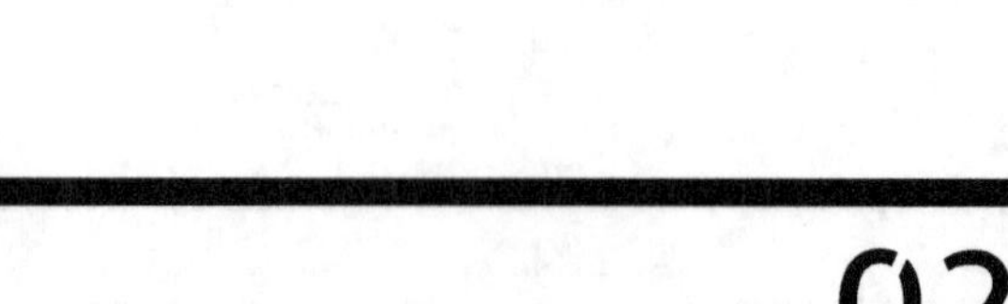

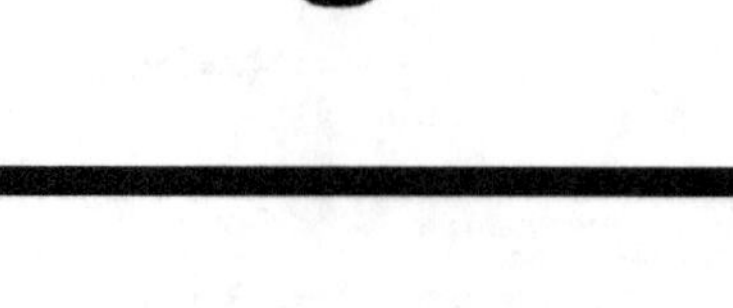

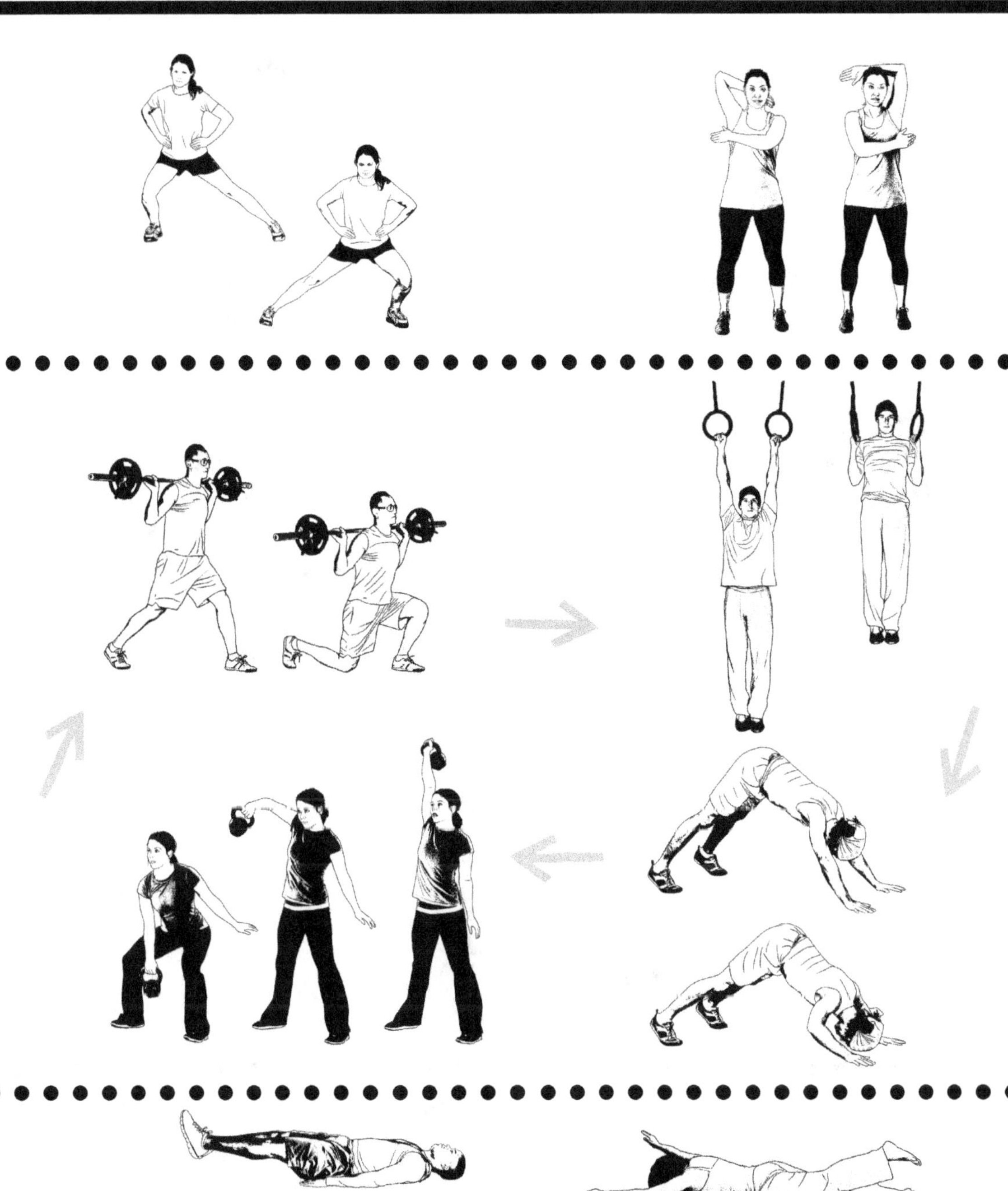

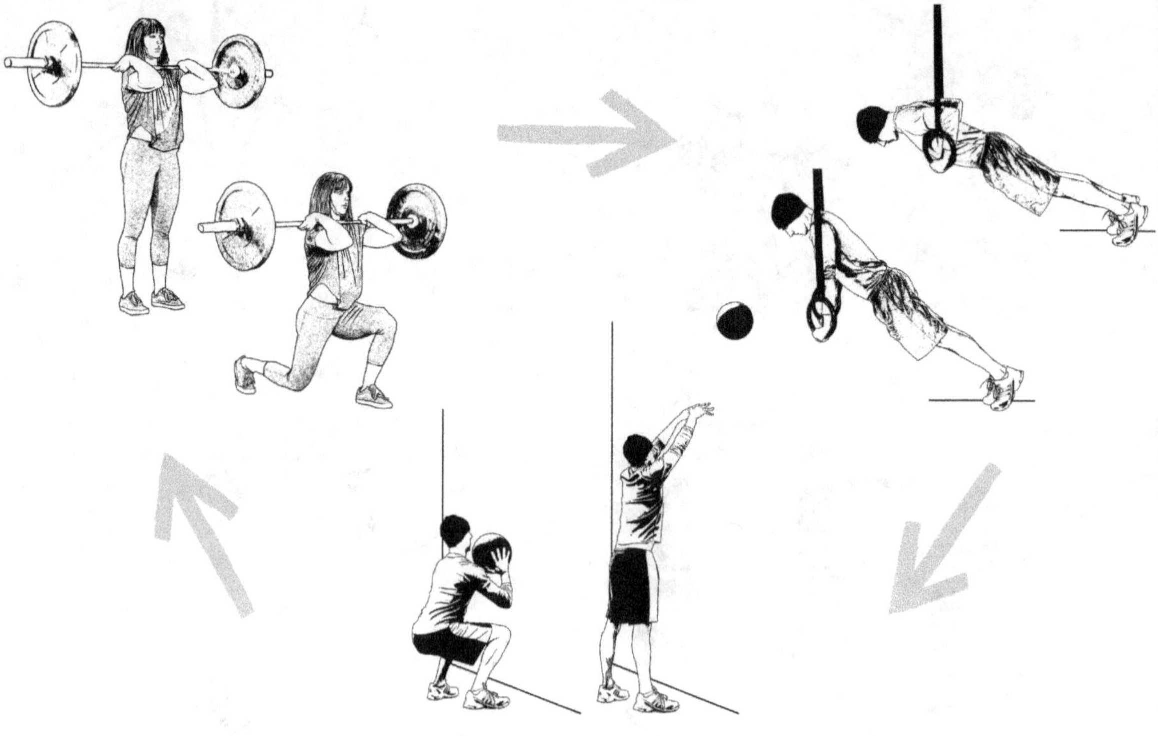

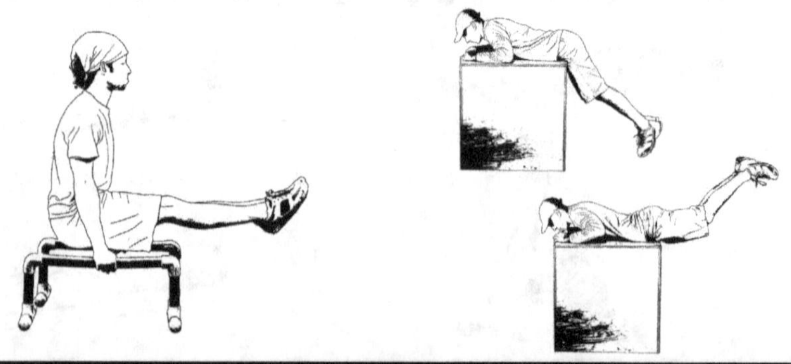

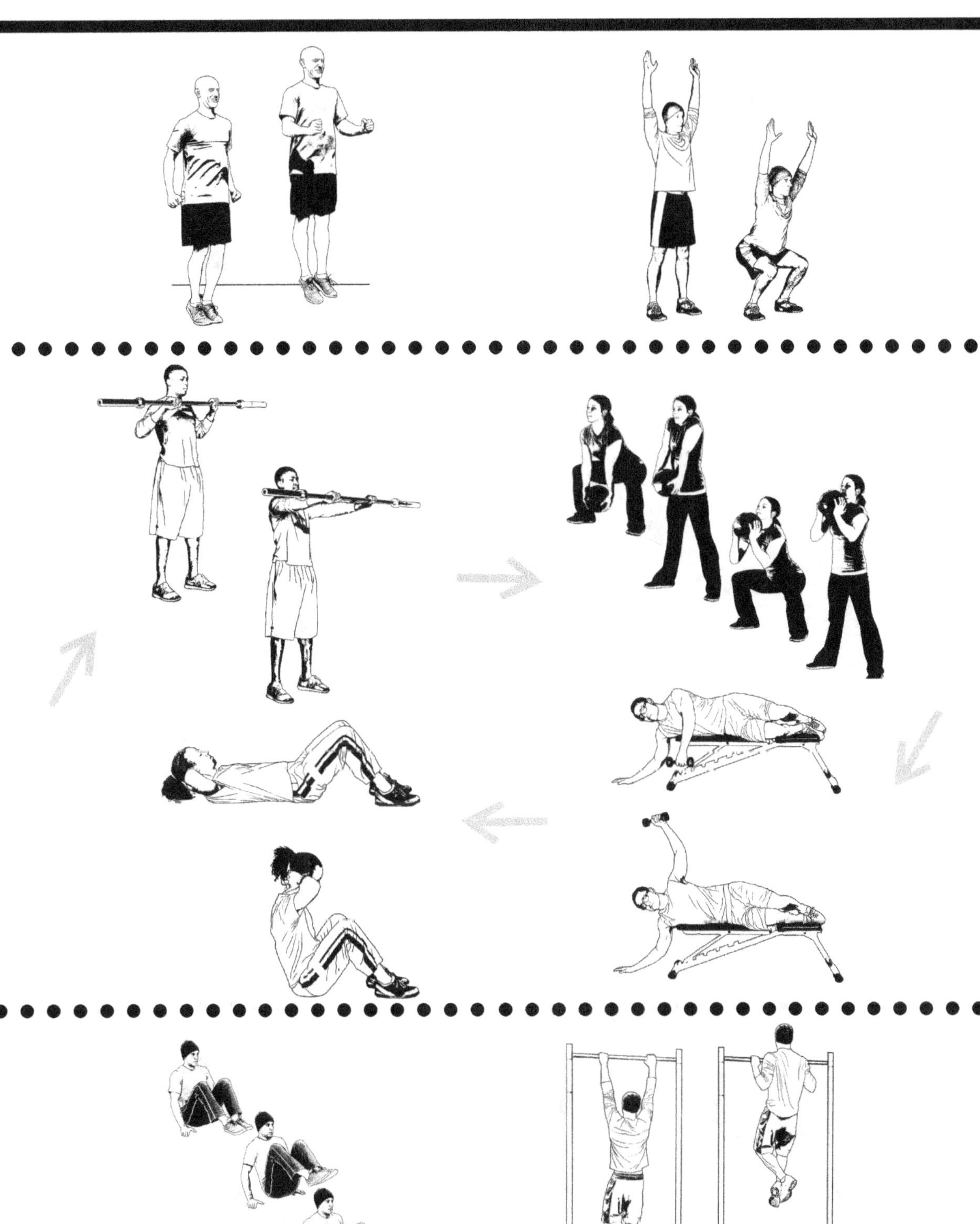

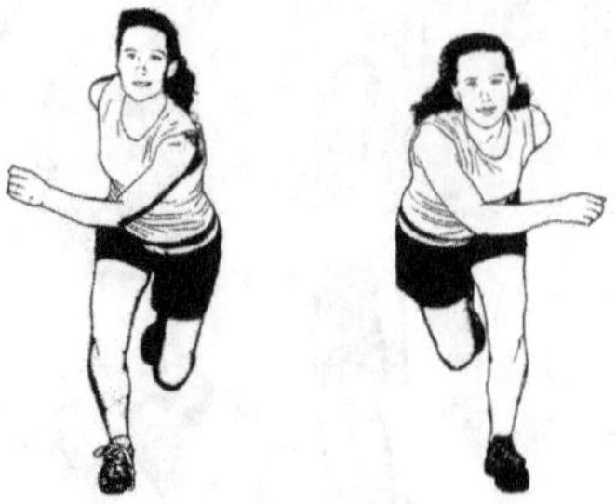

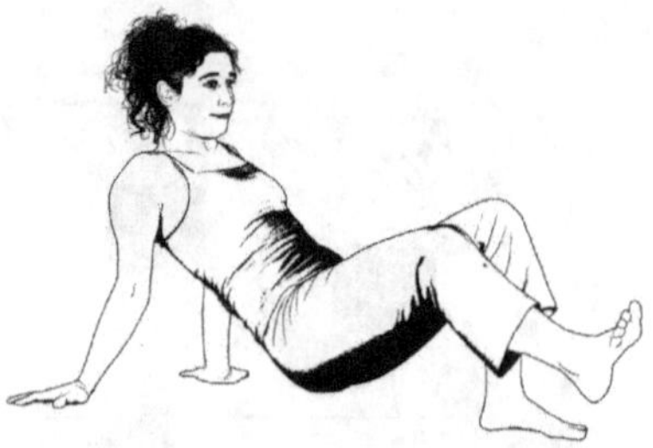

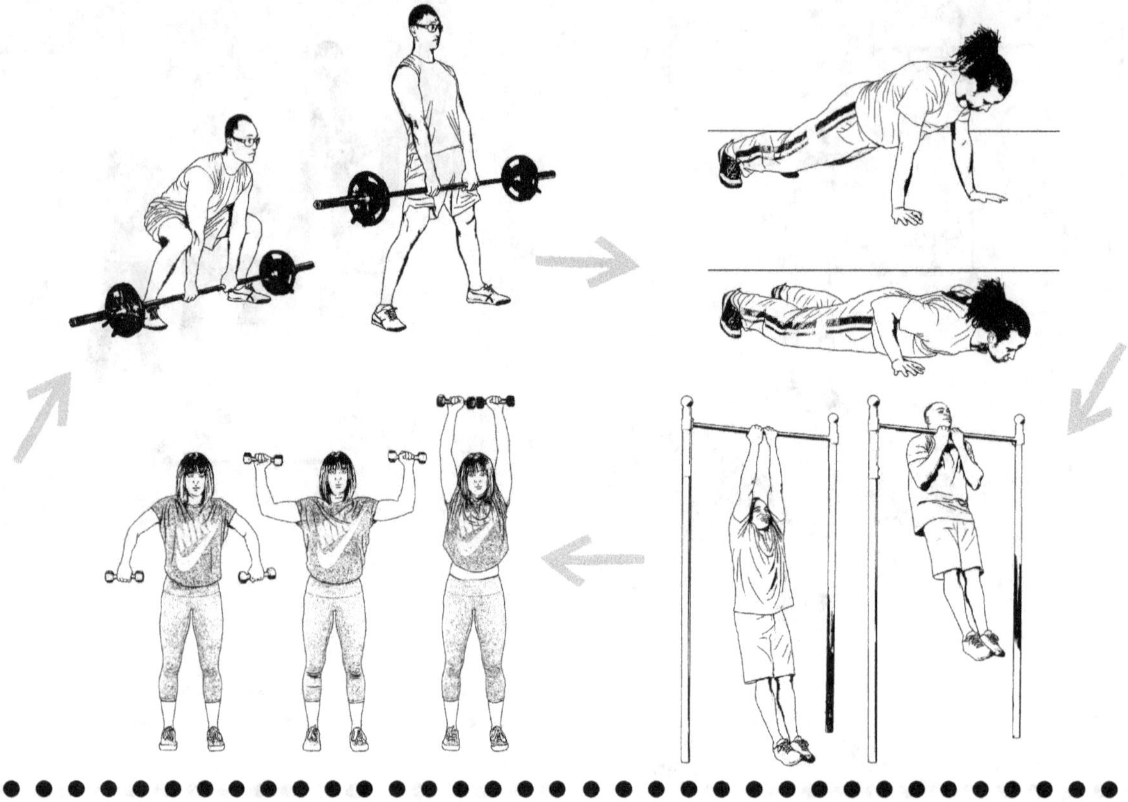

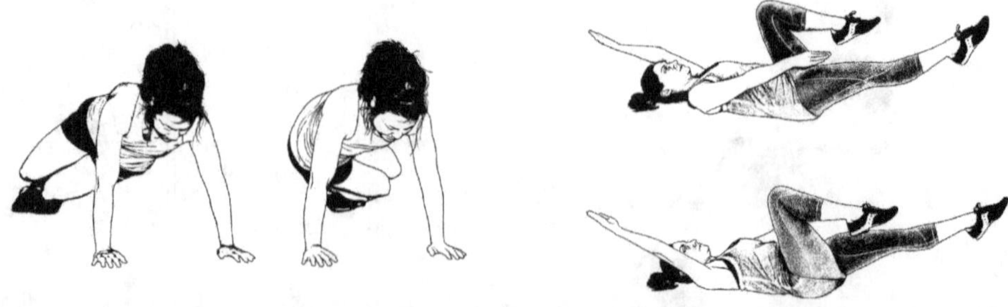

SIDE A

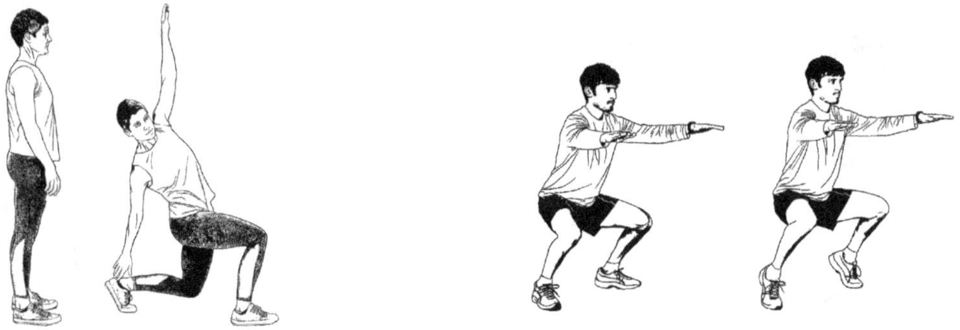

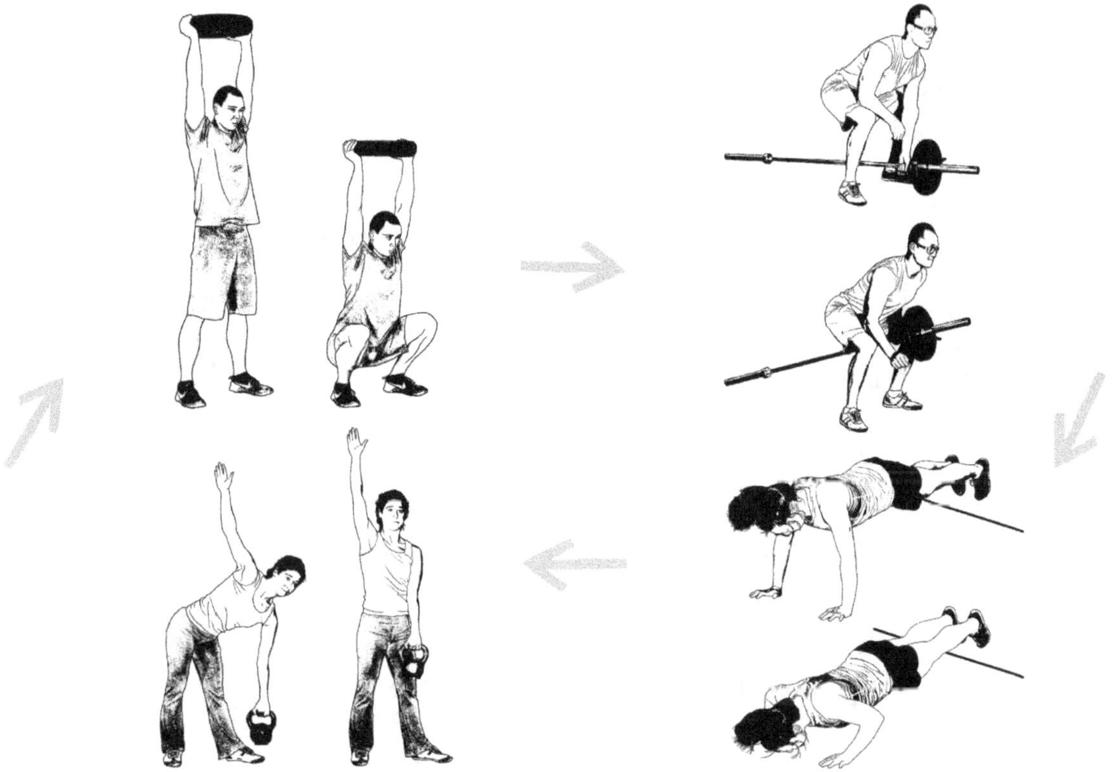

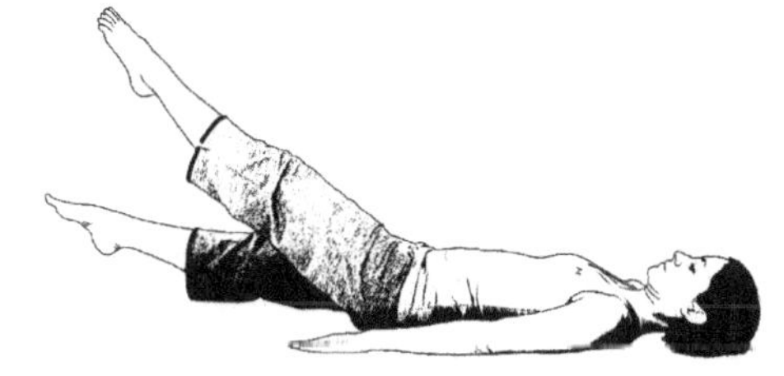

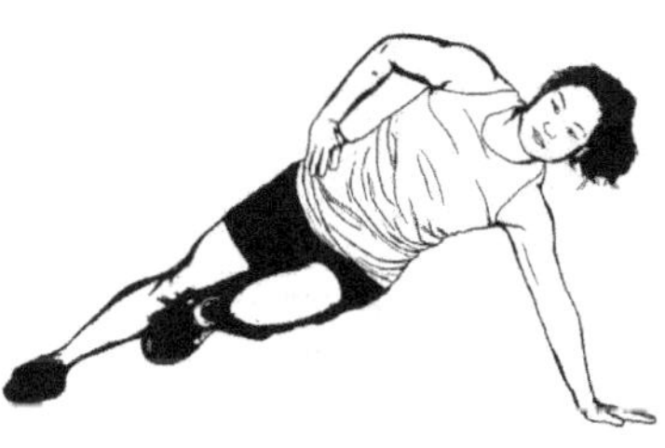

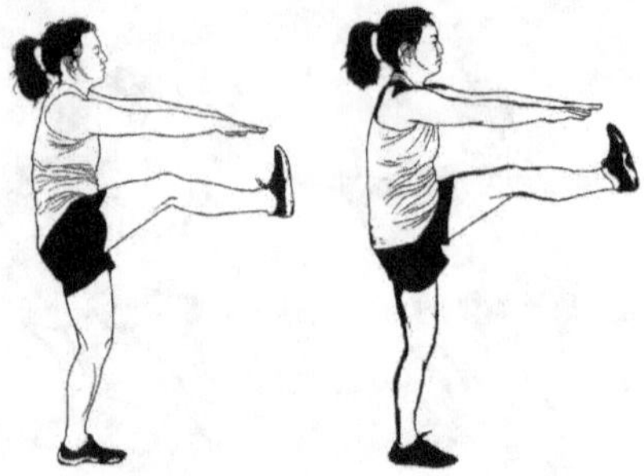

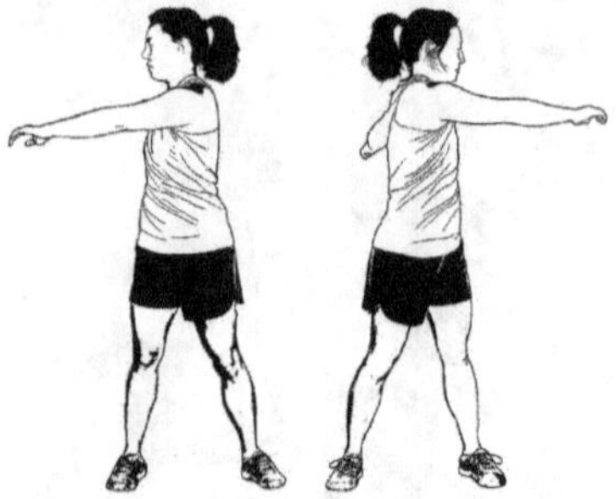

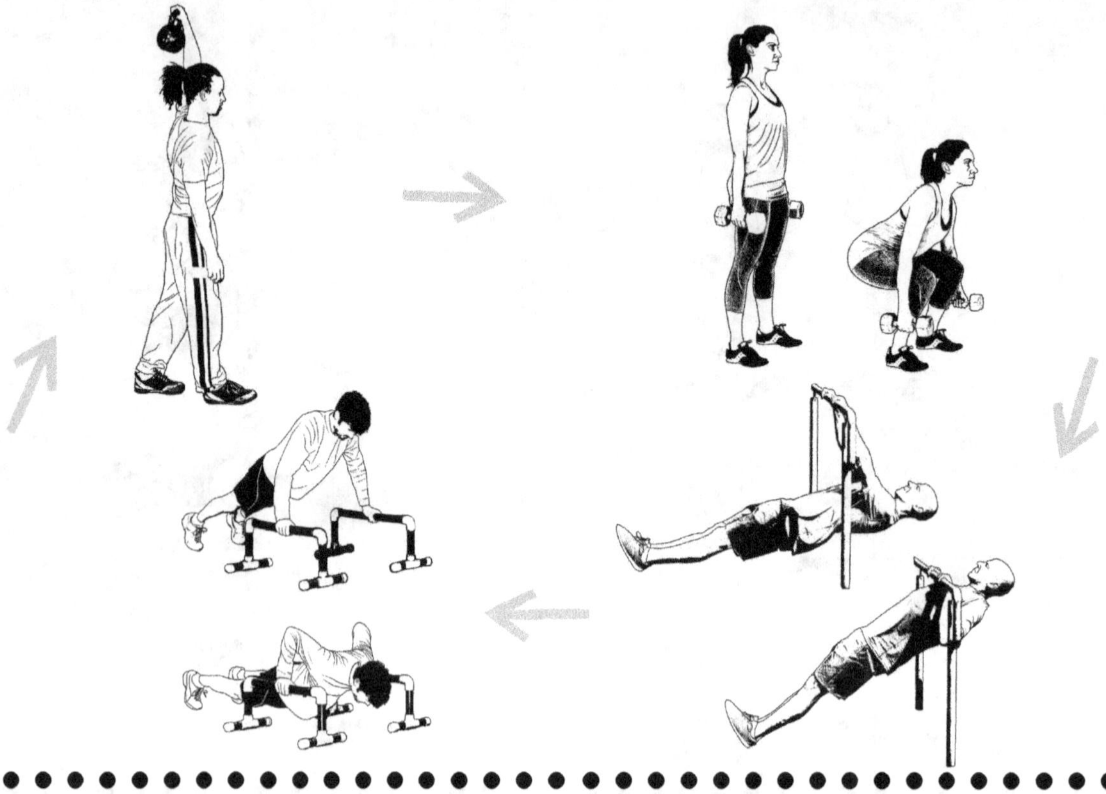

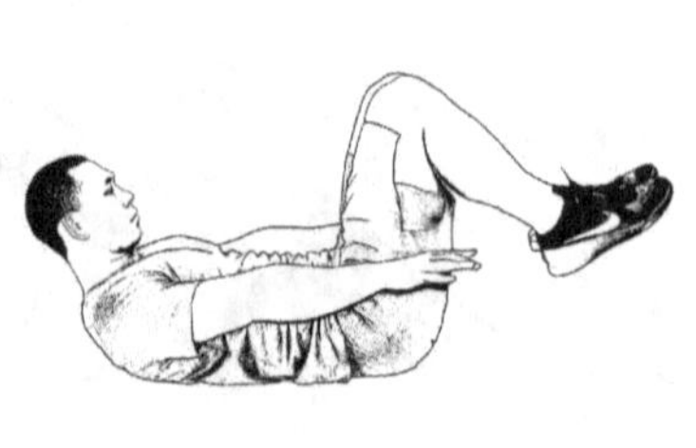

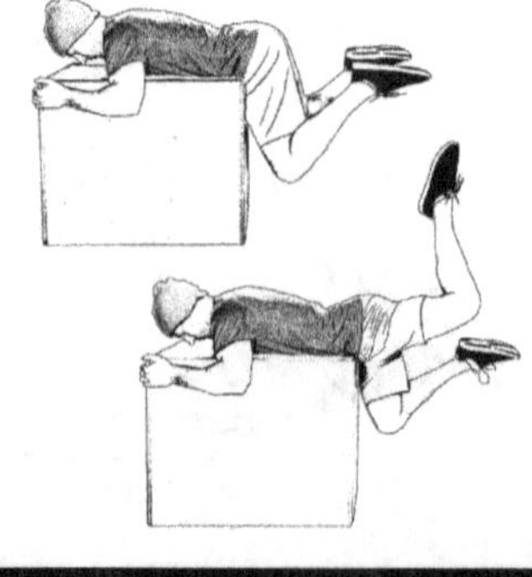

SIDE A

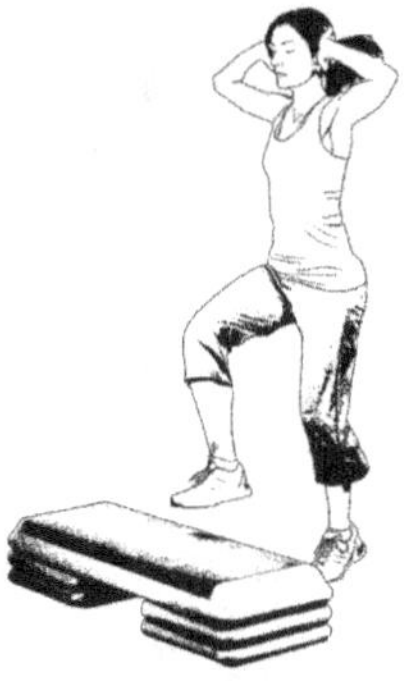

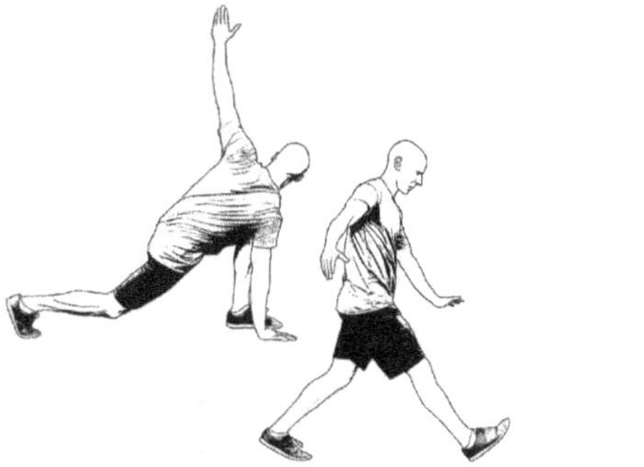

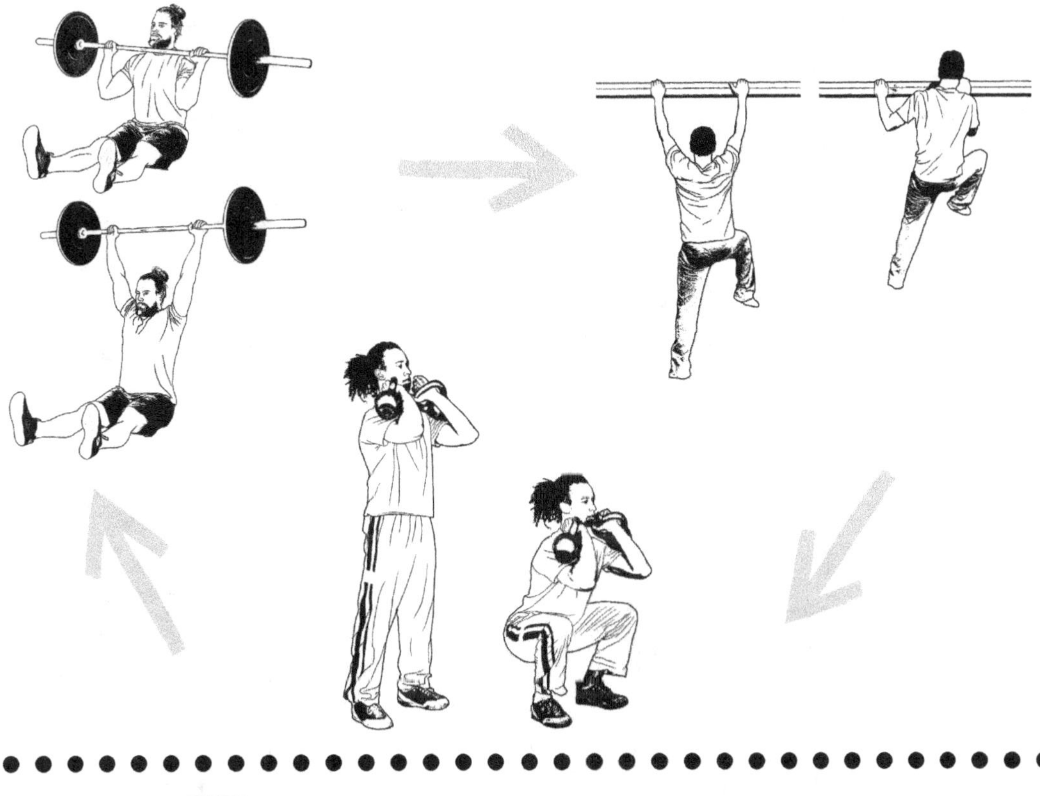

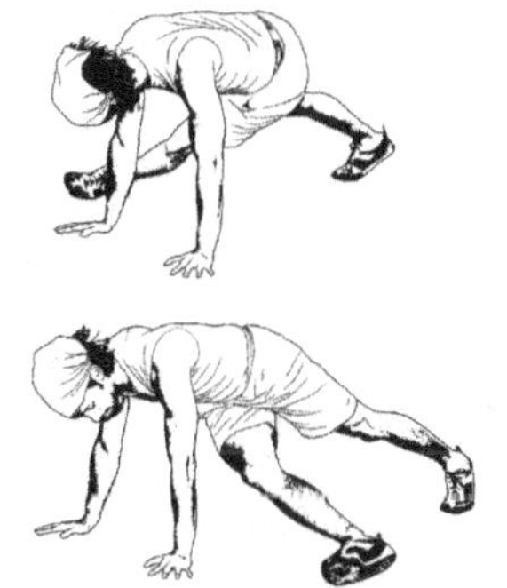

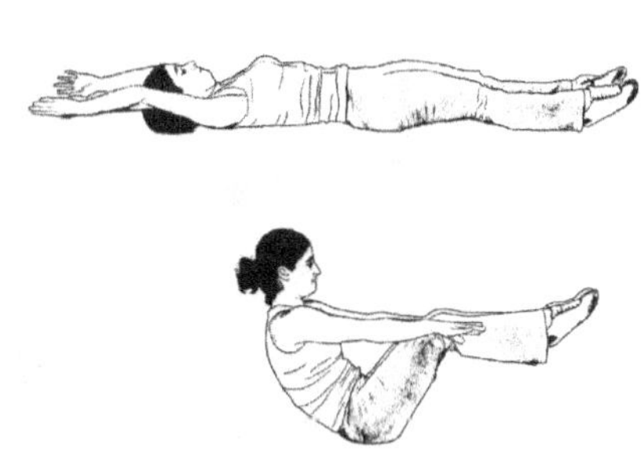

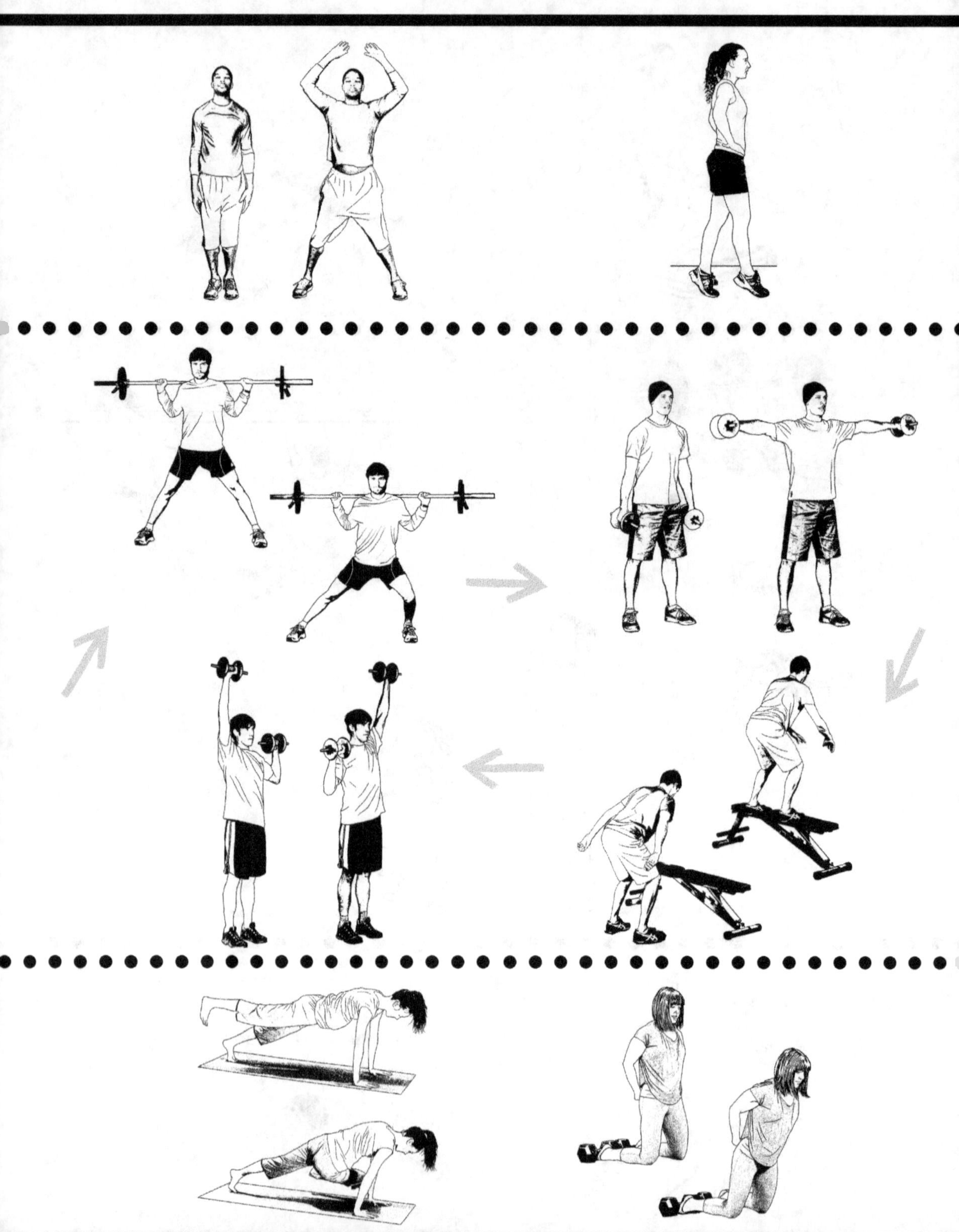

SIDE A

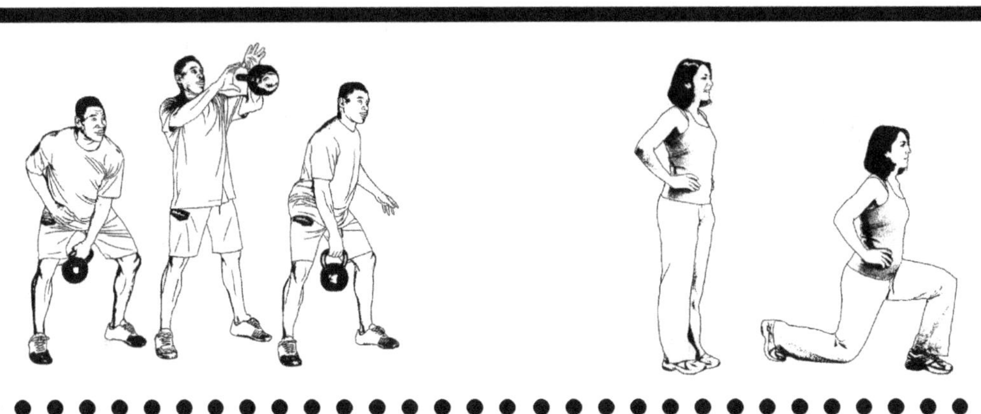

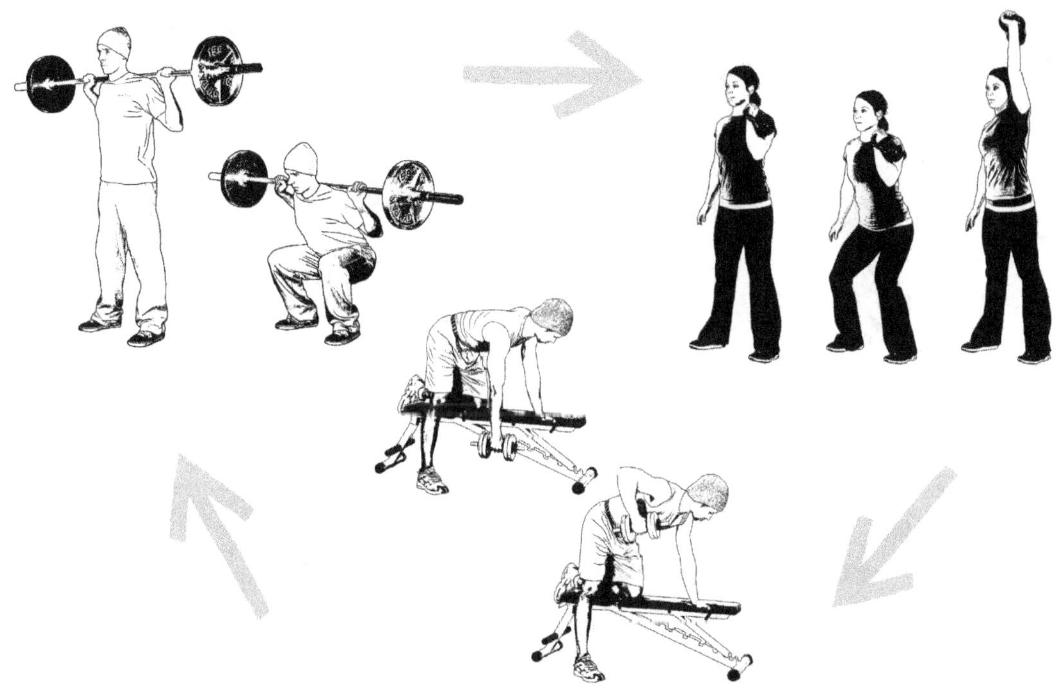

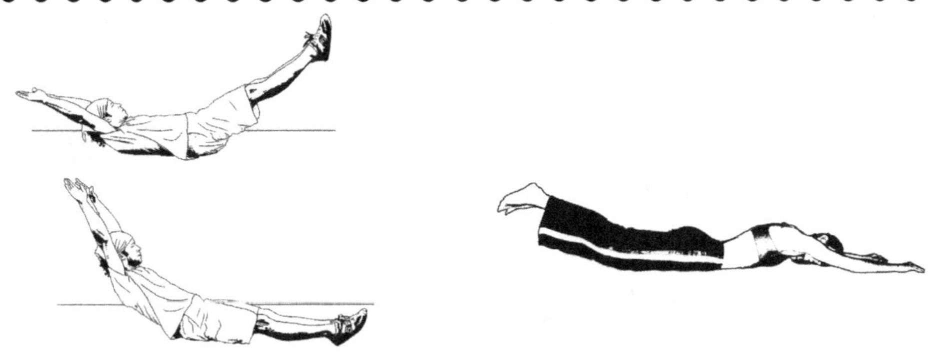

SIDE A

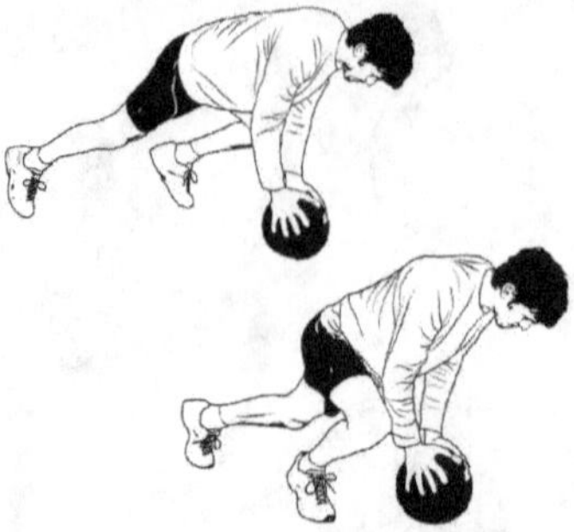

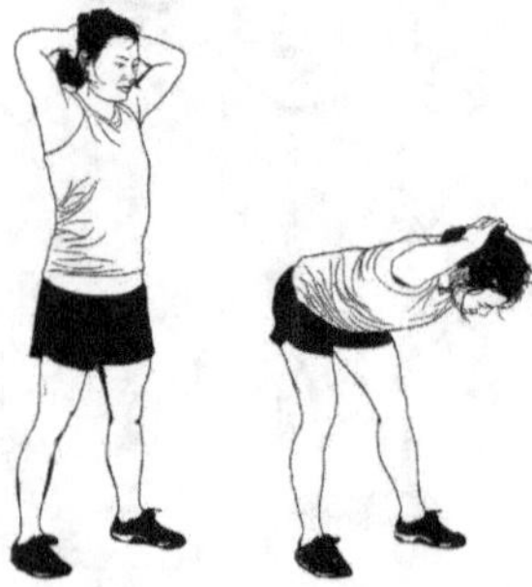

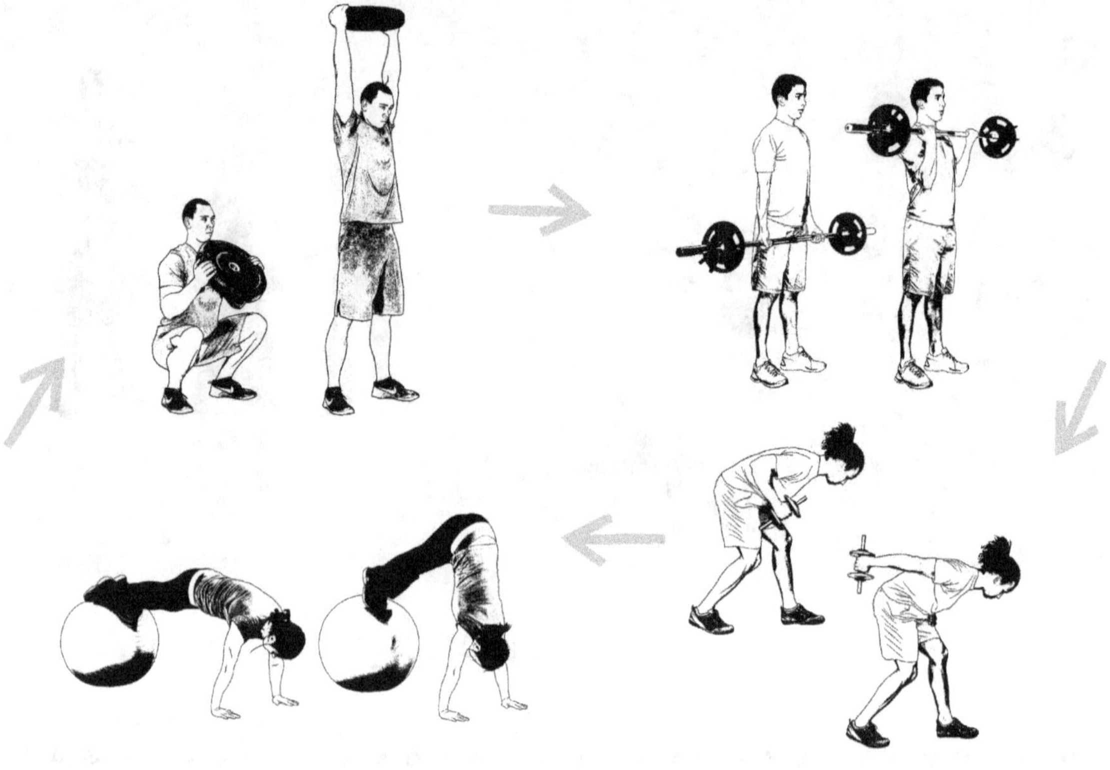

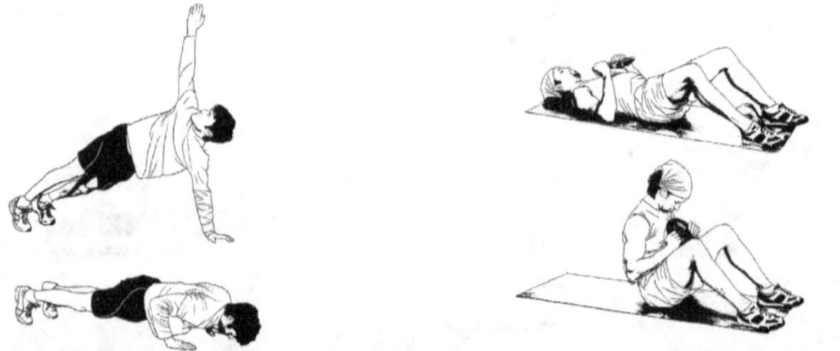

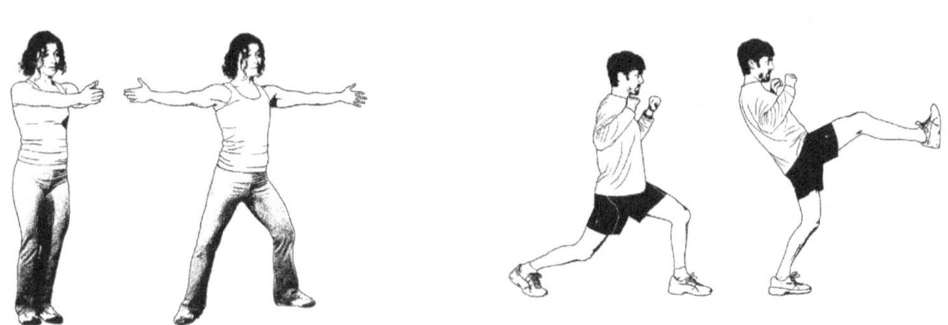

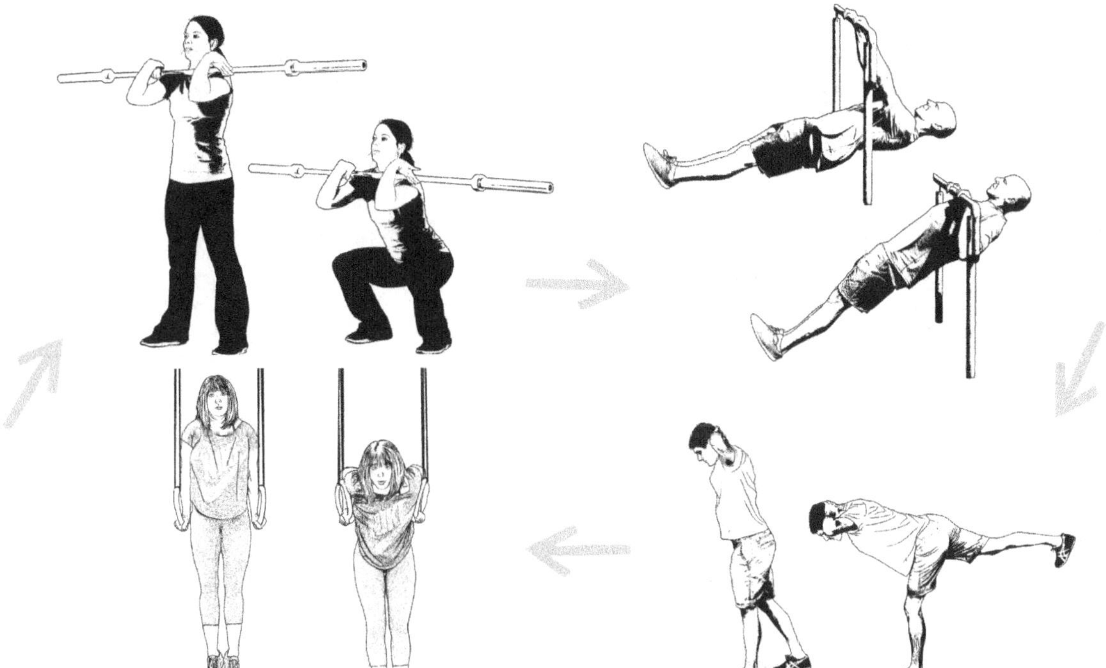

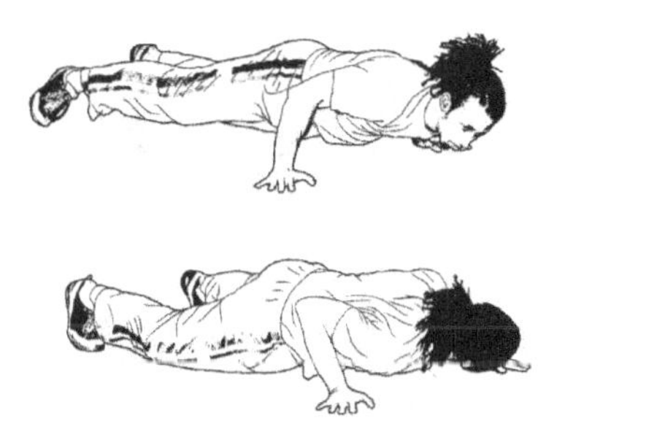

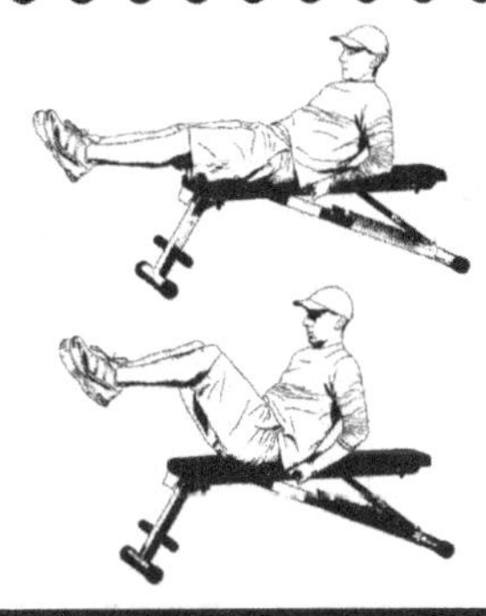

SIDE A

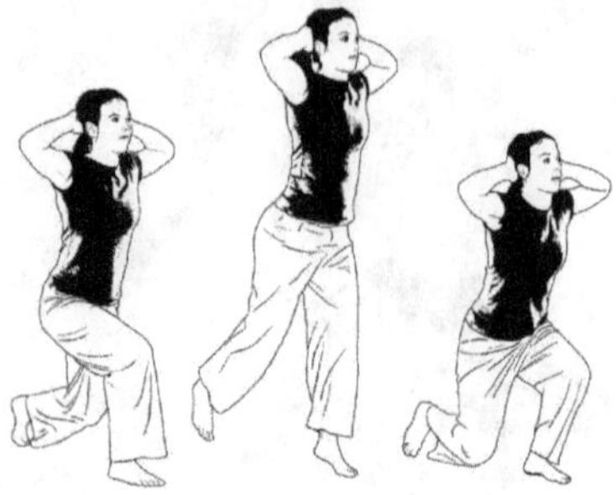

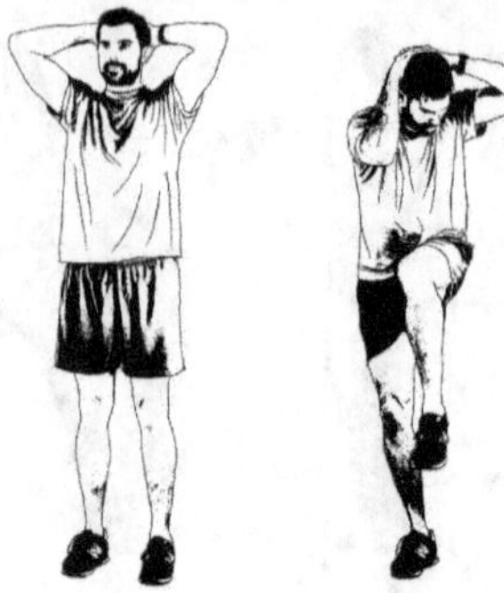

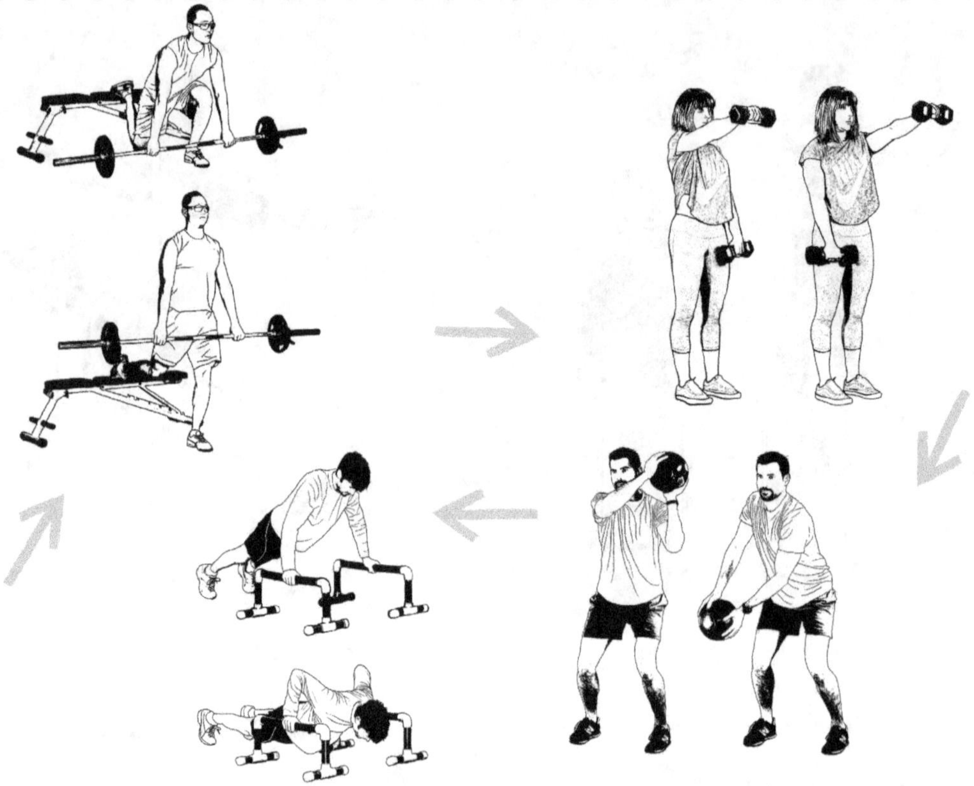

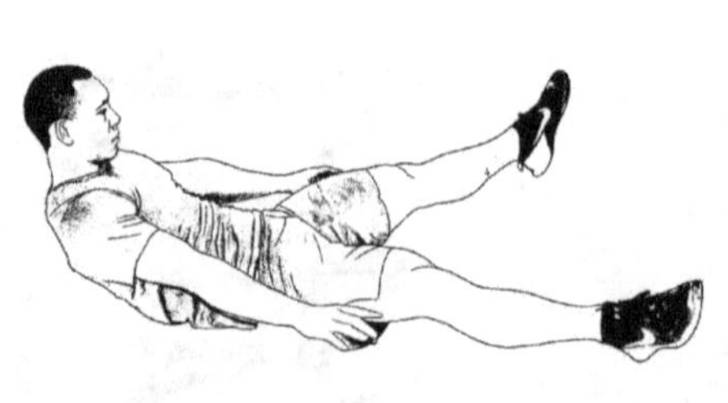

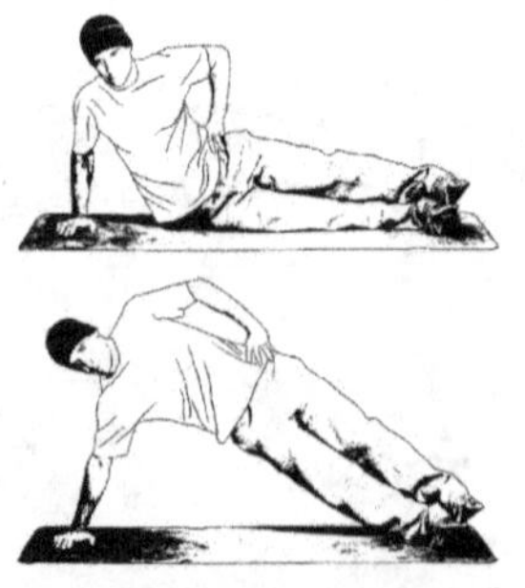

SIDE A

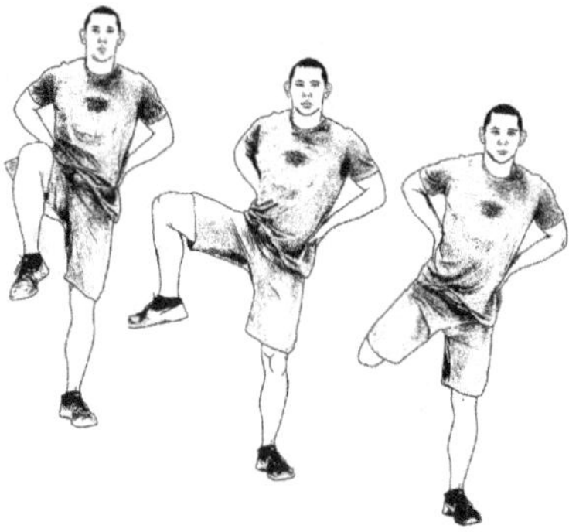

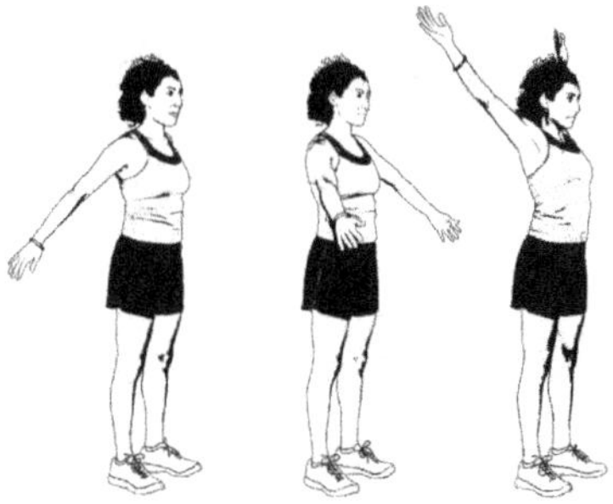

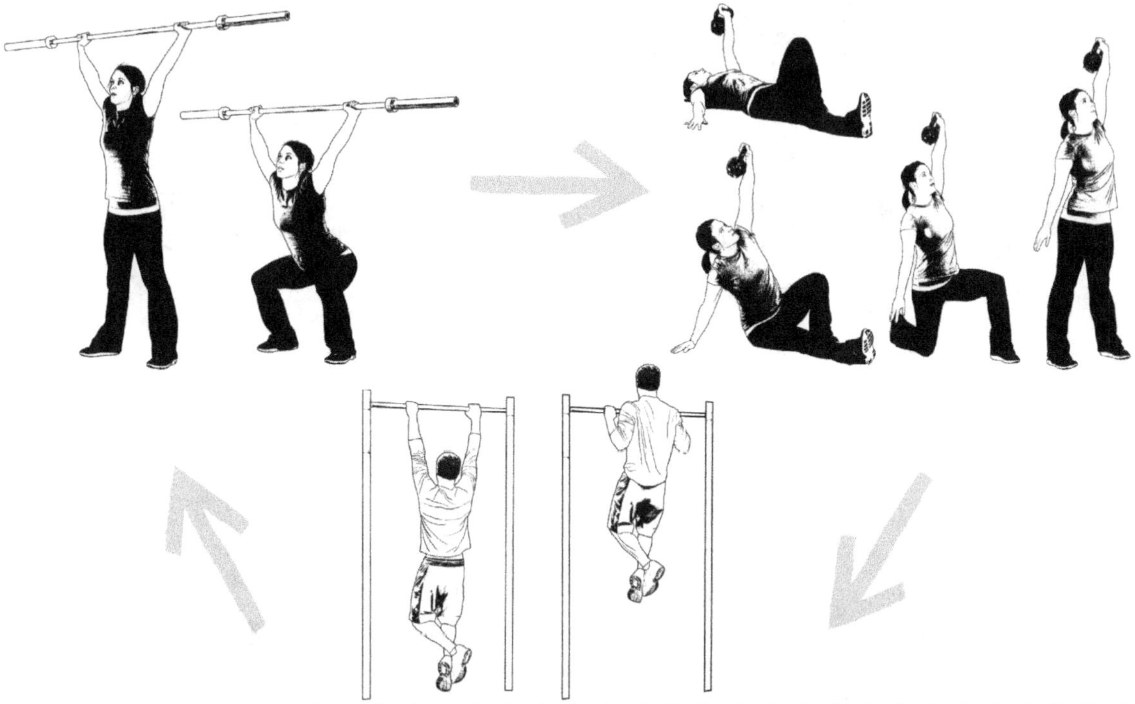

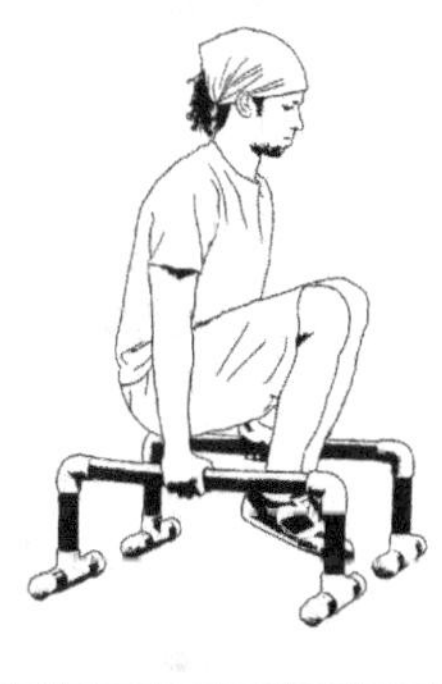

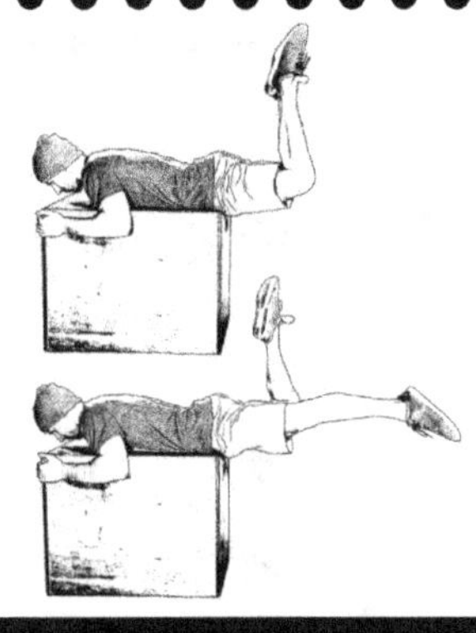

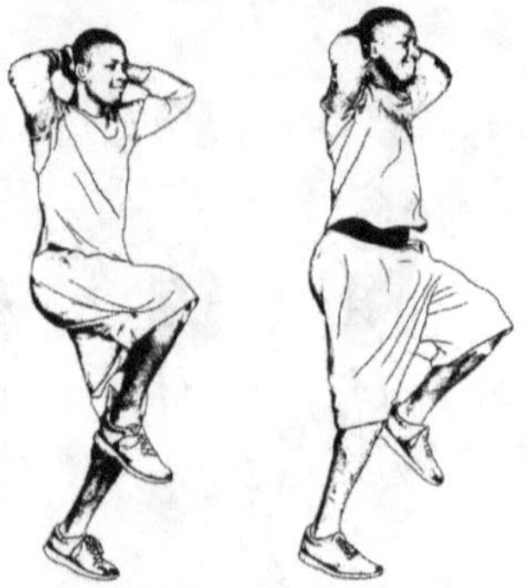

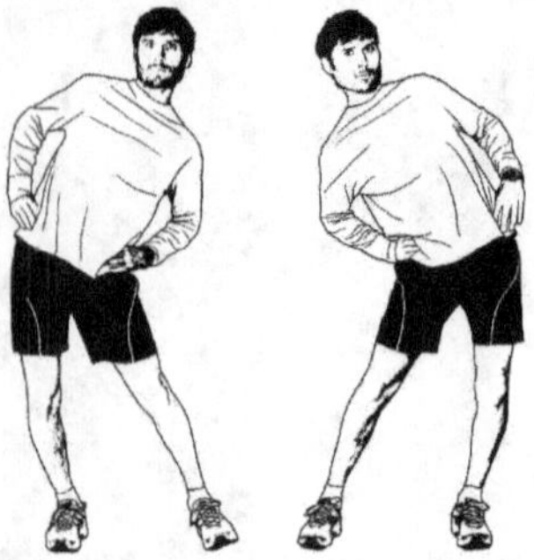

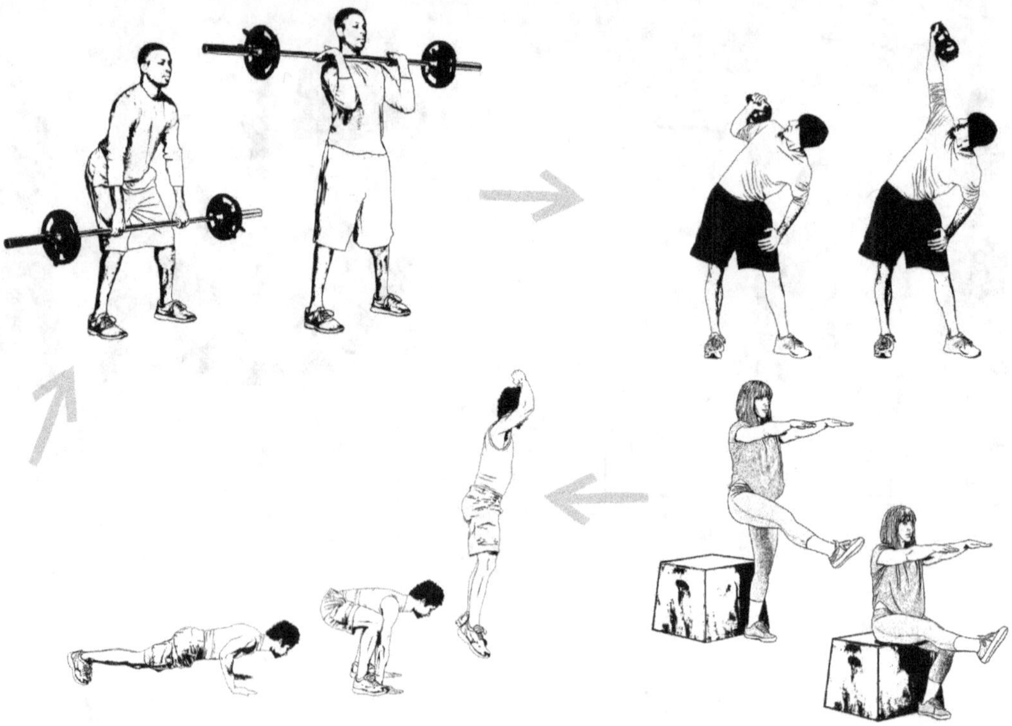

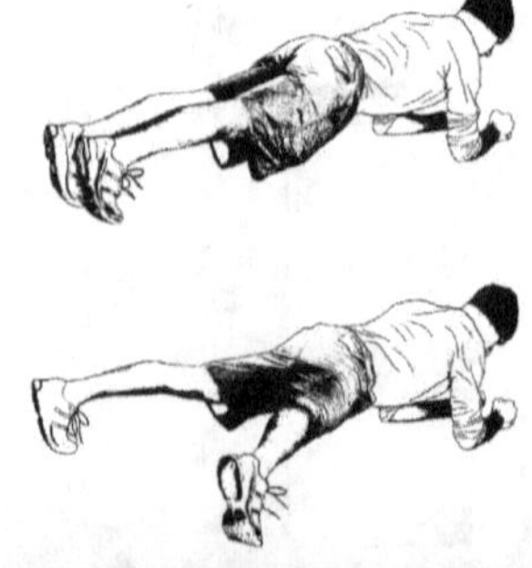
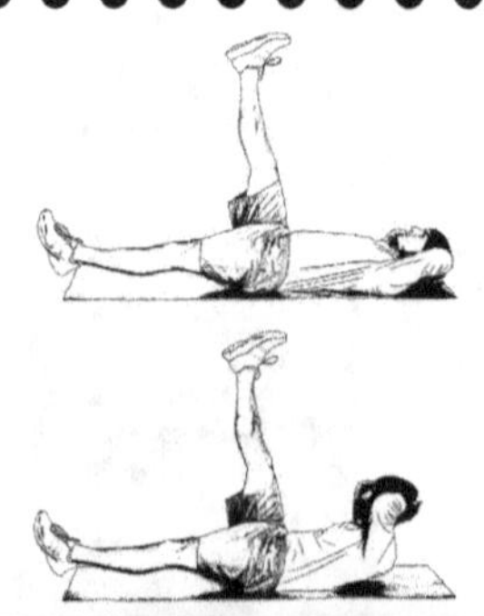

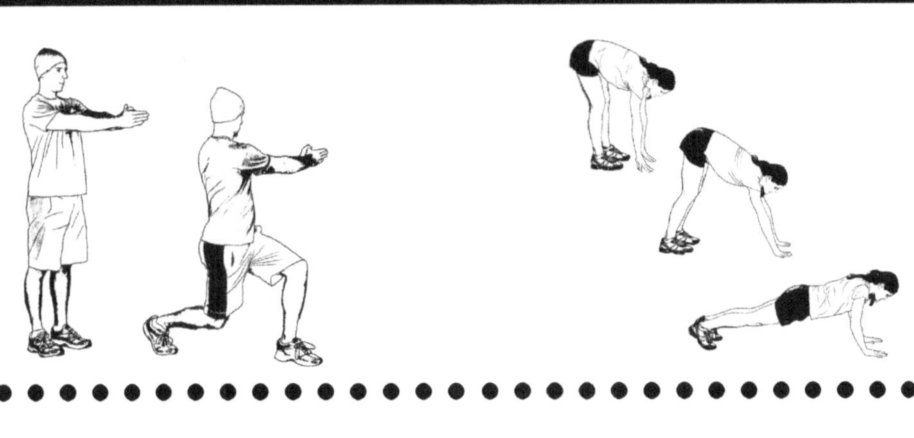

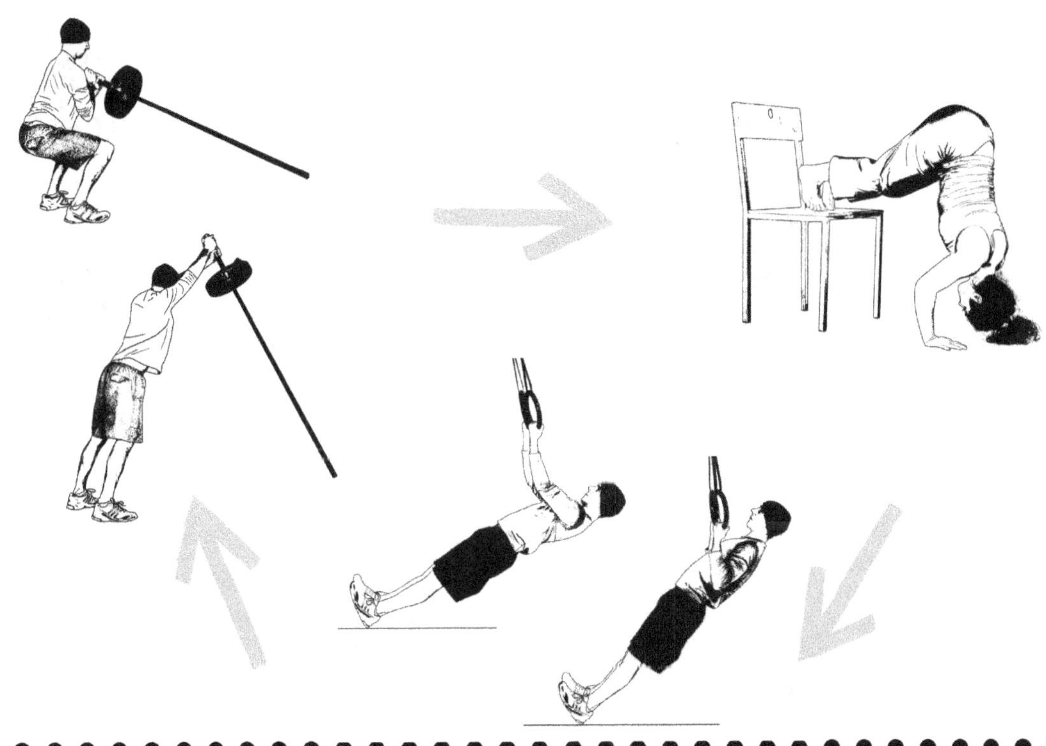

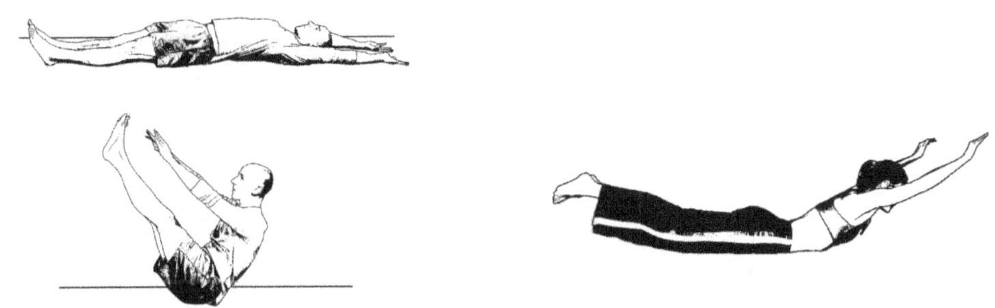

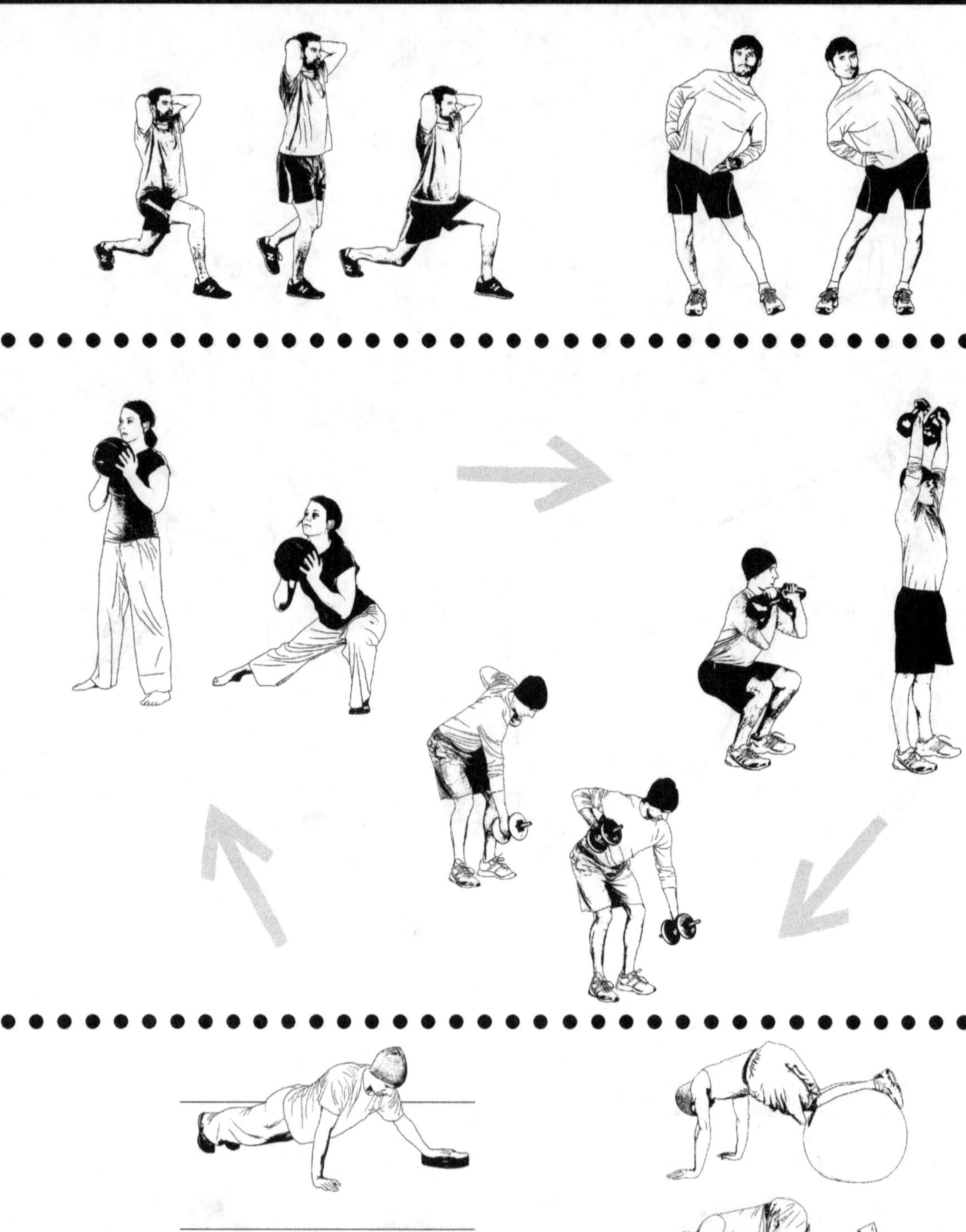

SIDE A

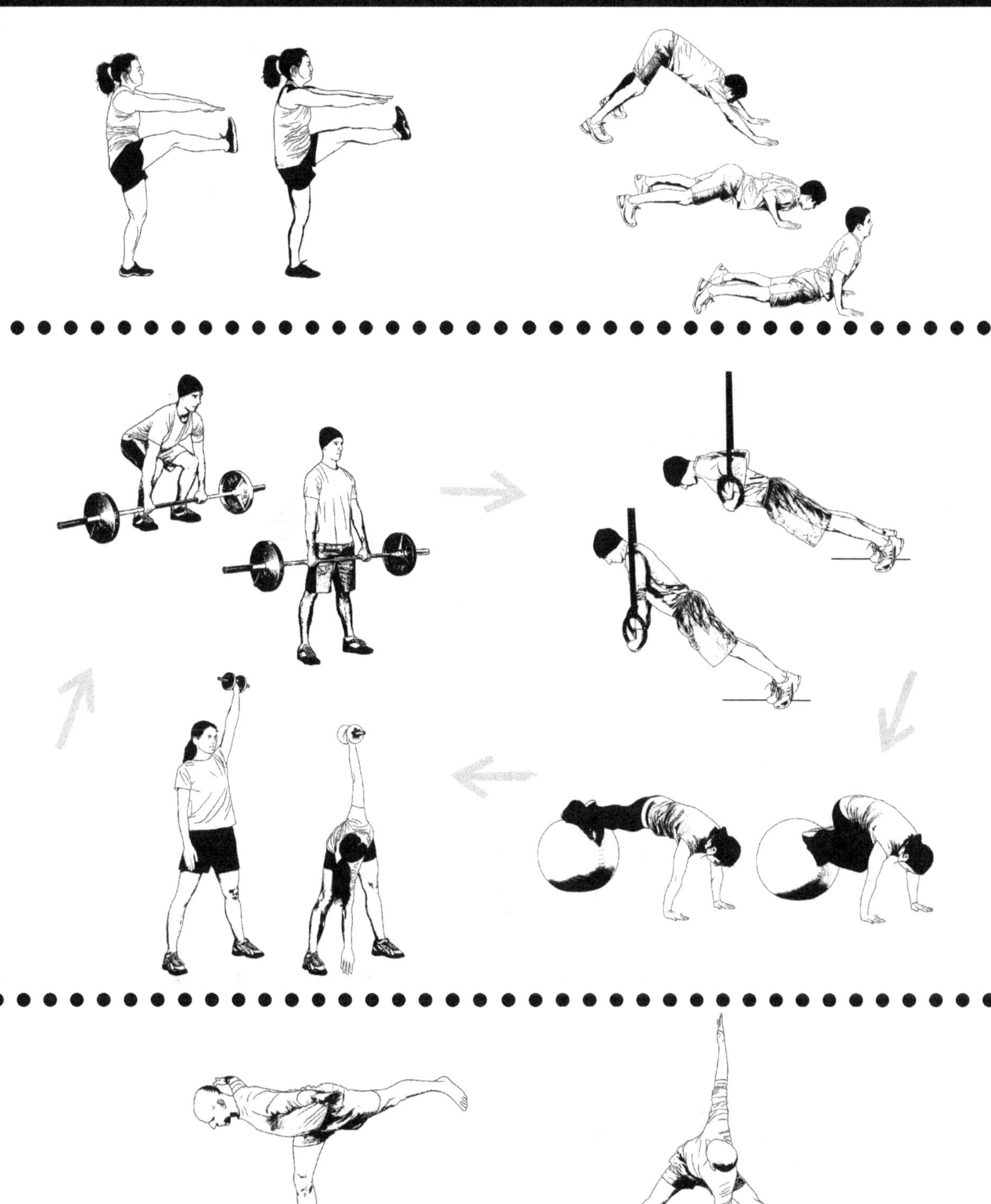

SIDE A

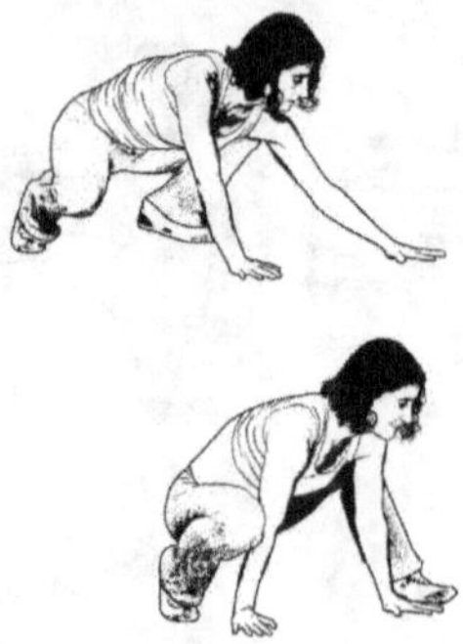

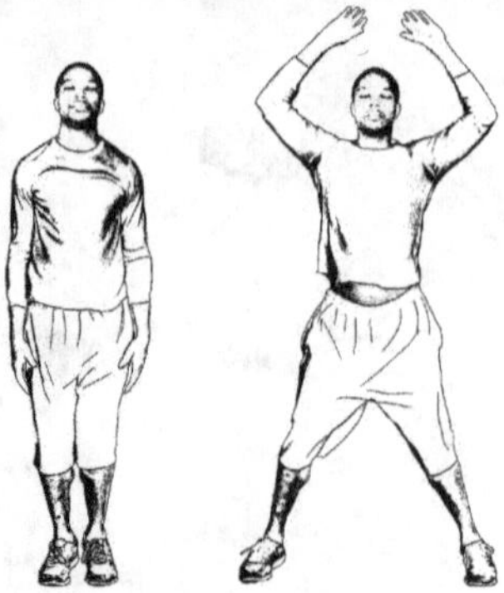

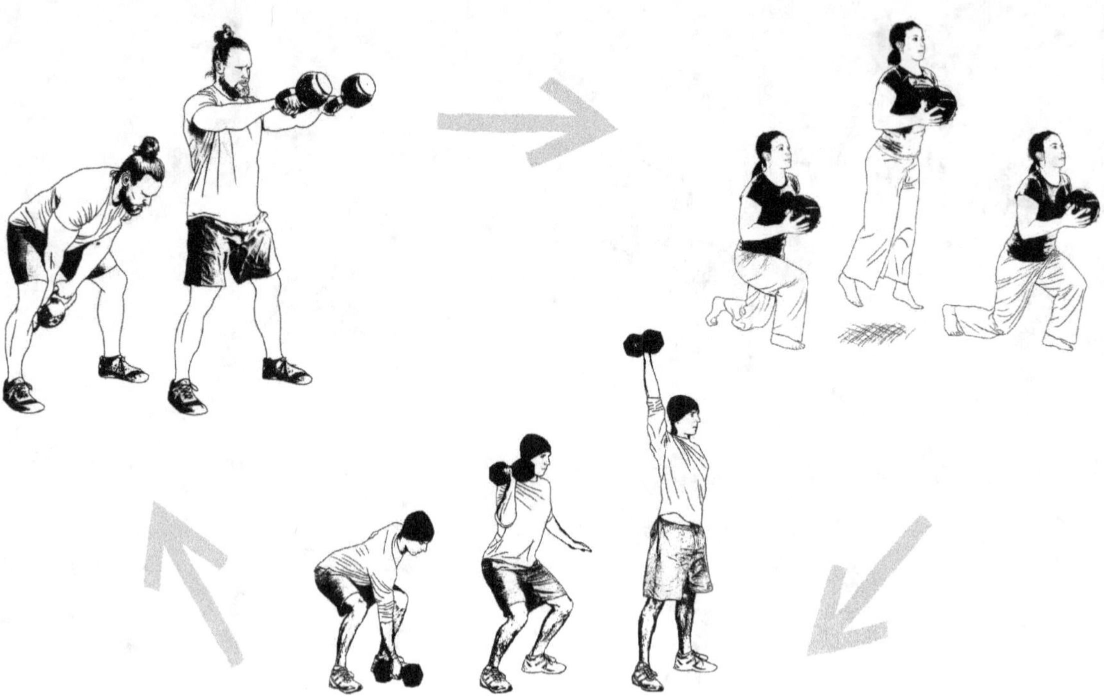

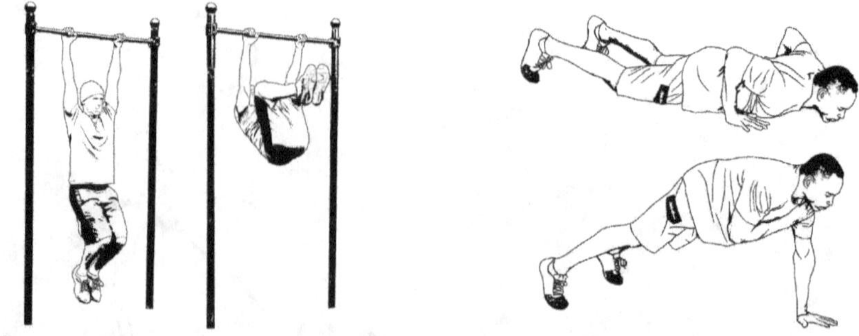

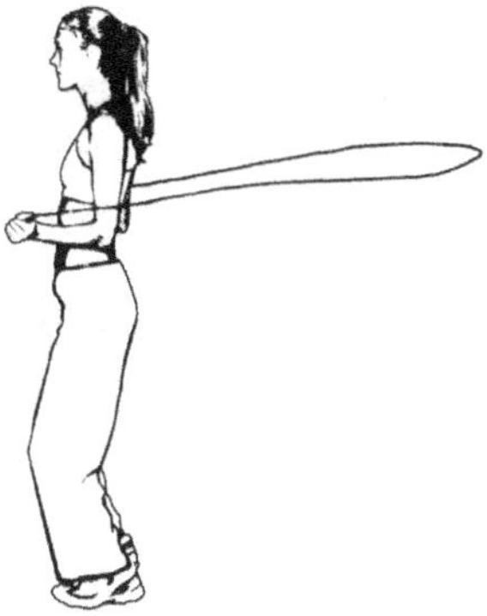

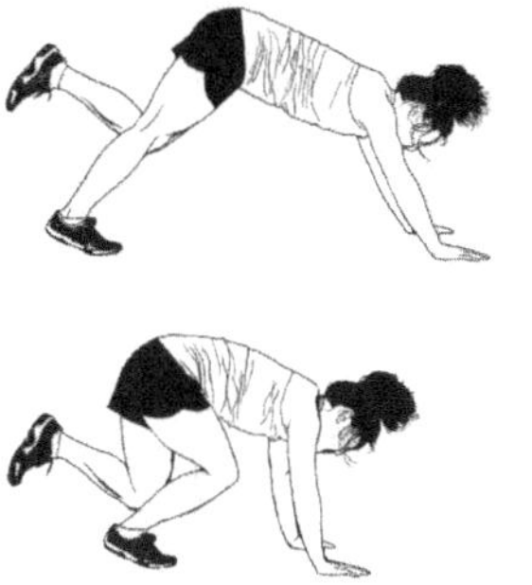

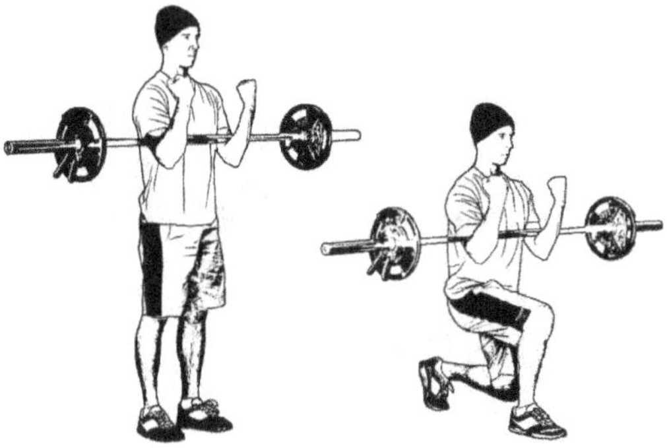

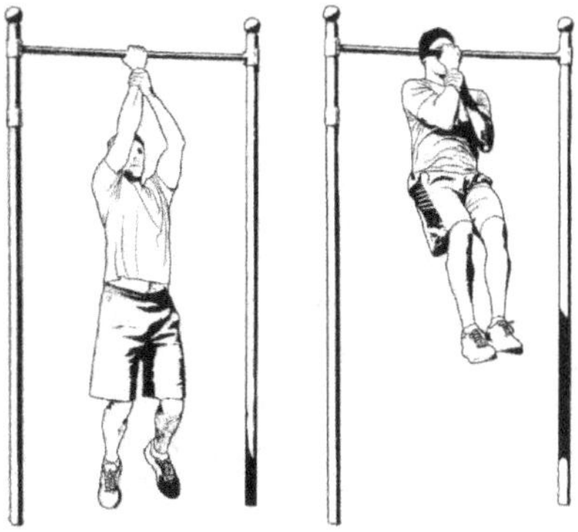

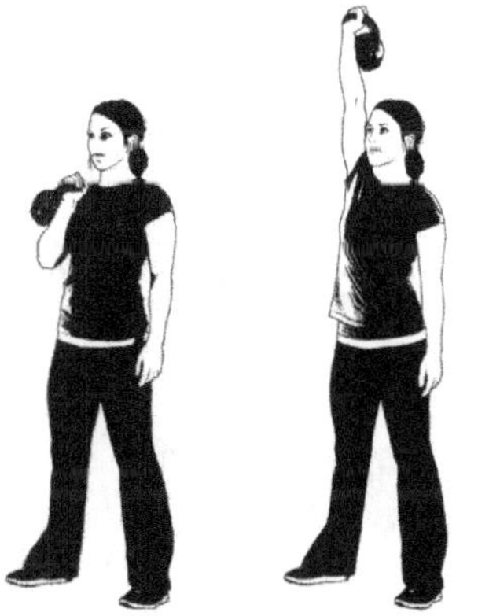

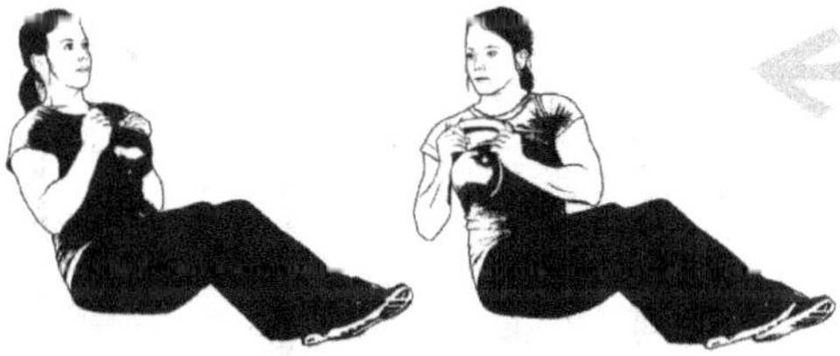

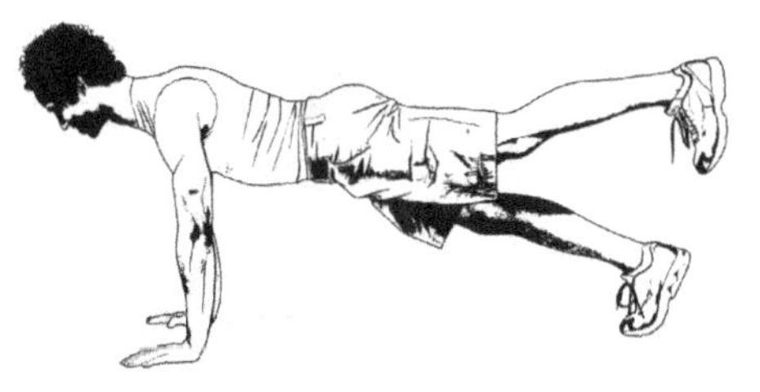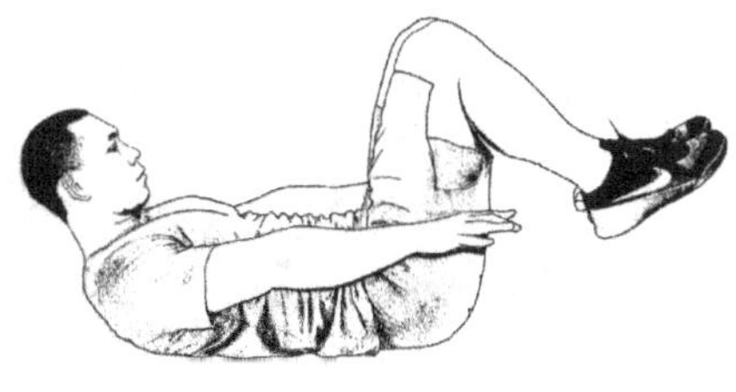

SIDE A

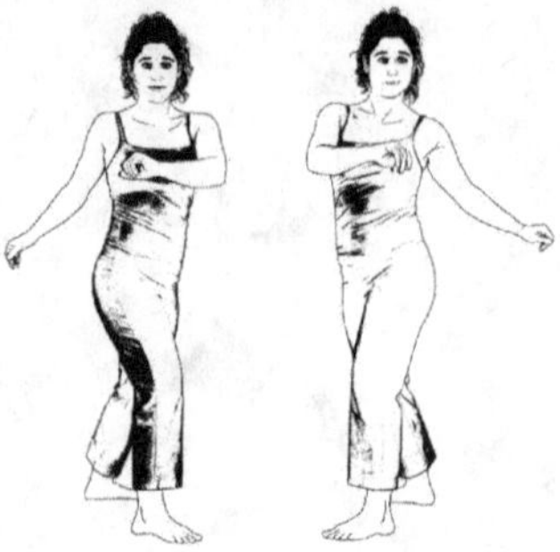

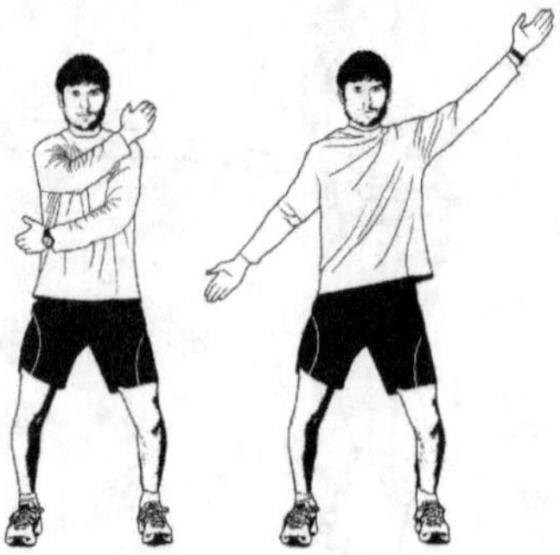

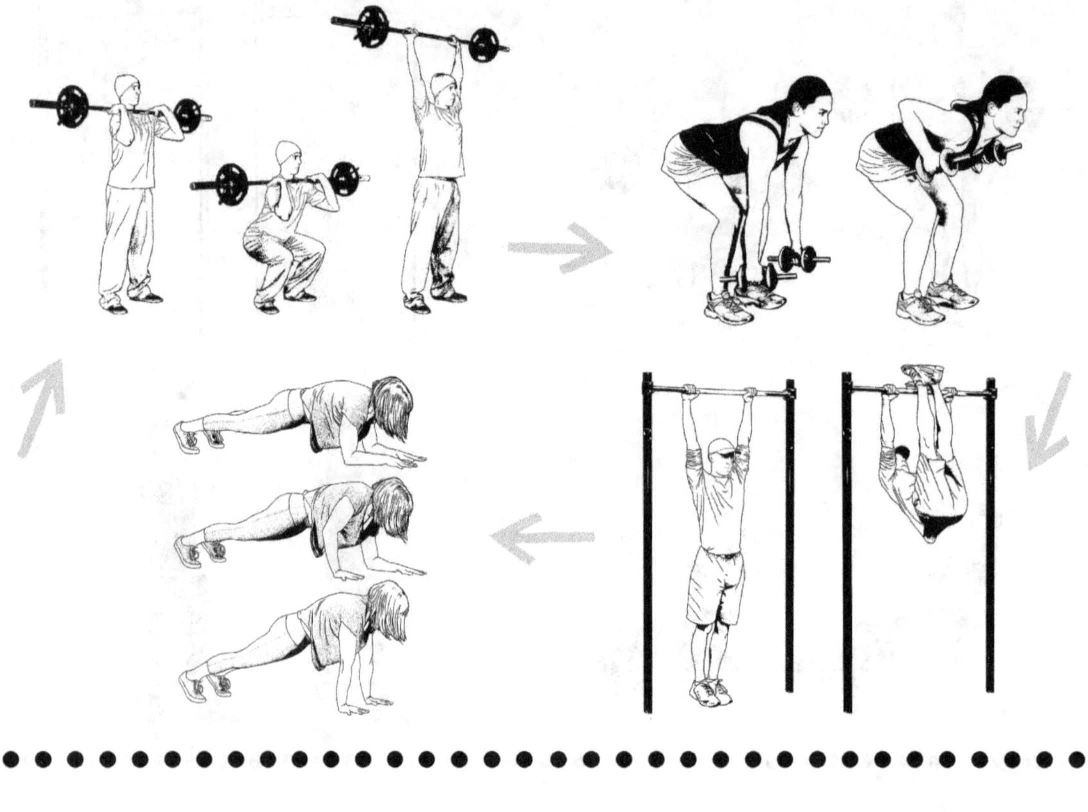

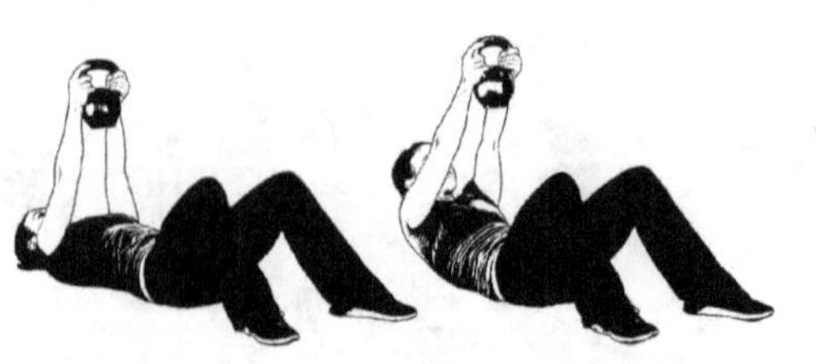

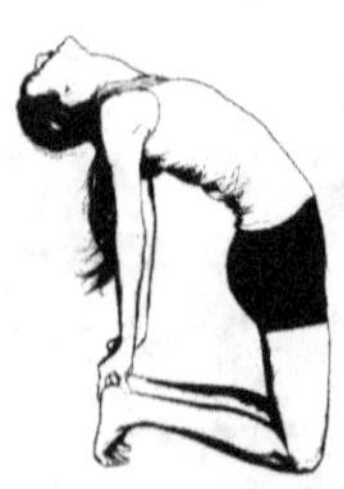

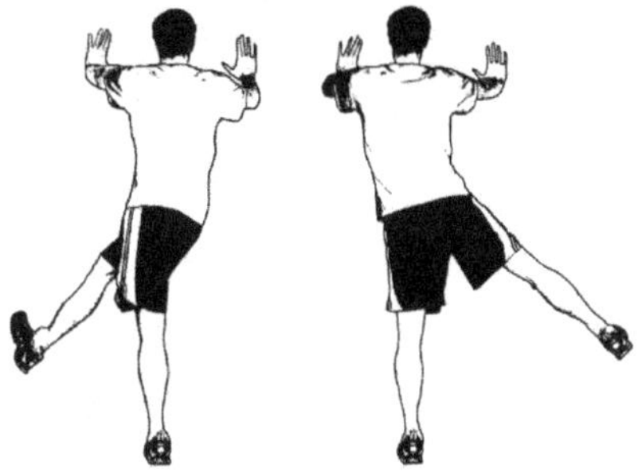

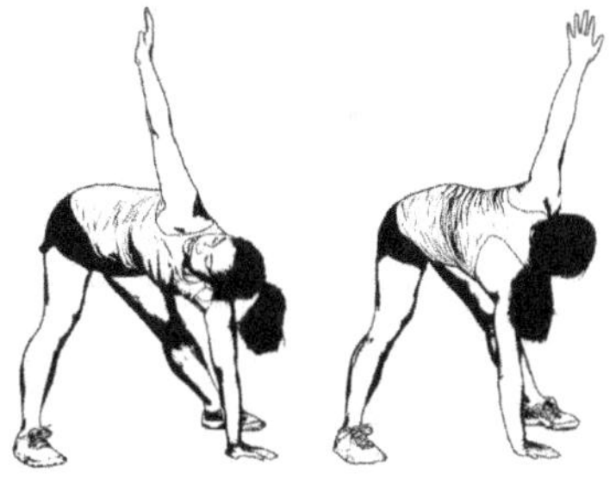

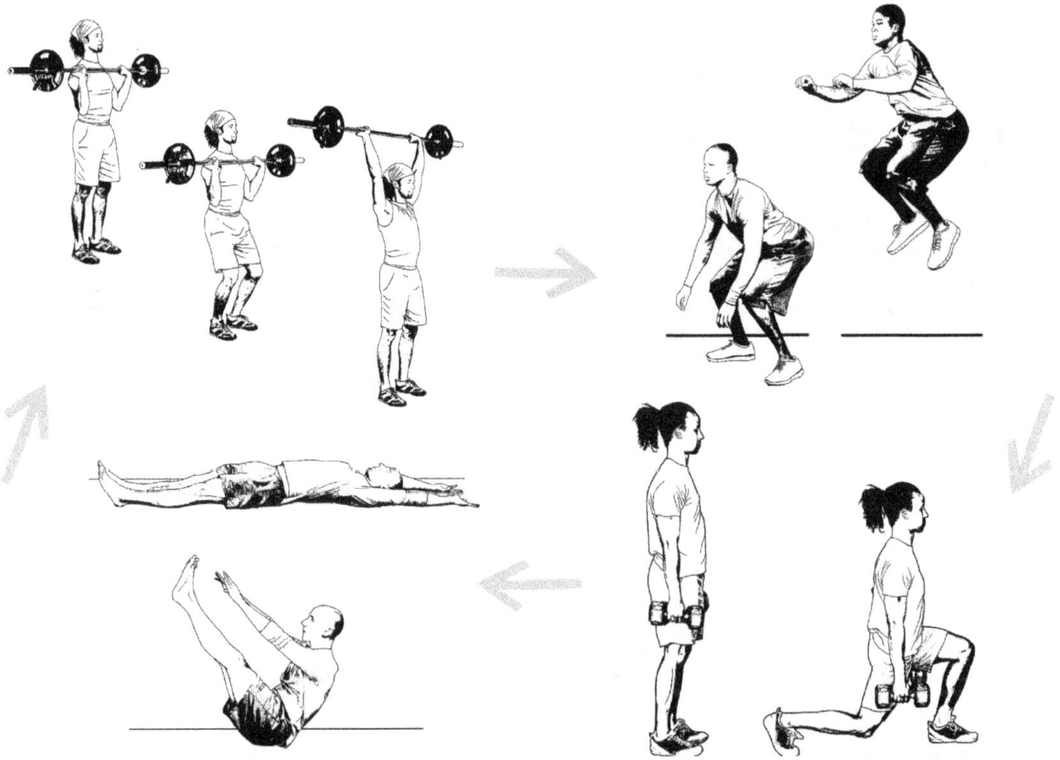

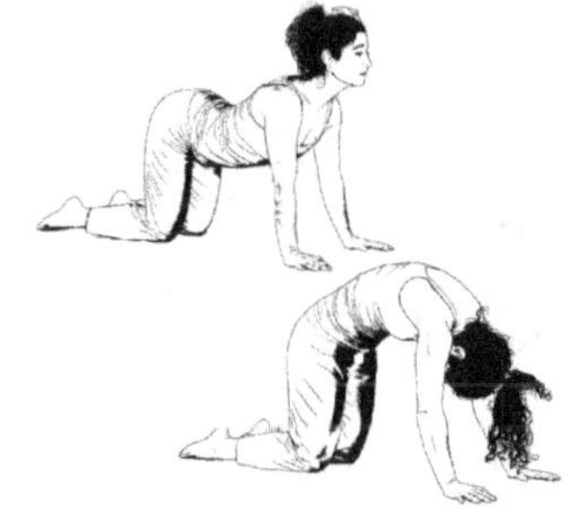

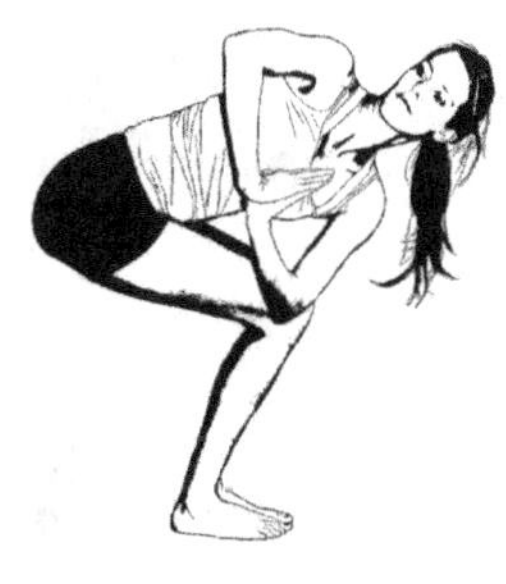

SIDE A

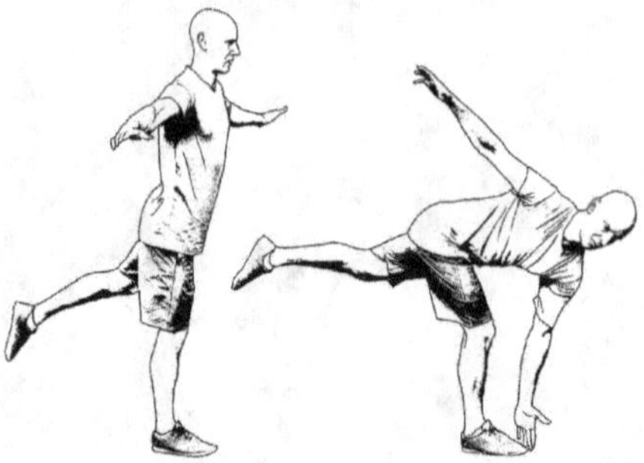

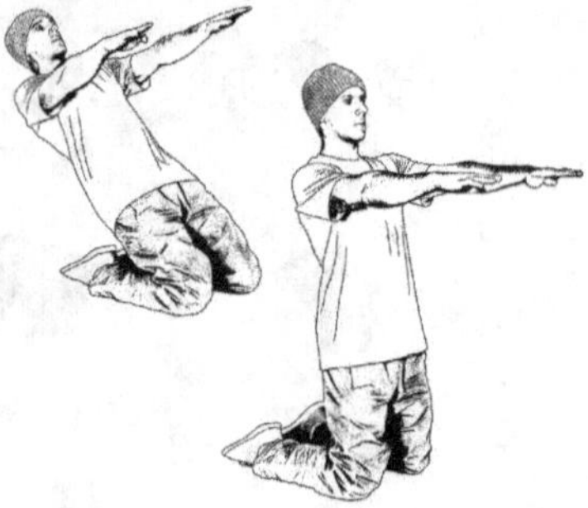

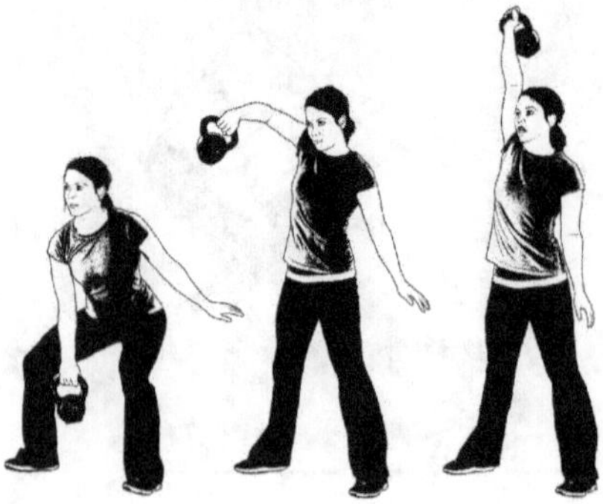

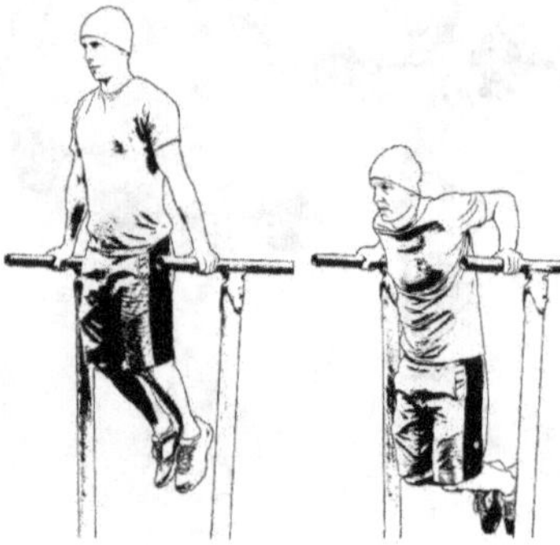

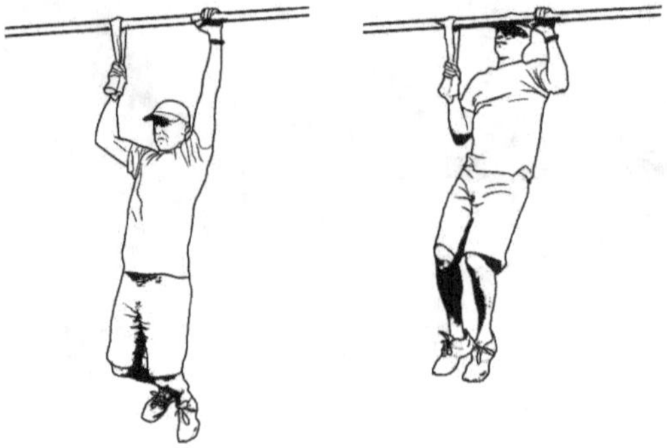

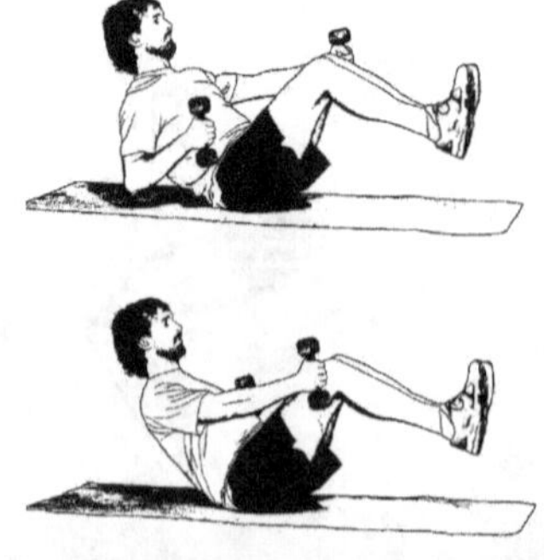

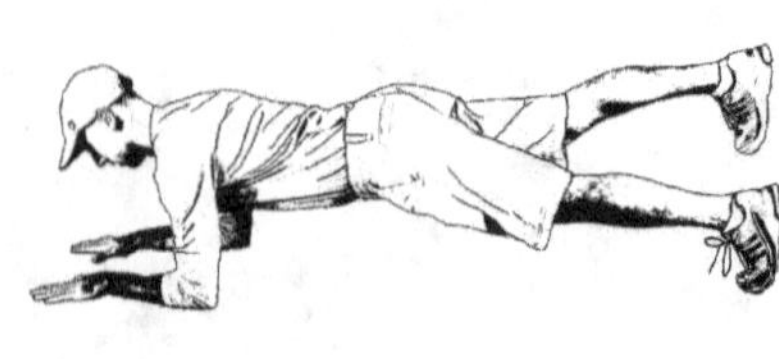

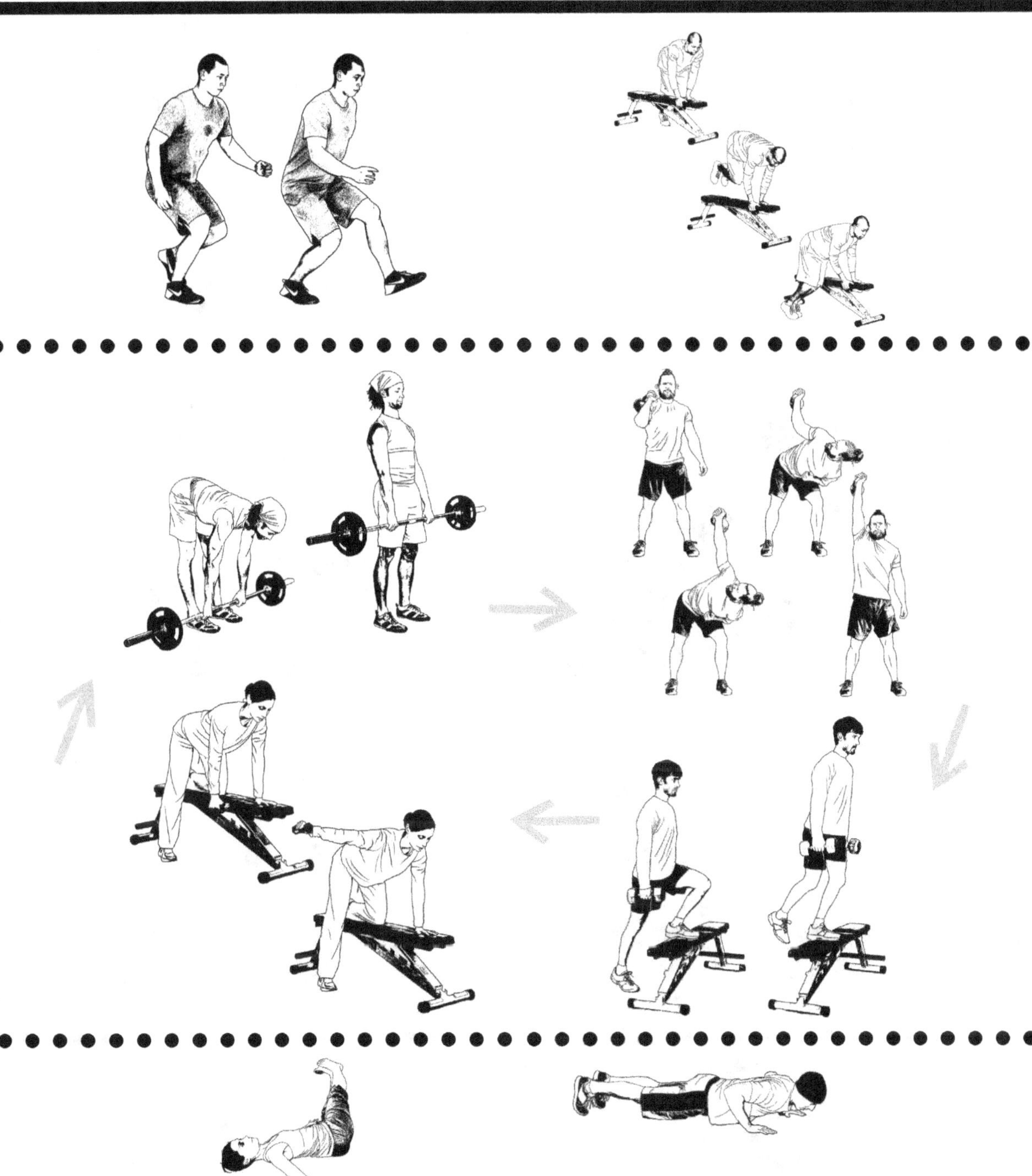

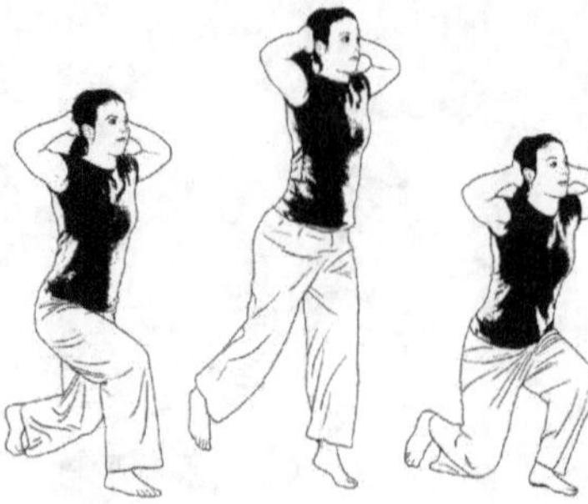

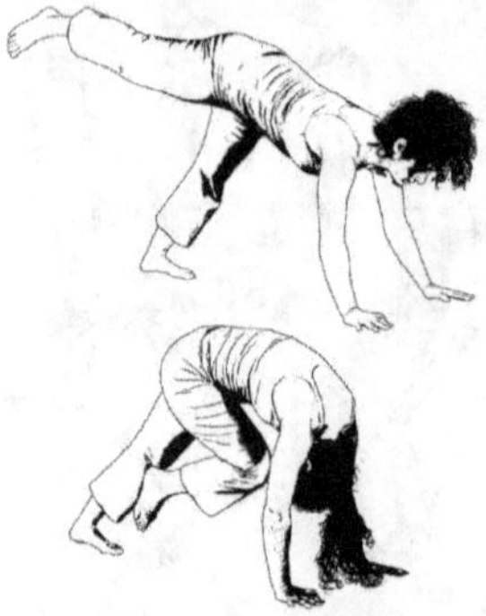

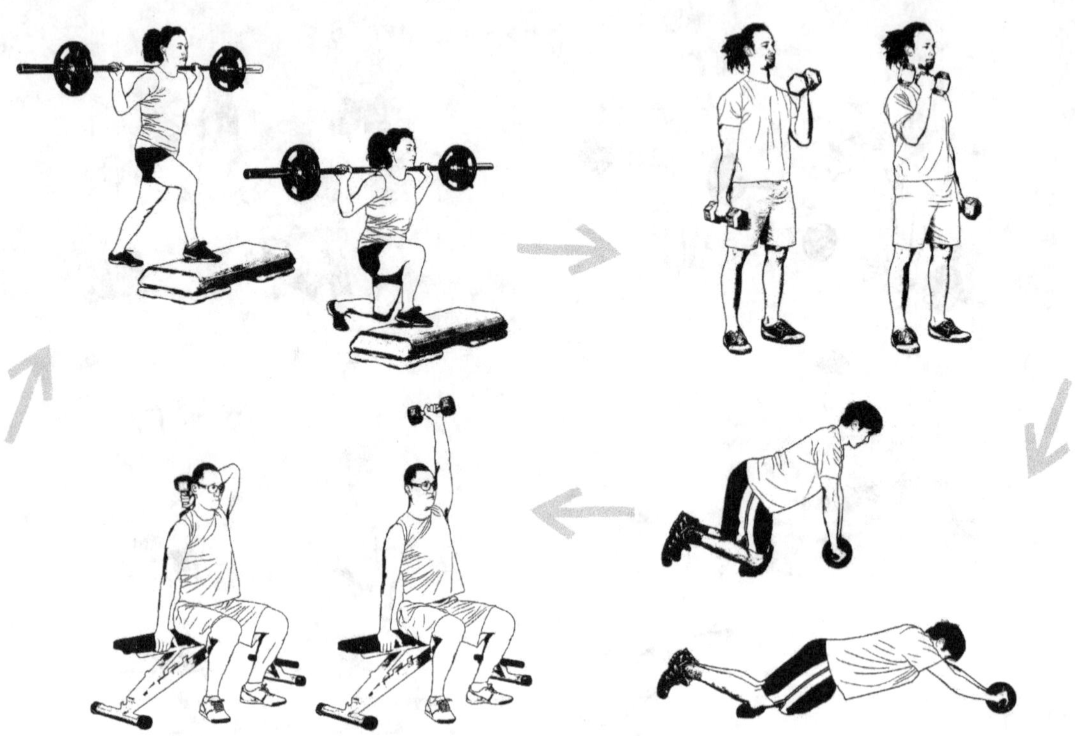

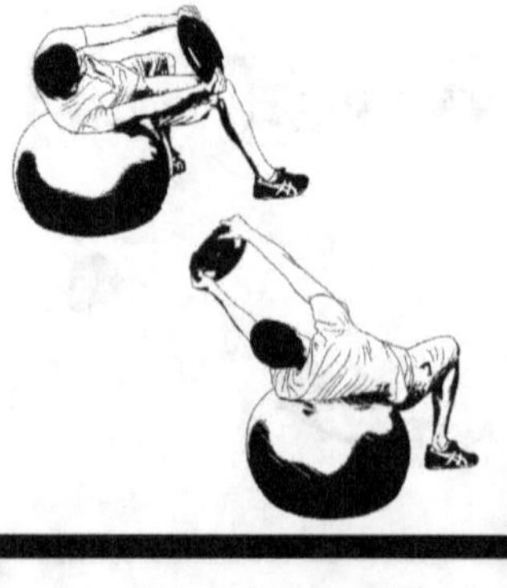

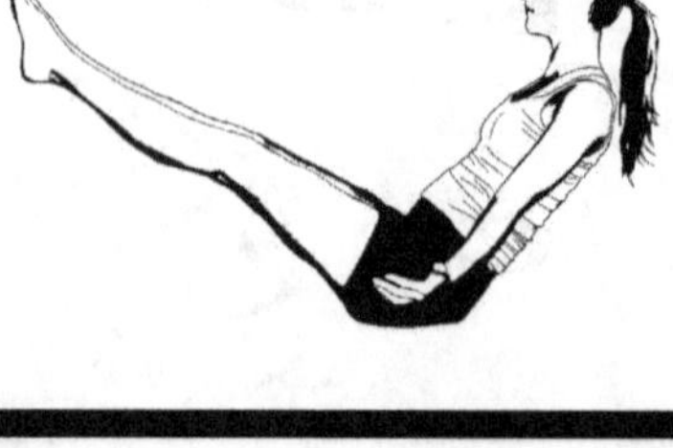

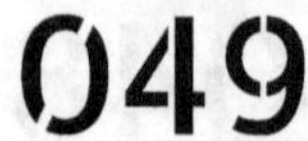

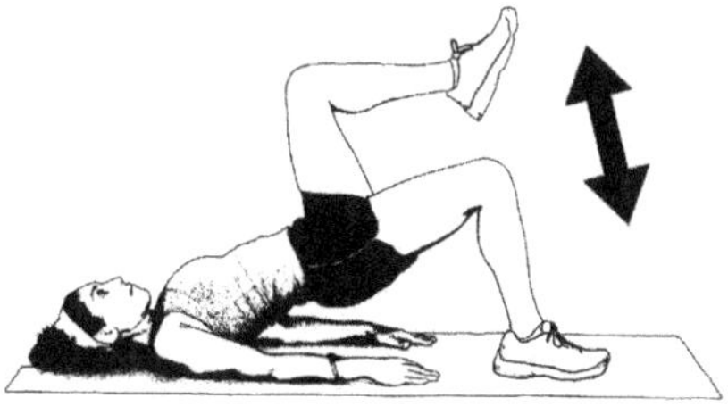

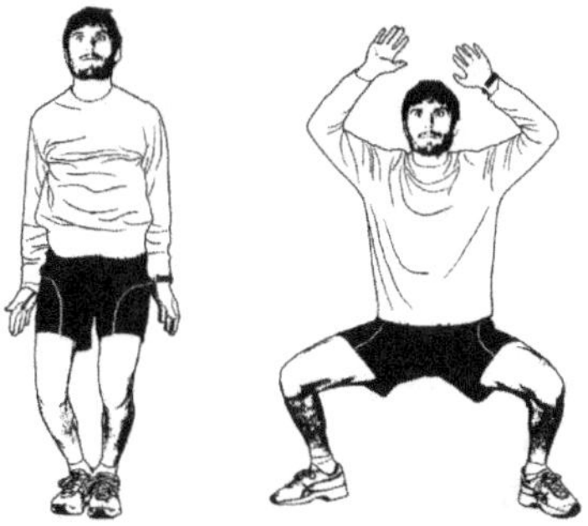

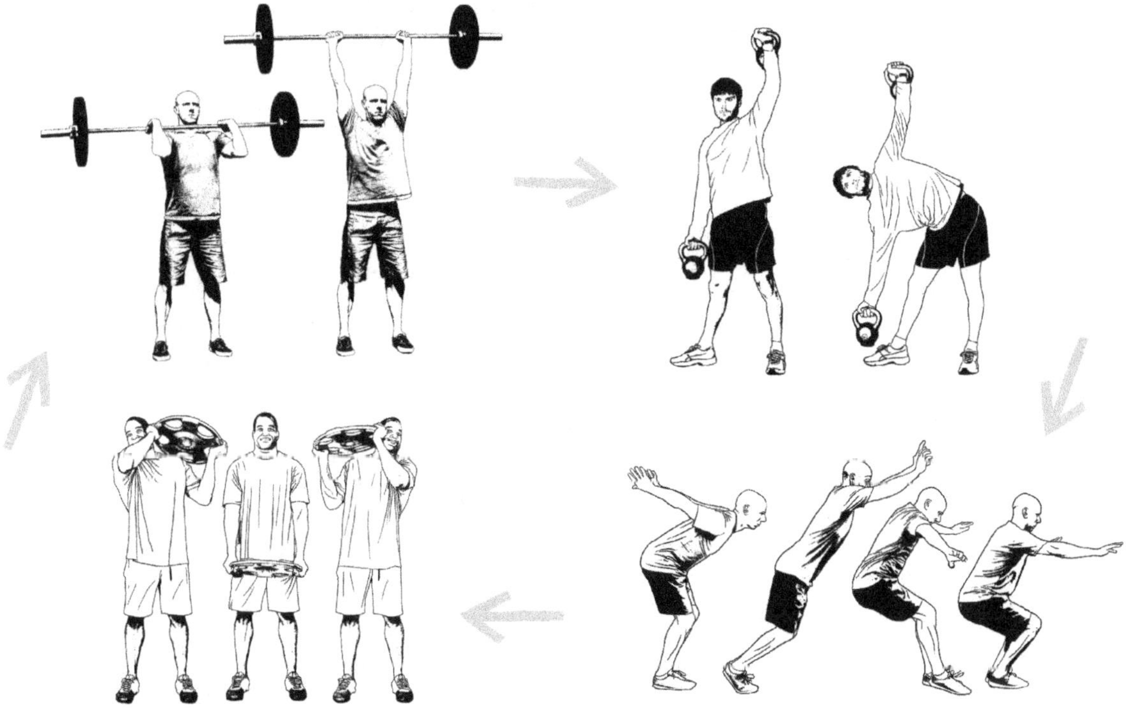

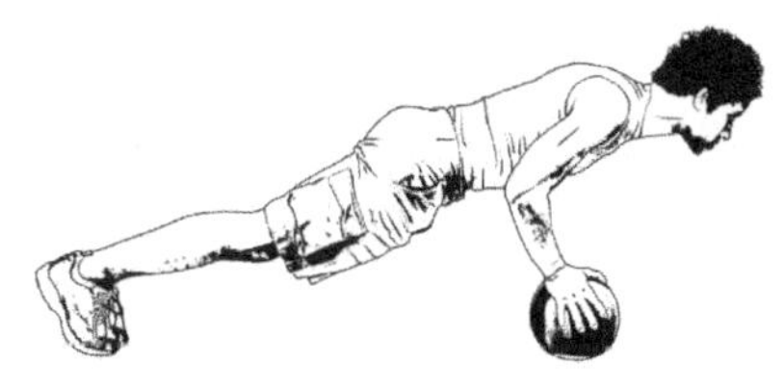

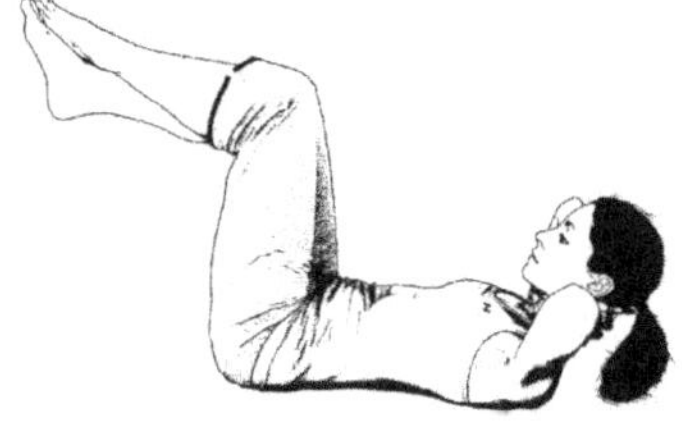

Side B

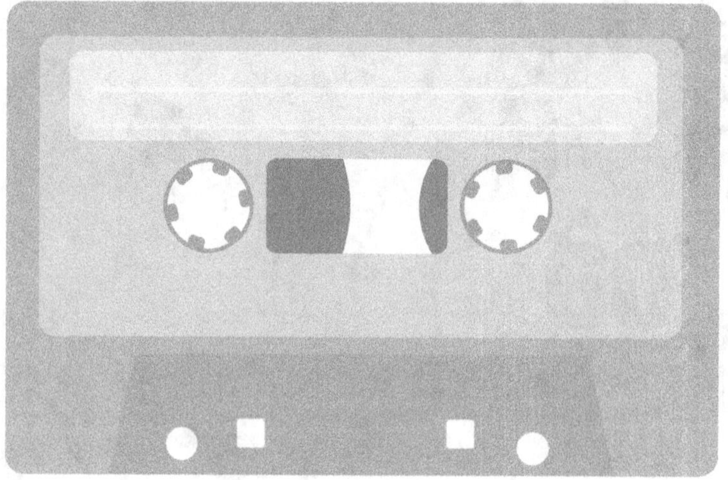

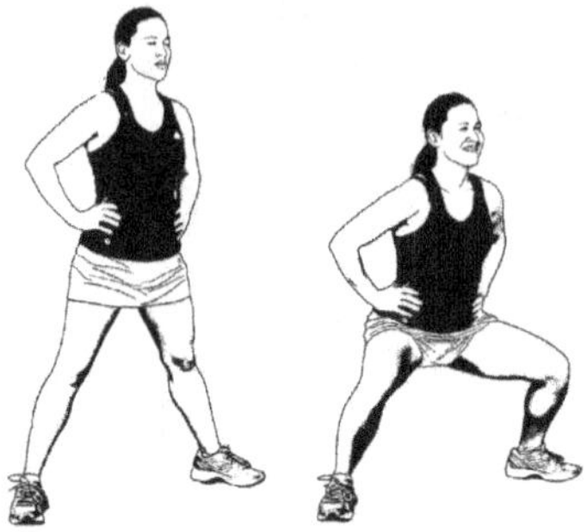

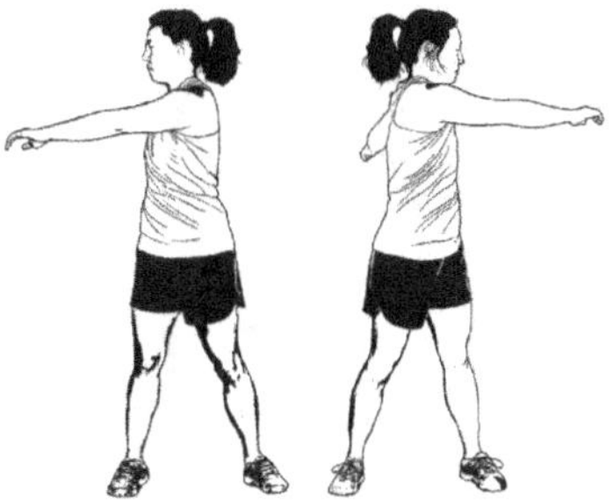

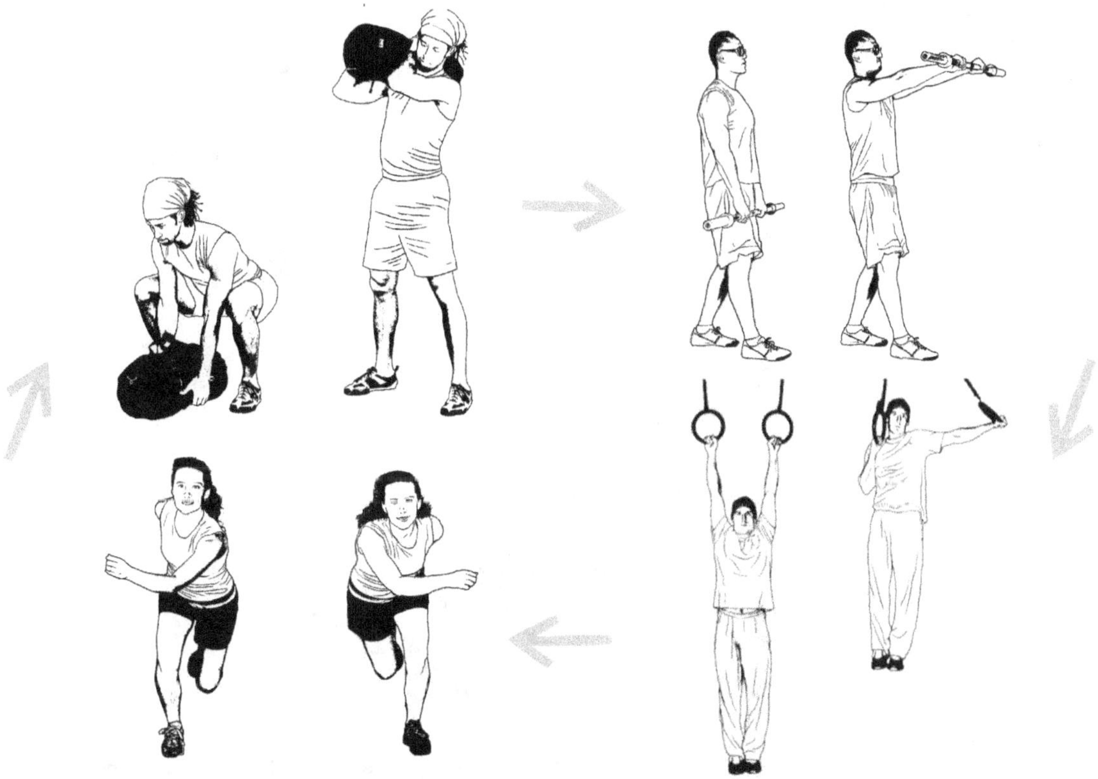

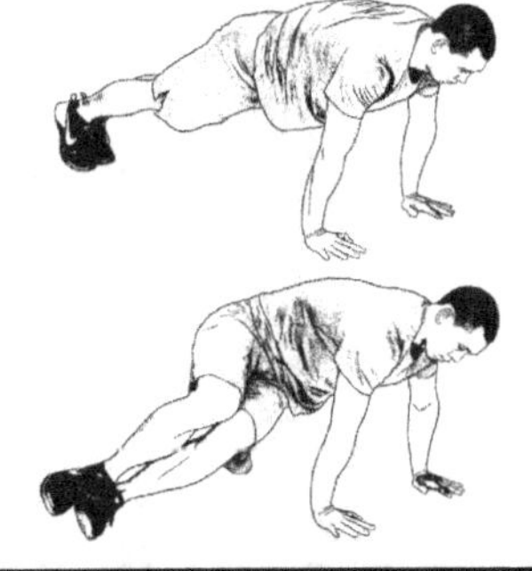
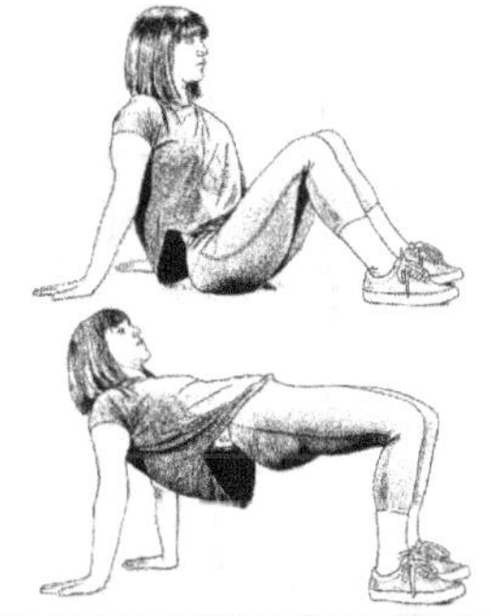

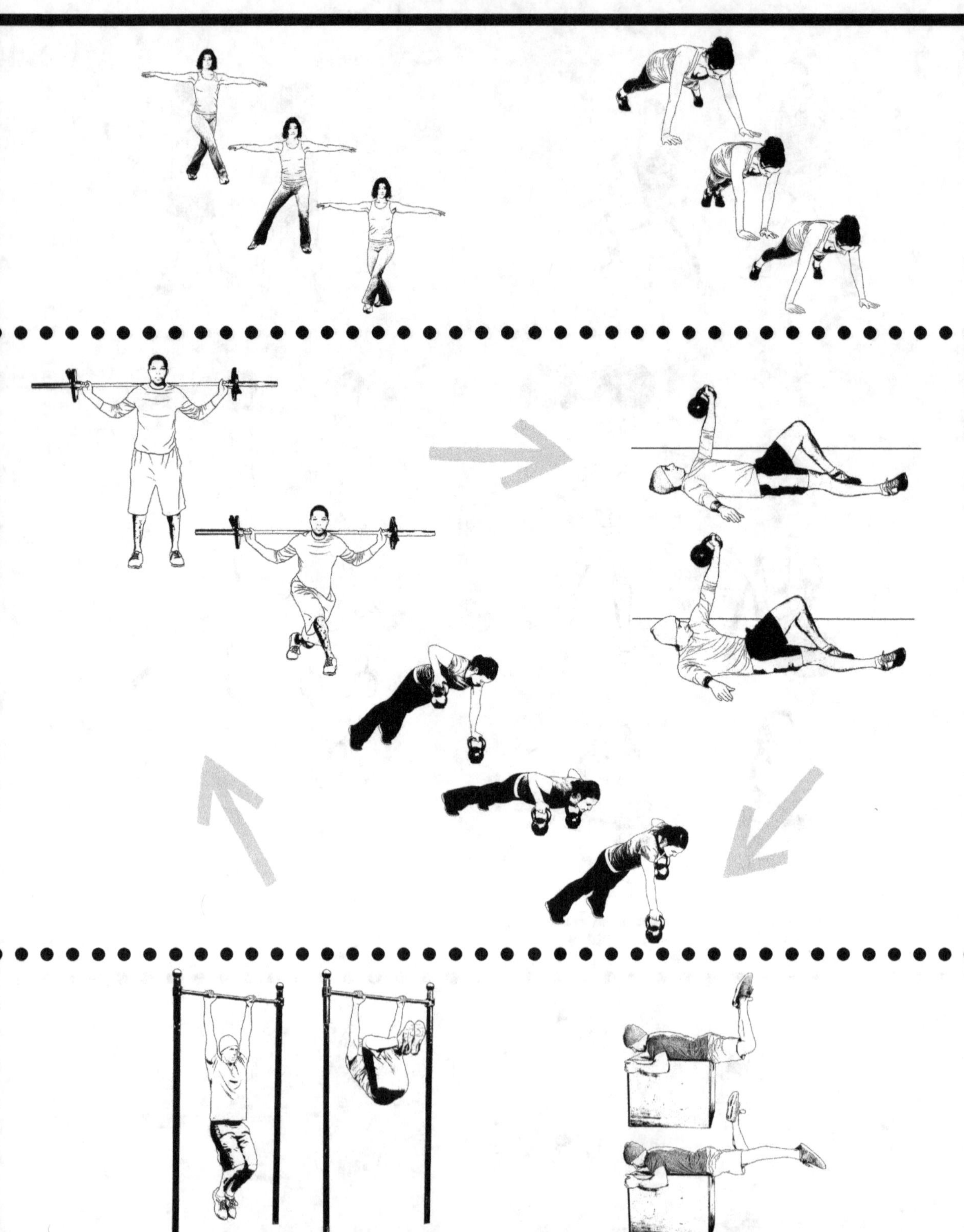

SIDE B

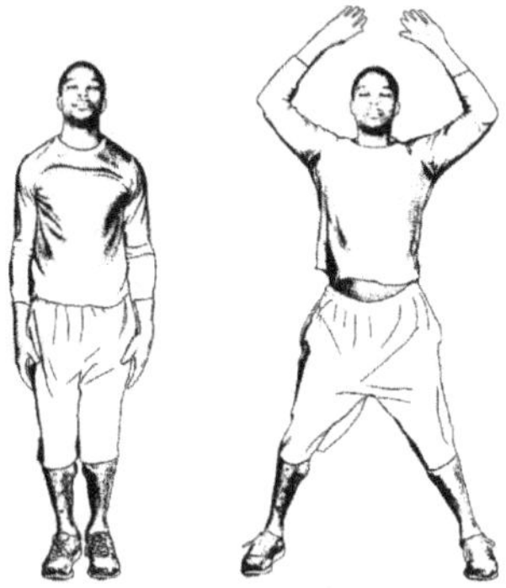

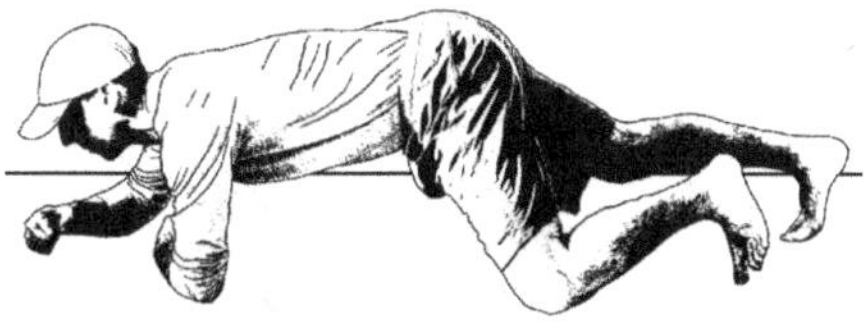

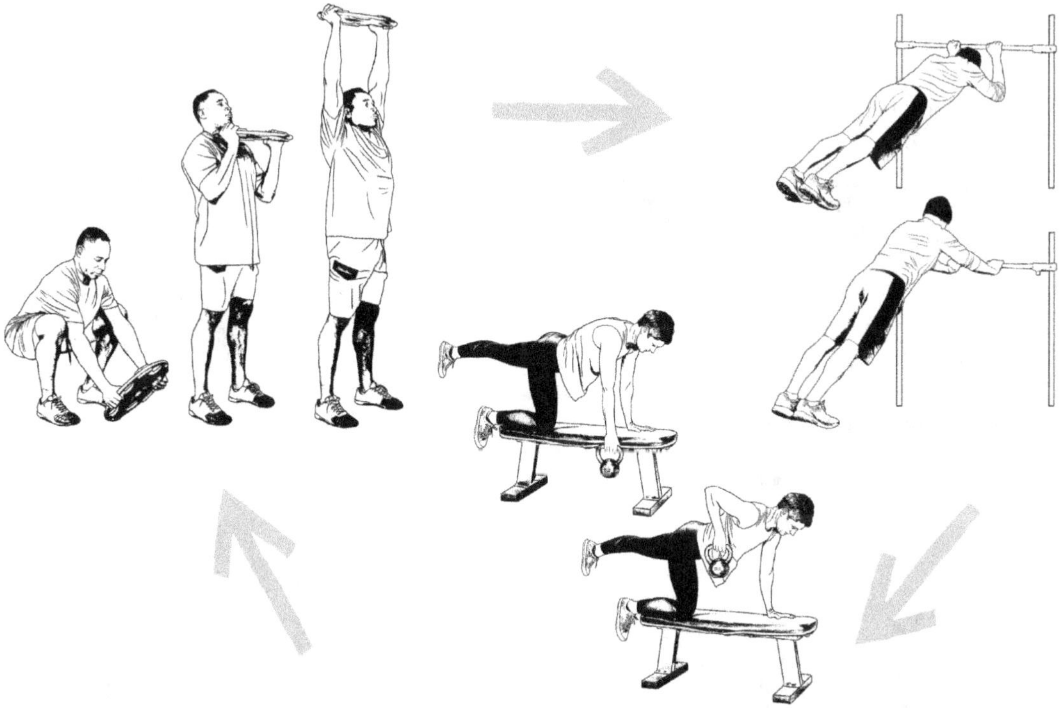

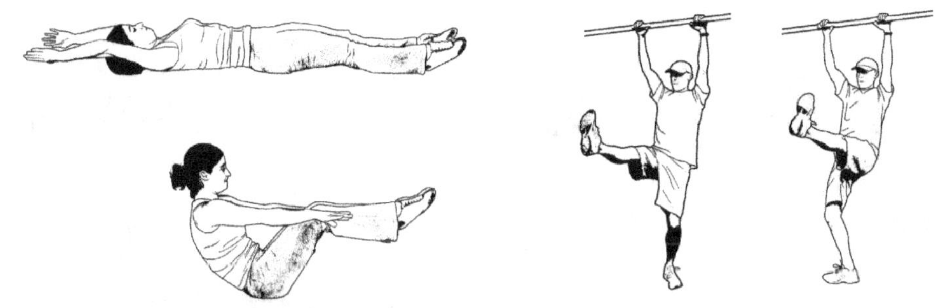

SIDE B

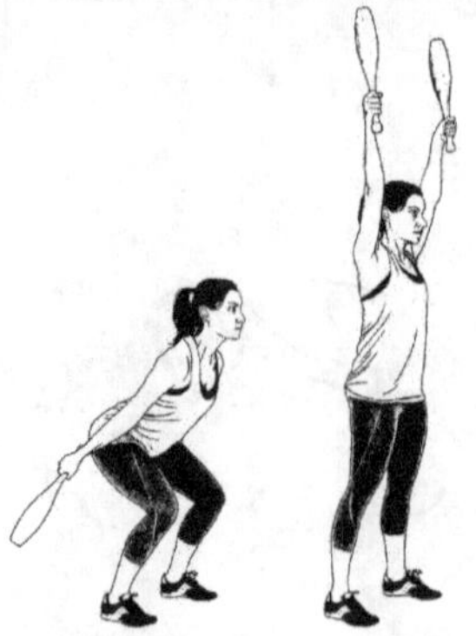

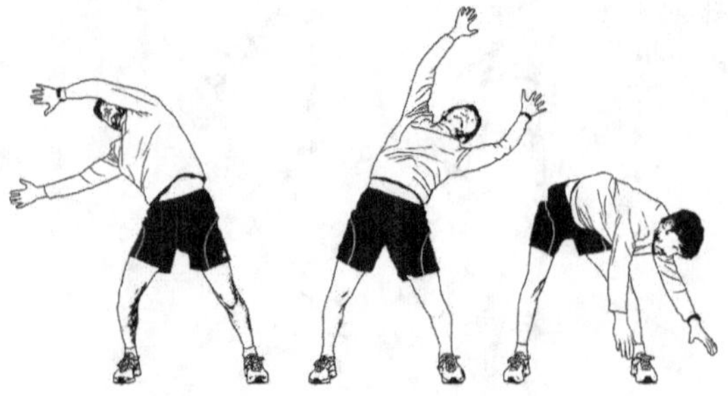

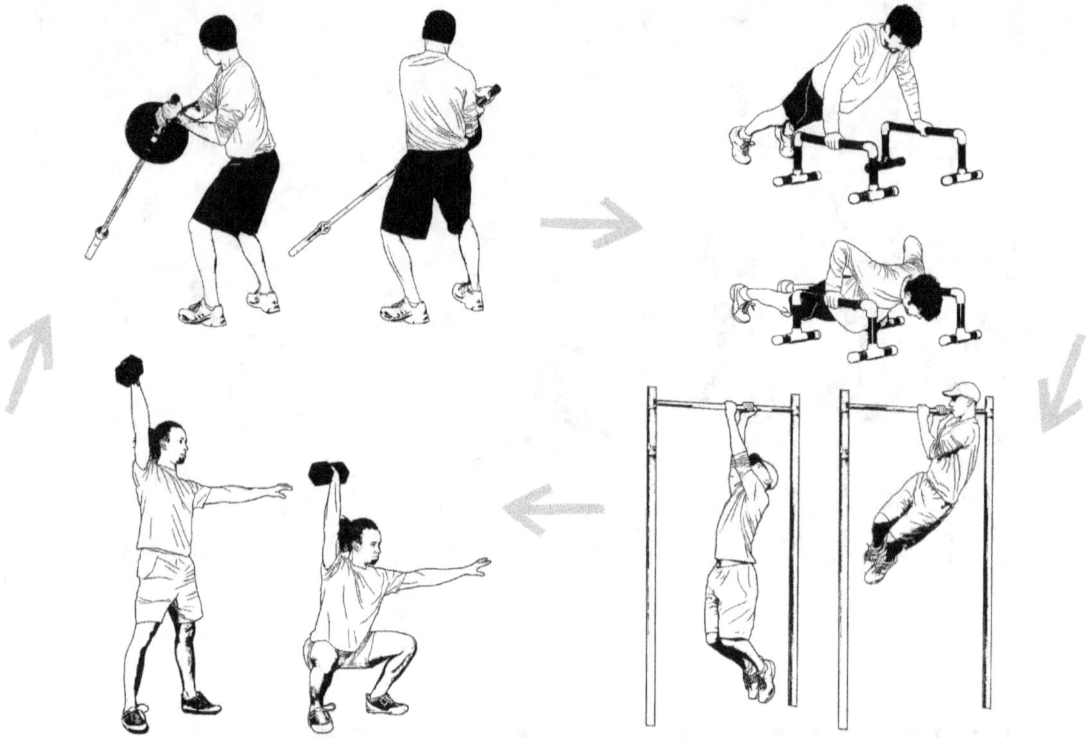

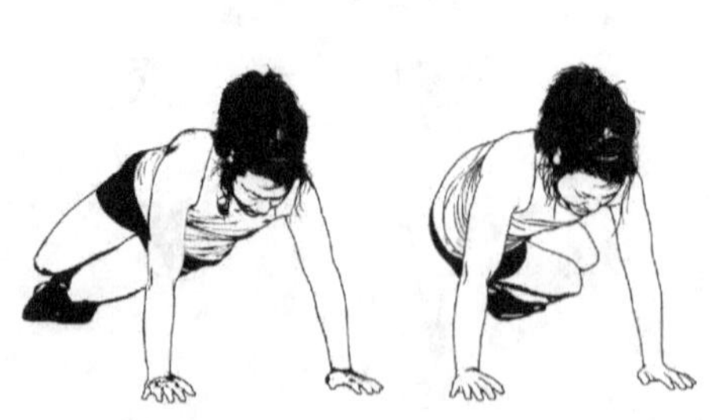

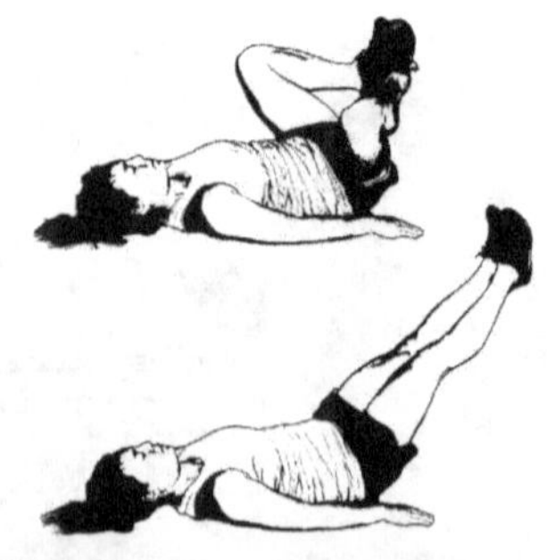

SIDE B

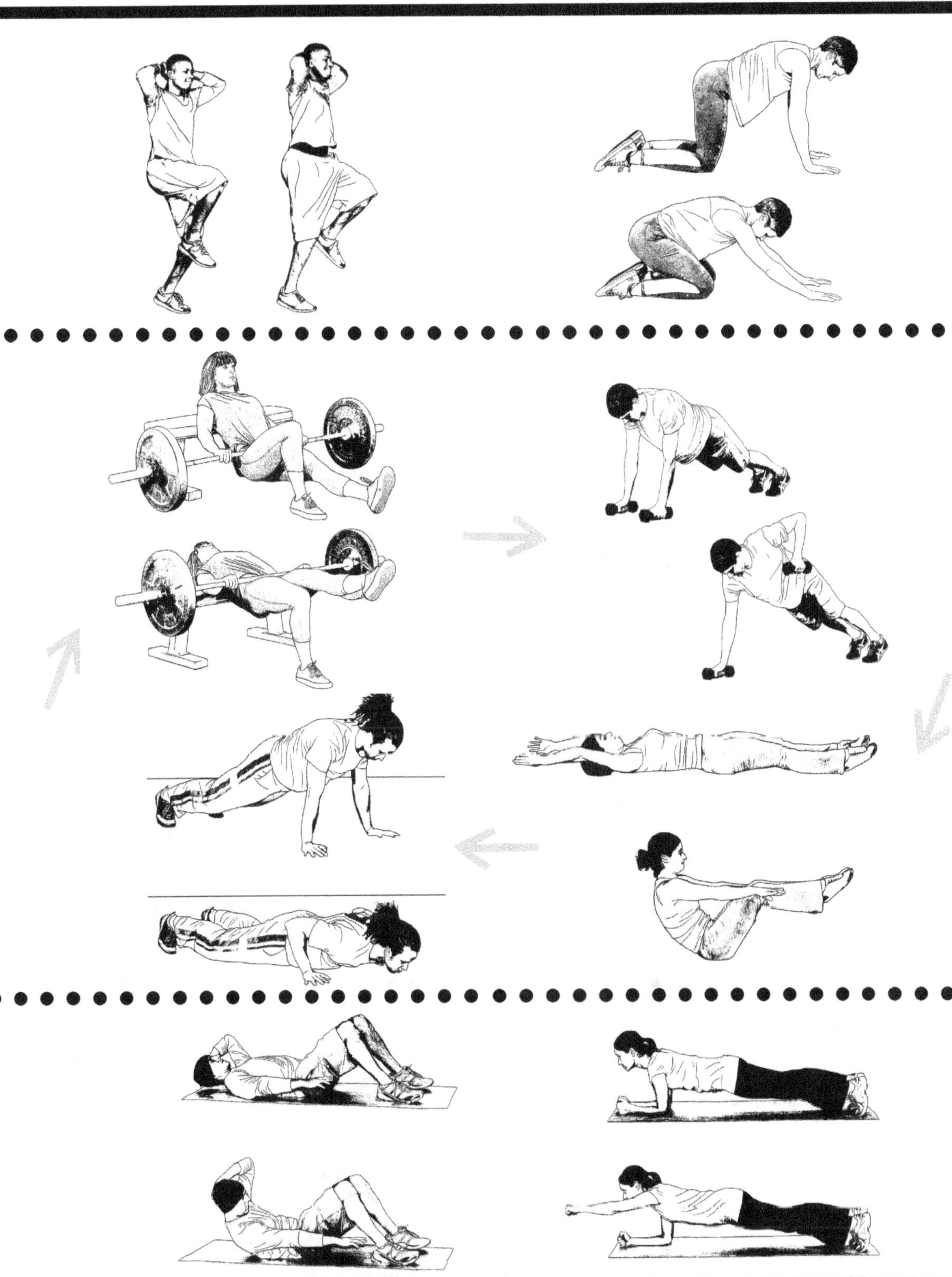

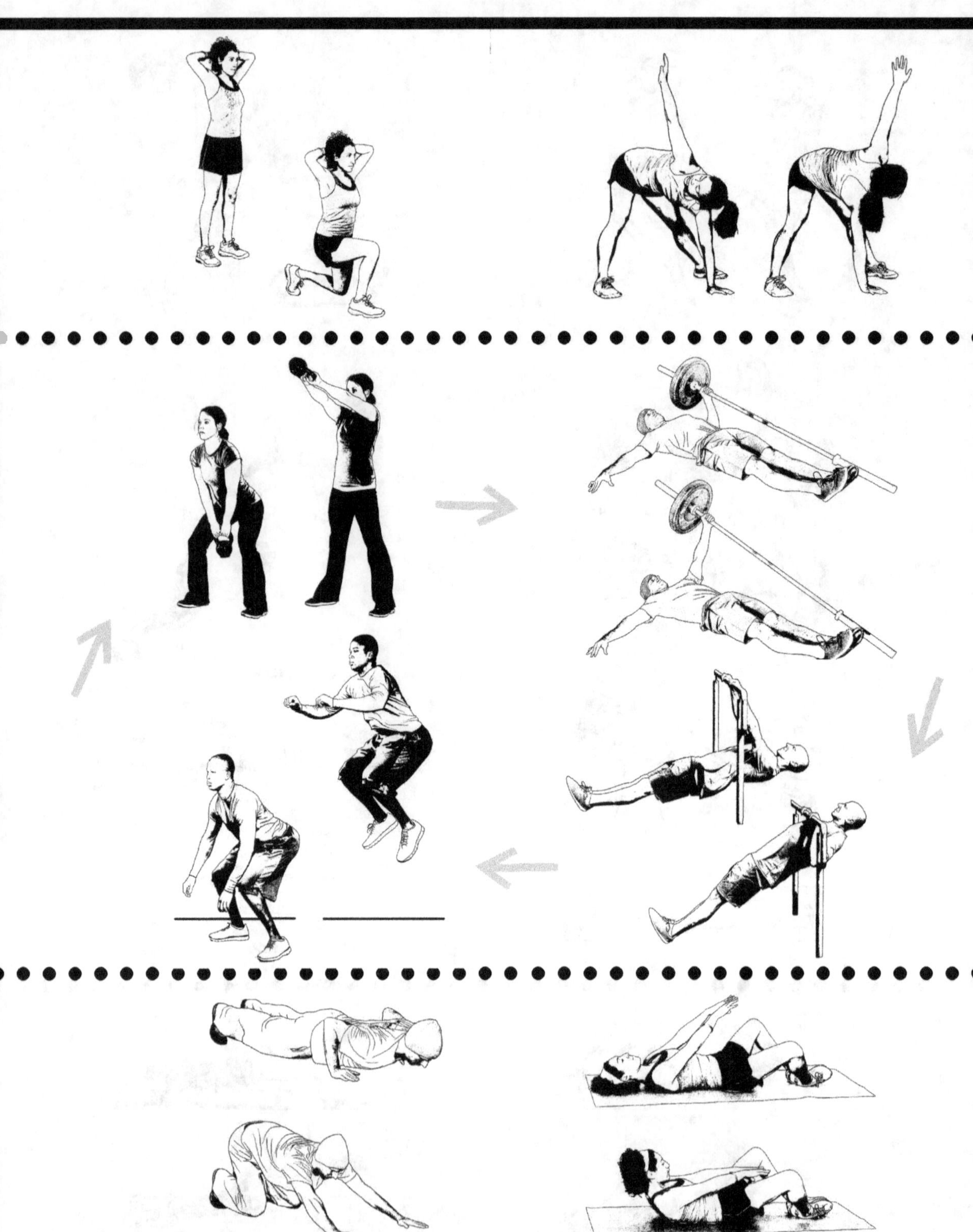

SIDE B

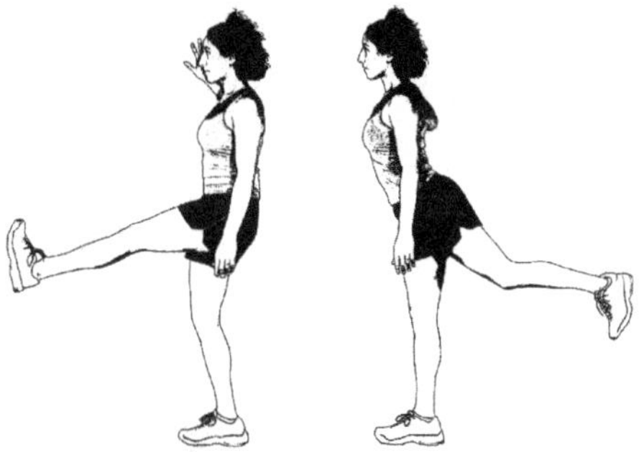

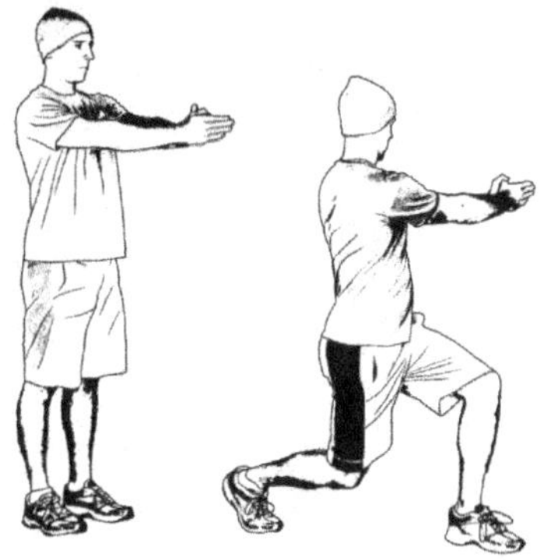

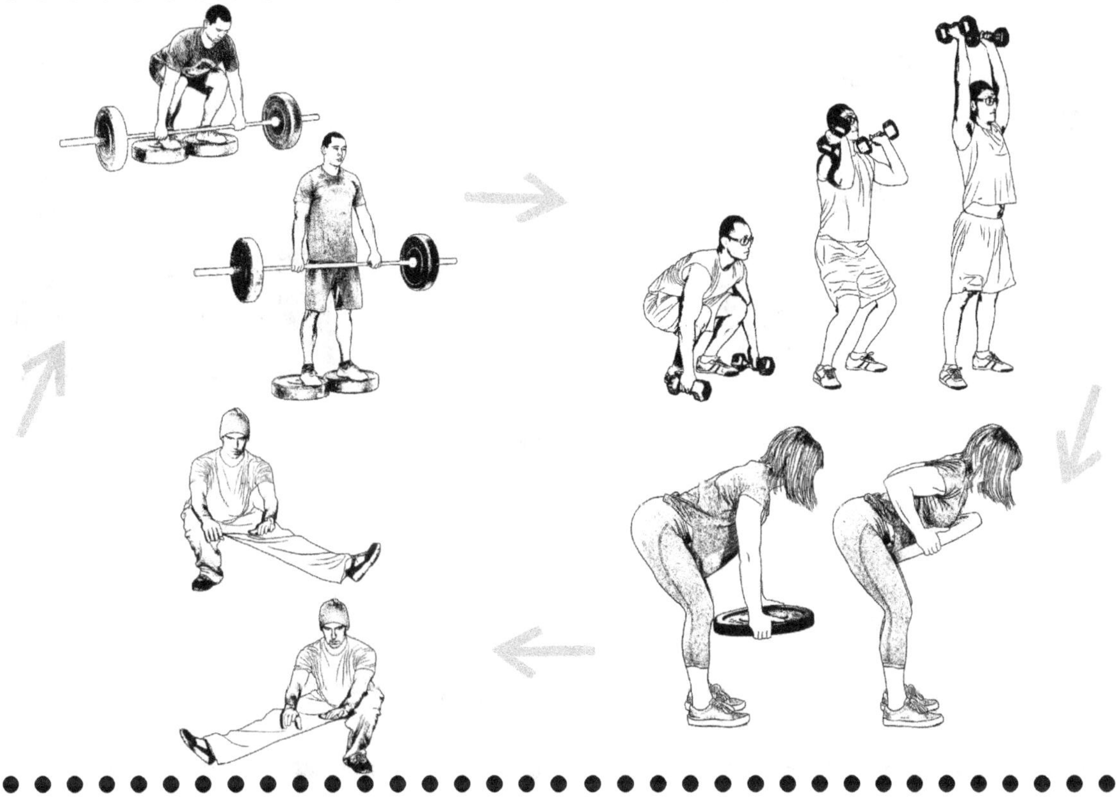

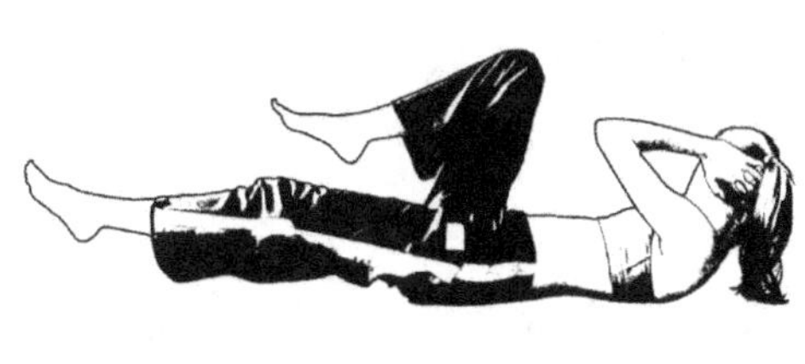

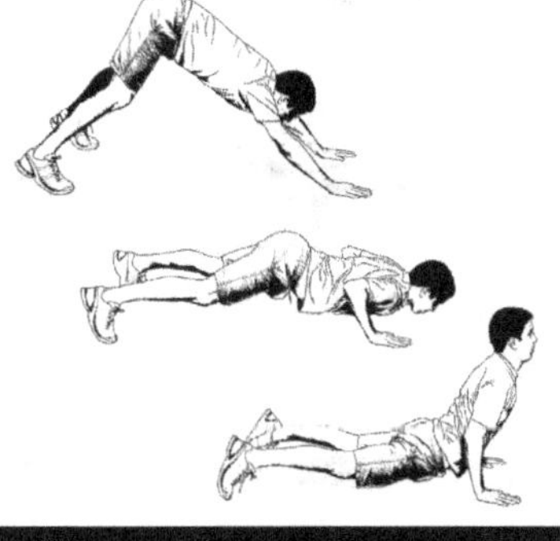

SIDE B

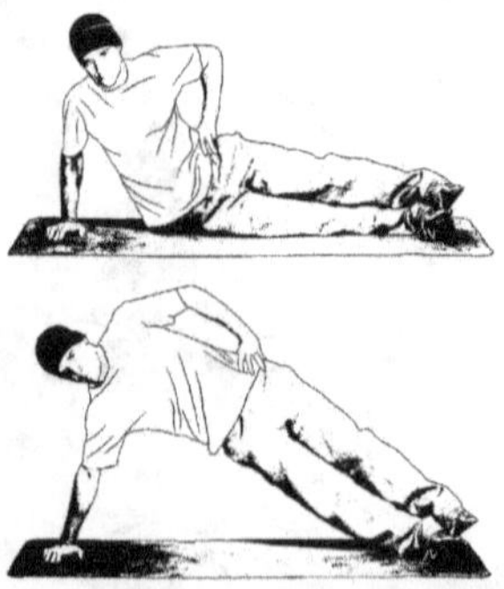

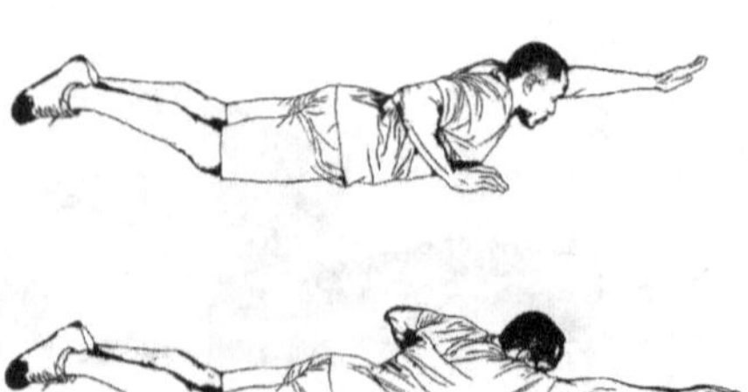

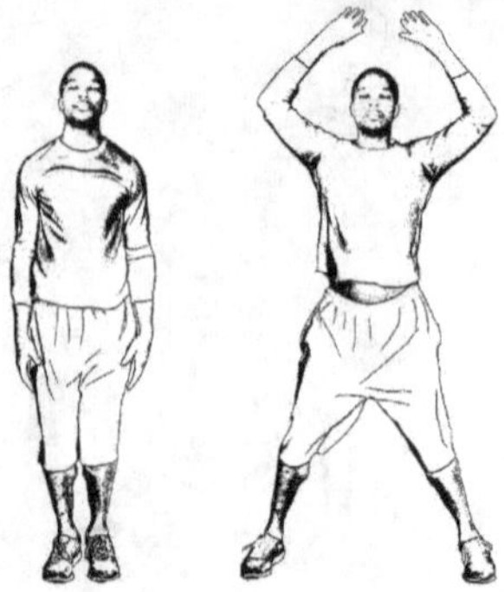

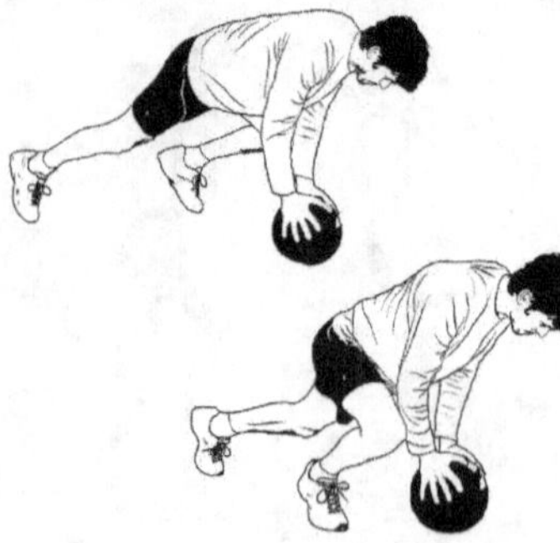

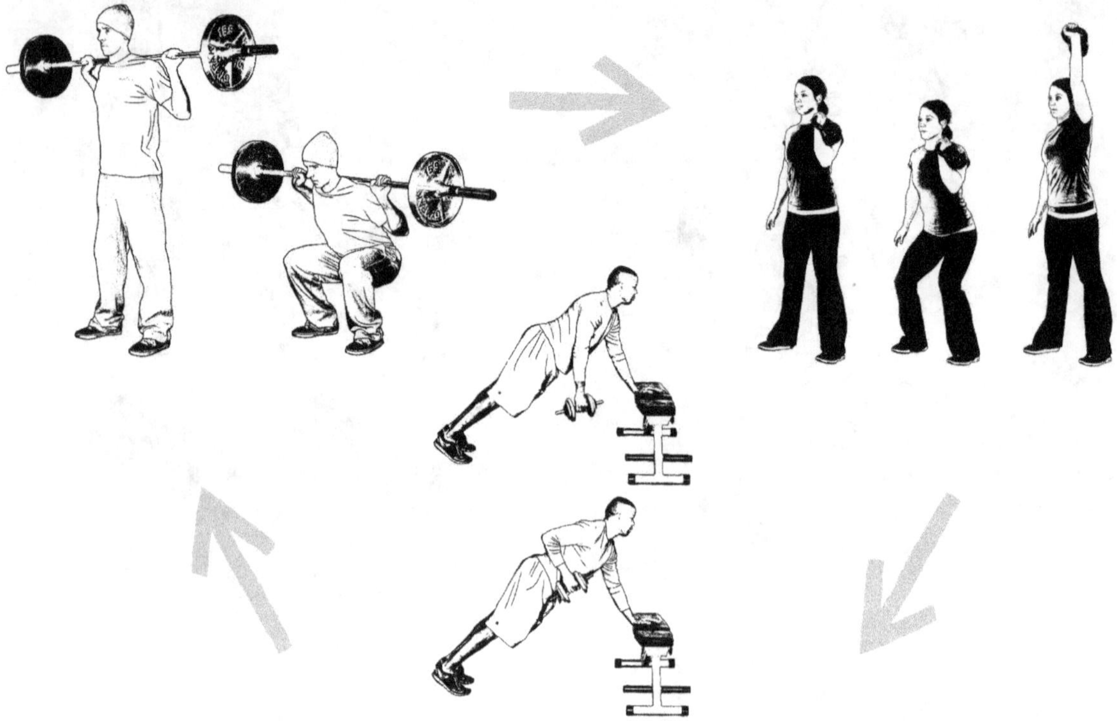

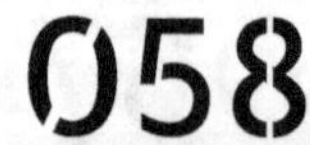

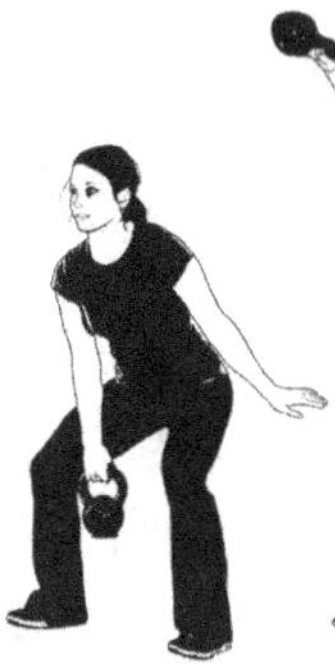

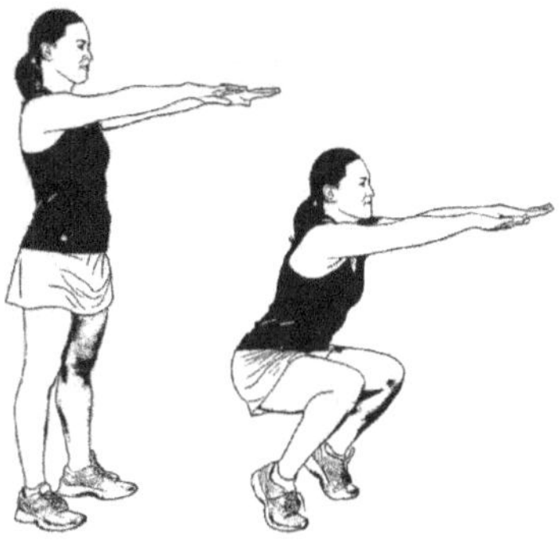

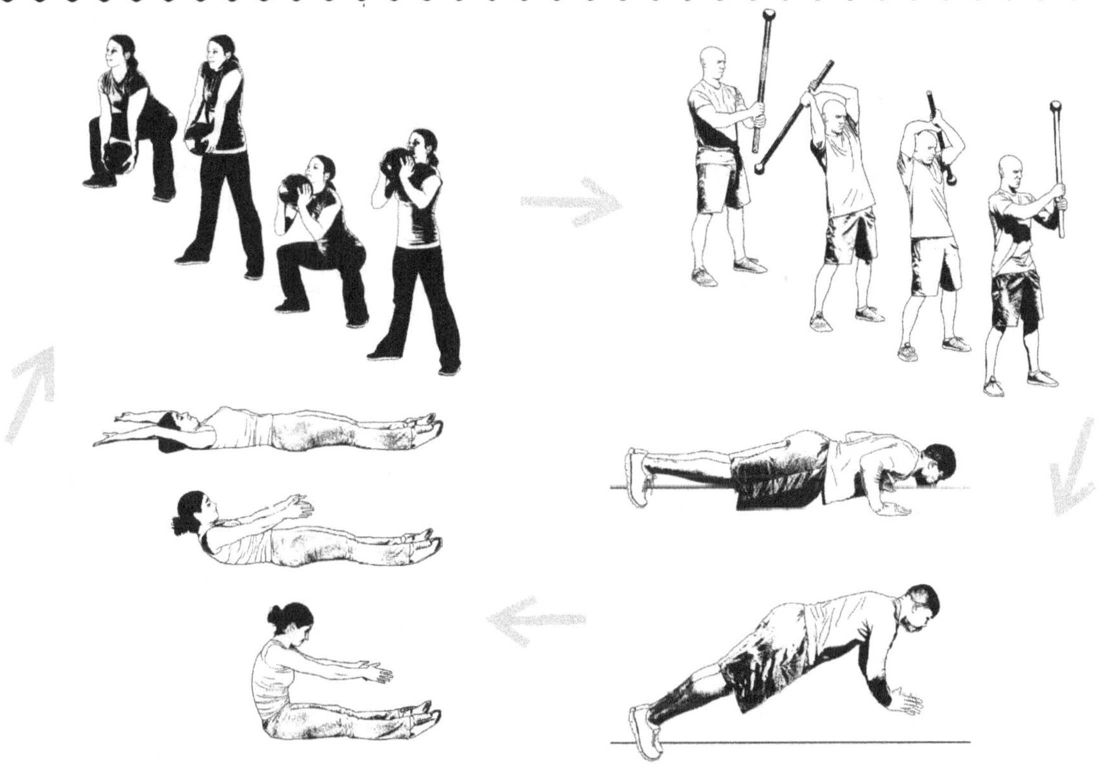

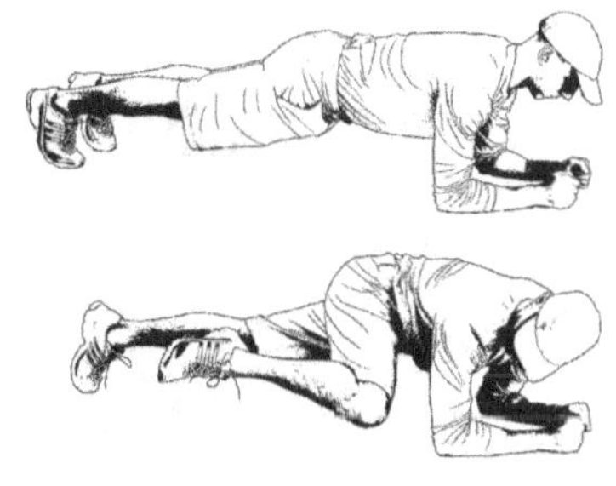

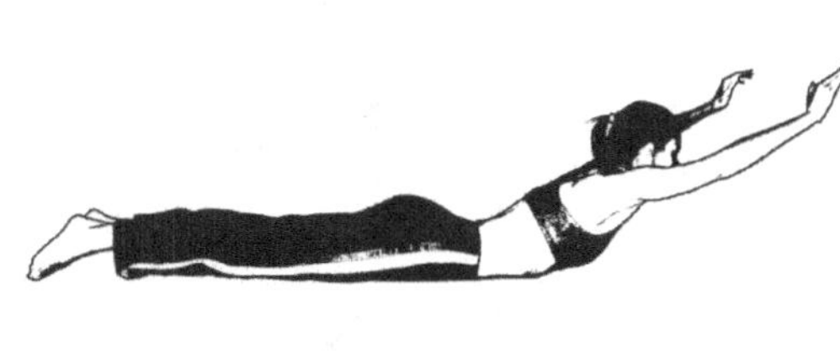

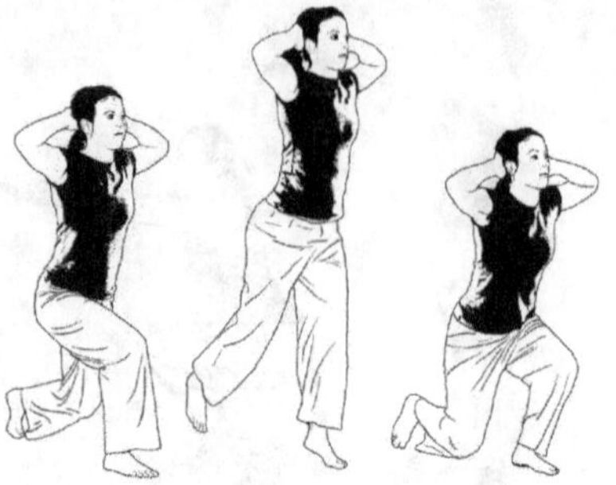

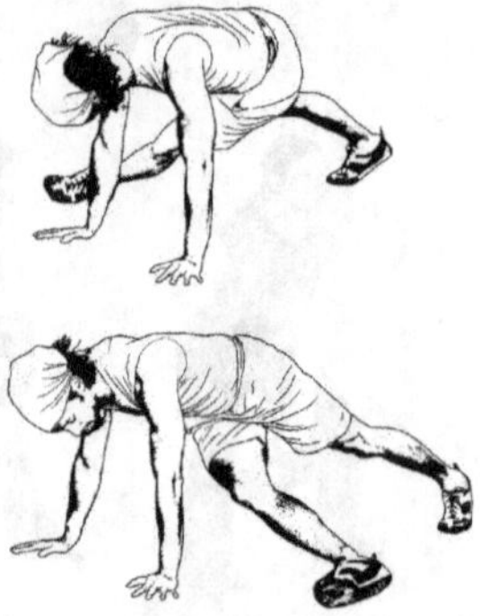

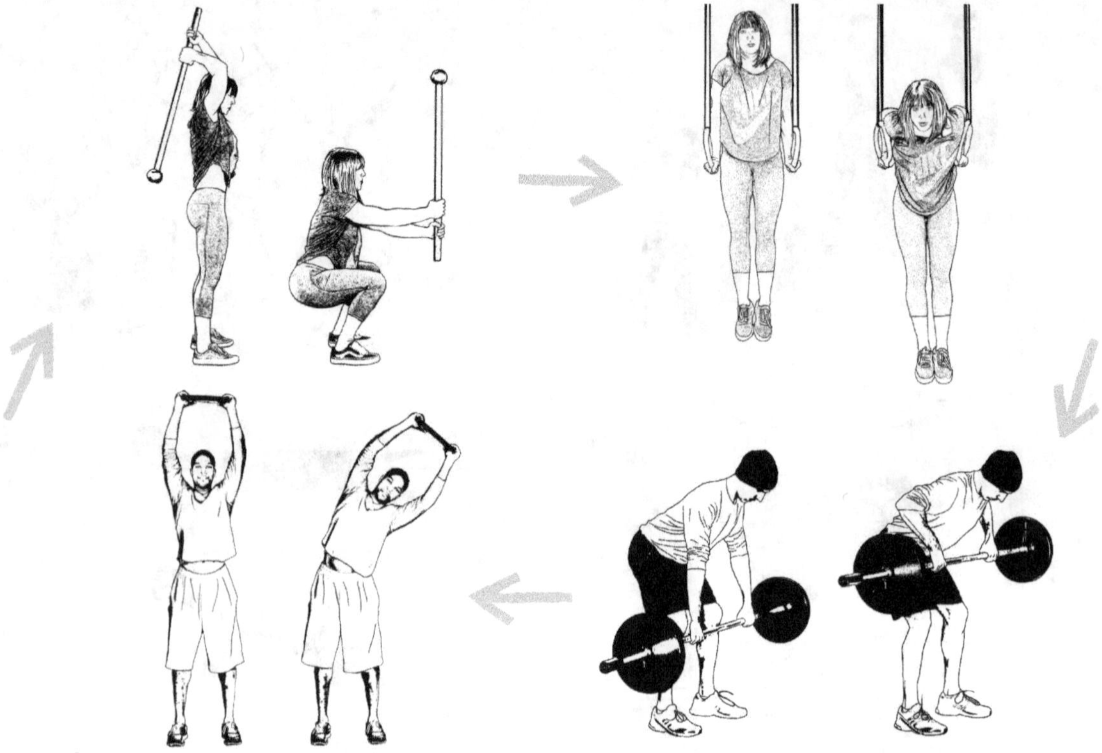

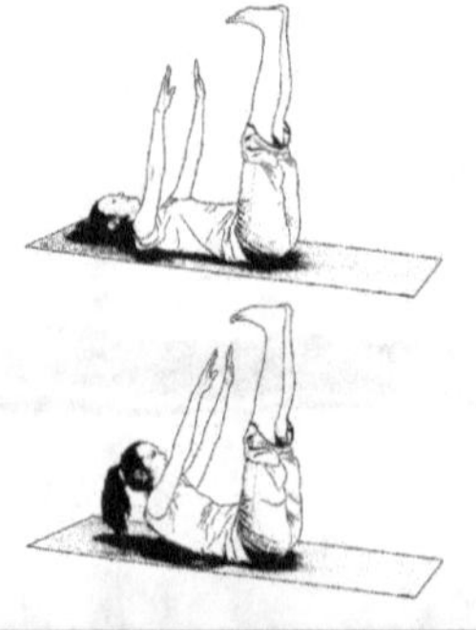
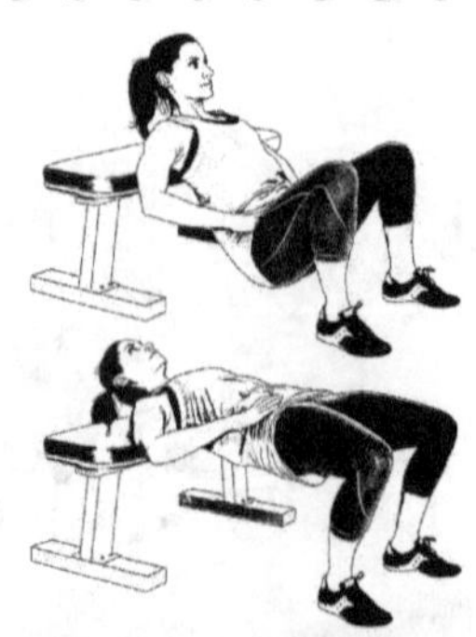

SIDE B

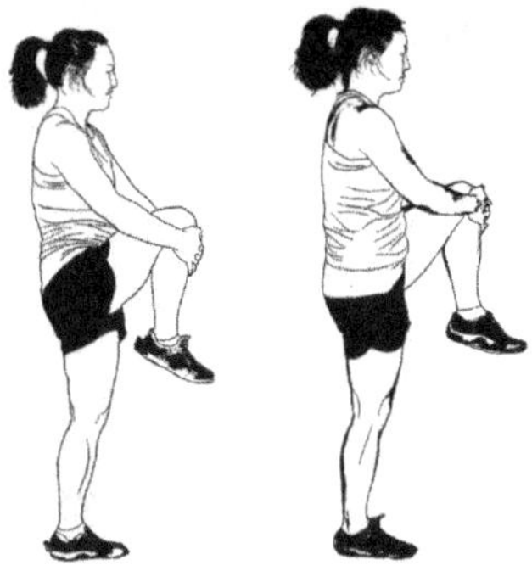

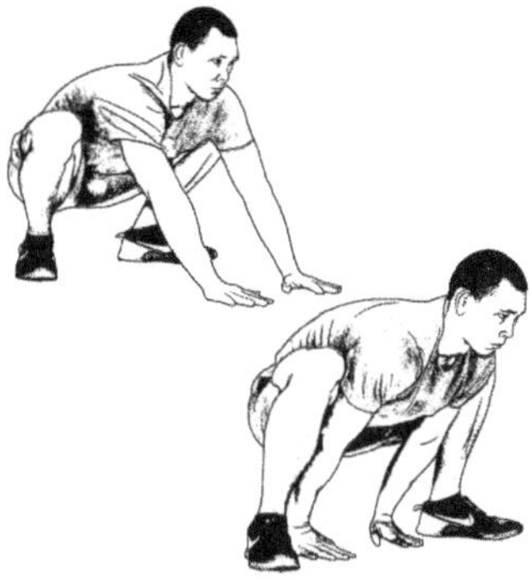

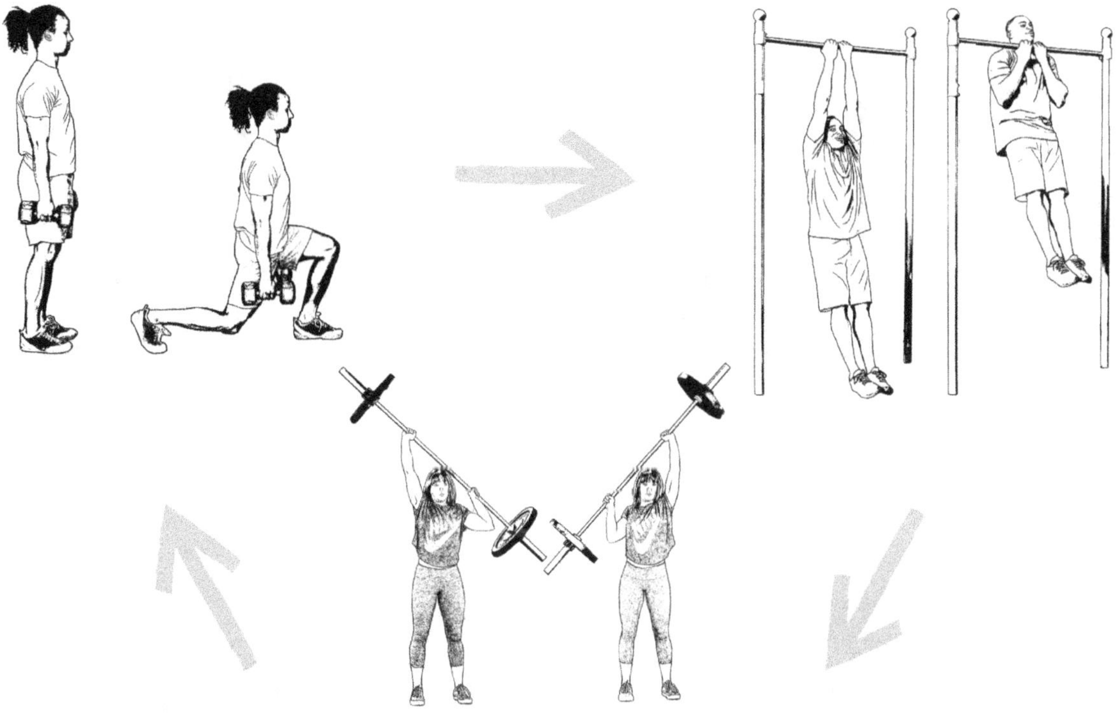

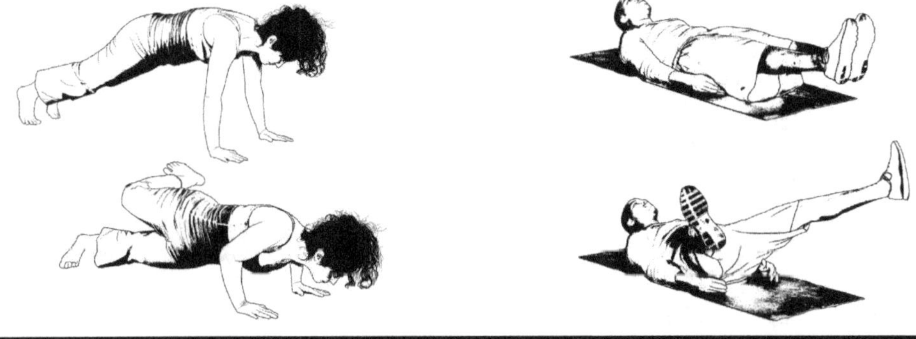

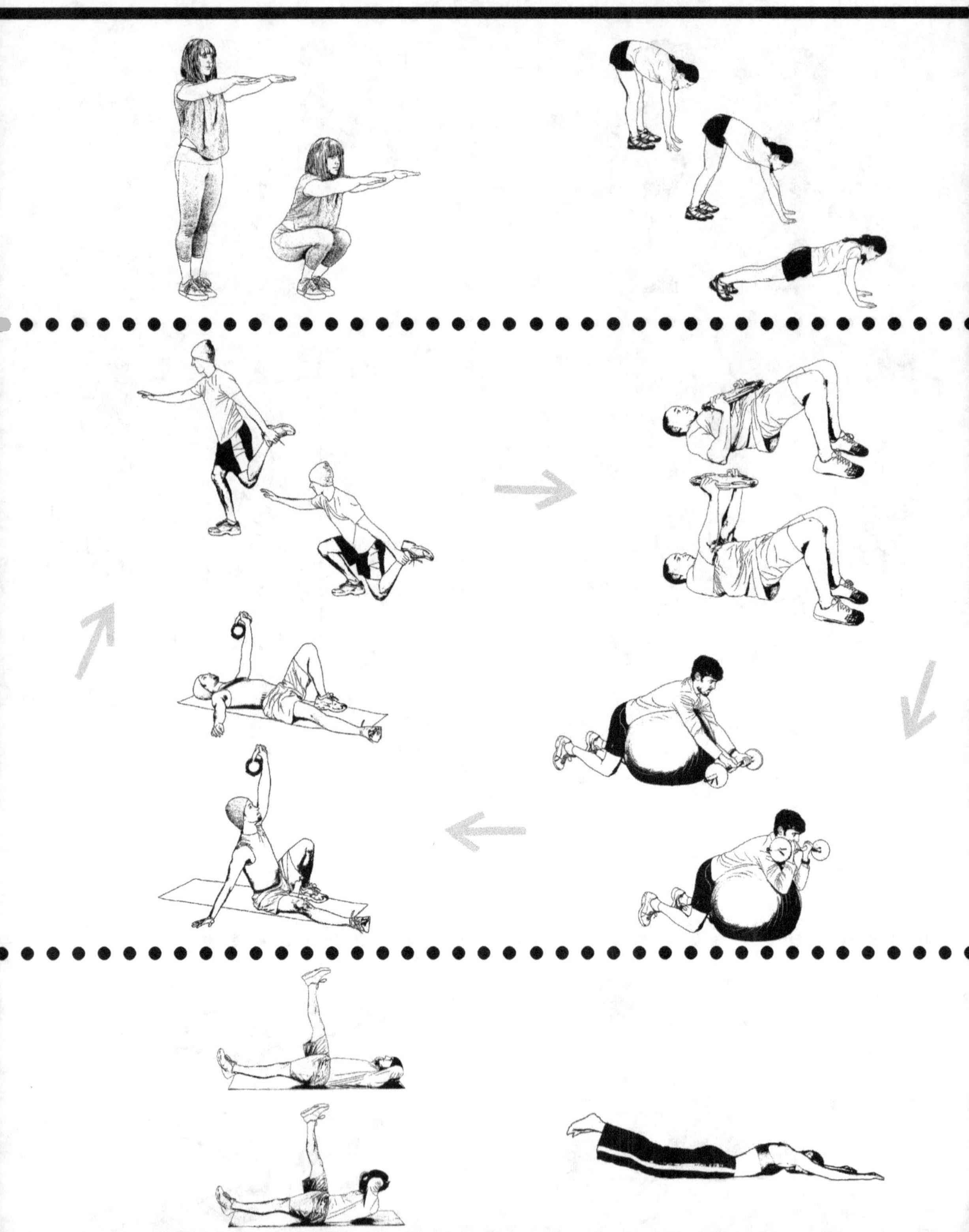

SIDE B

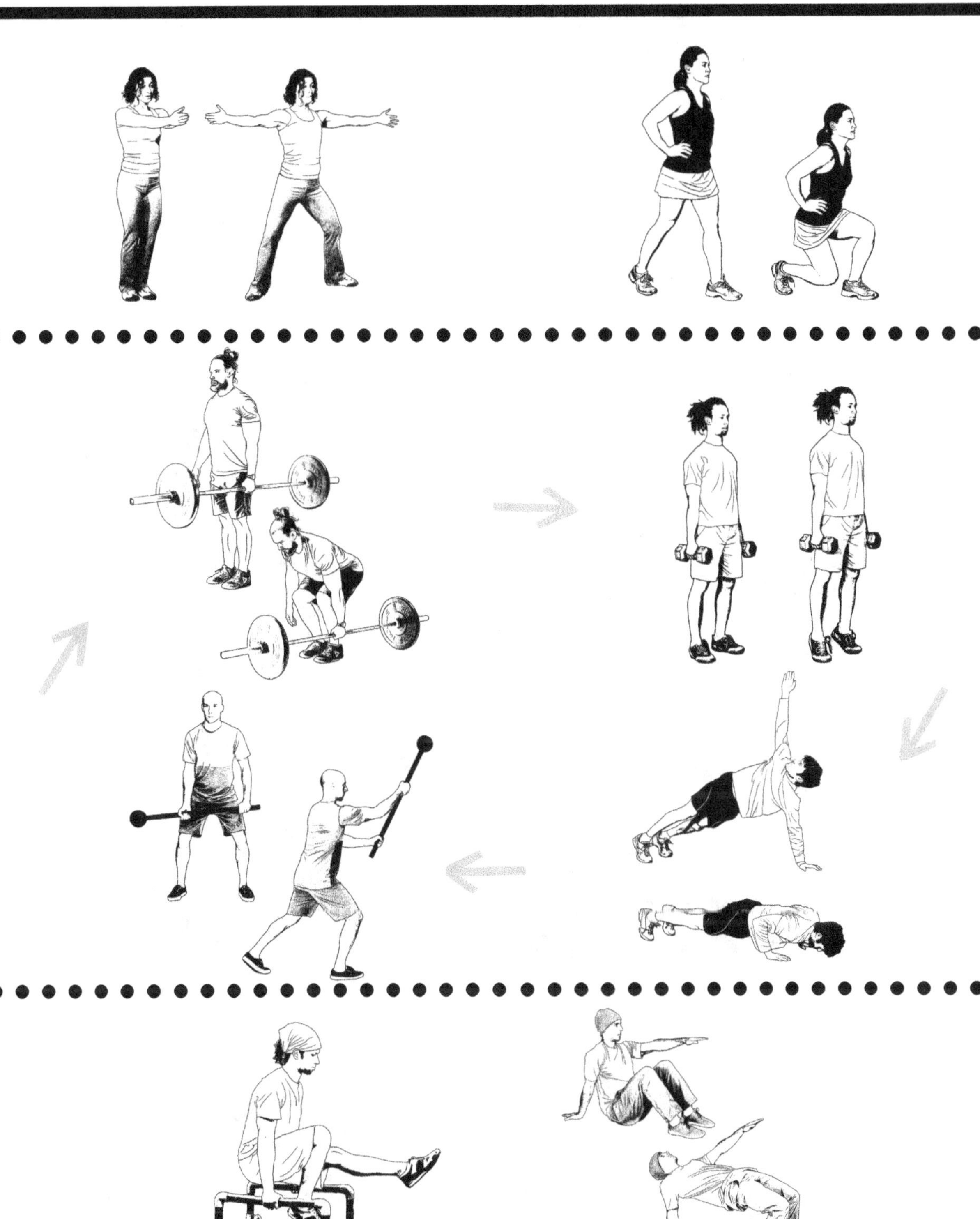

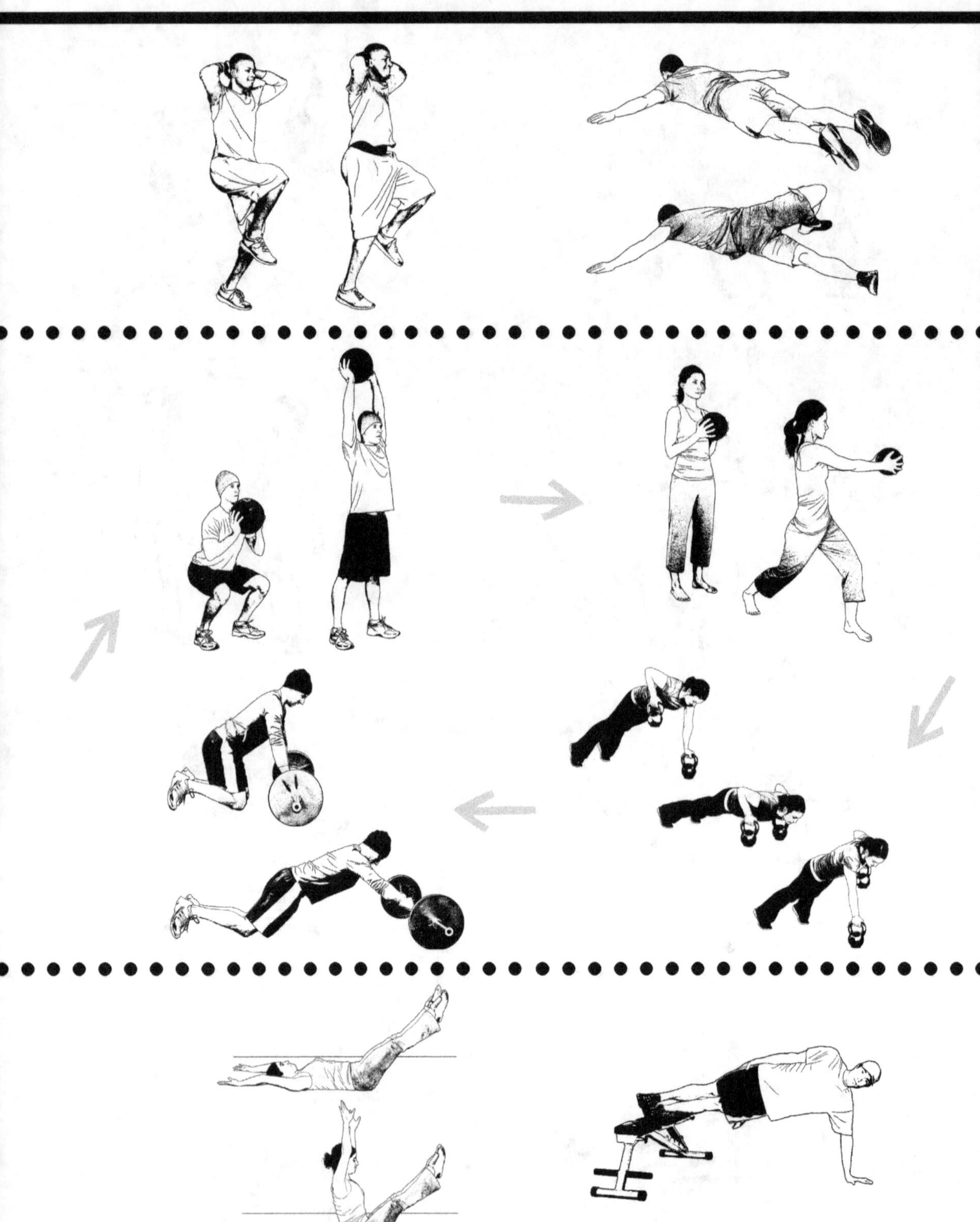

SIDE B

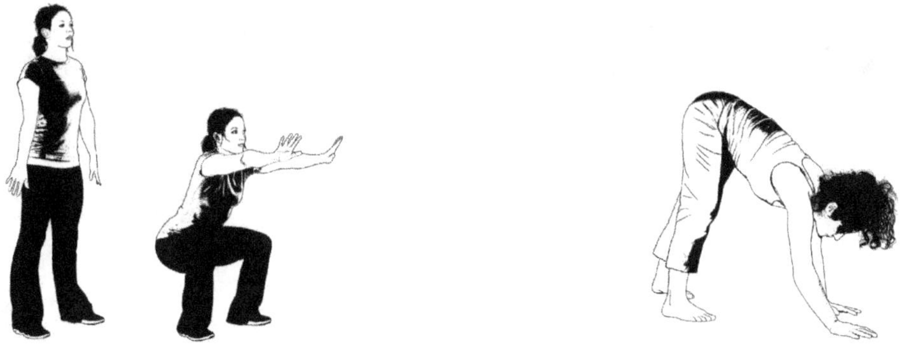

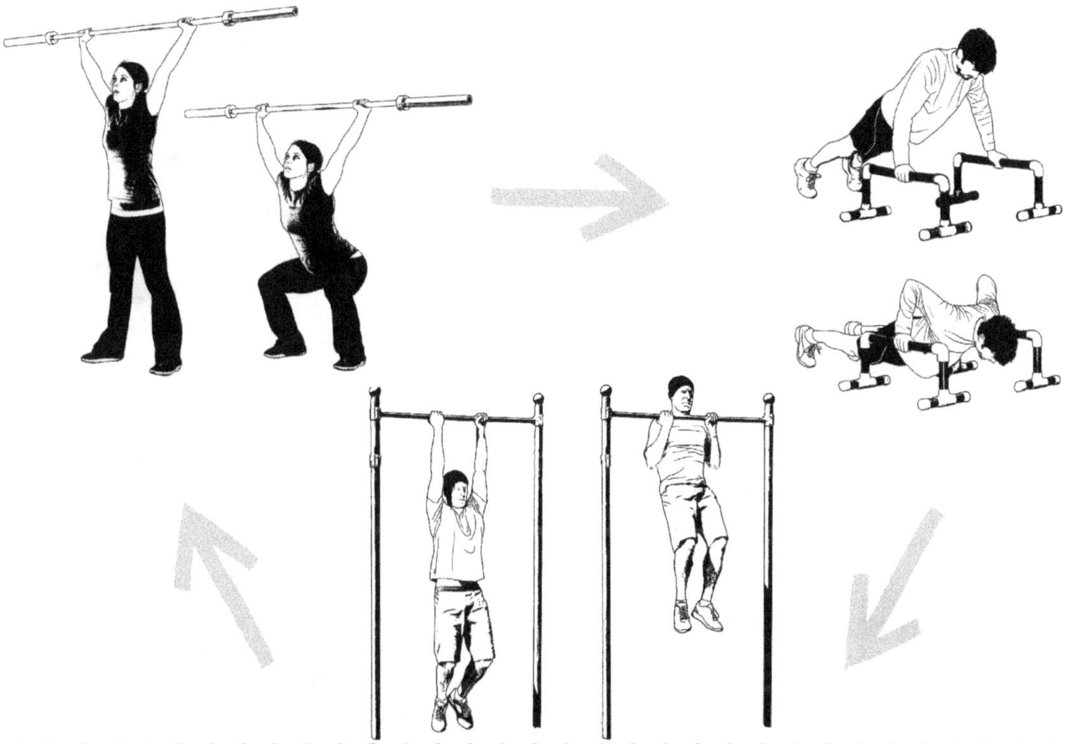

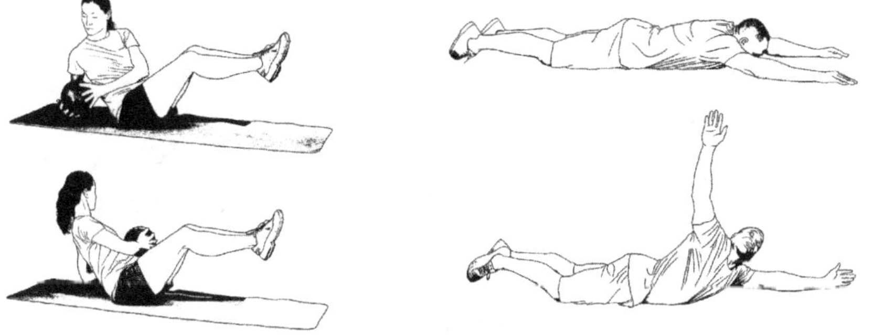

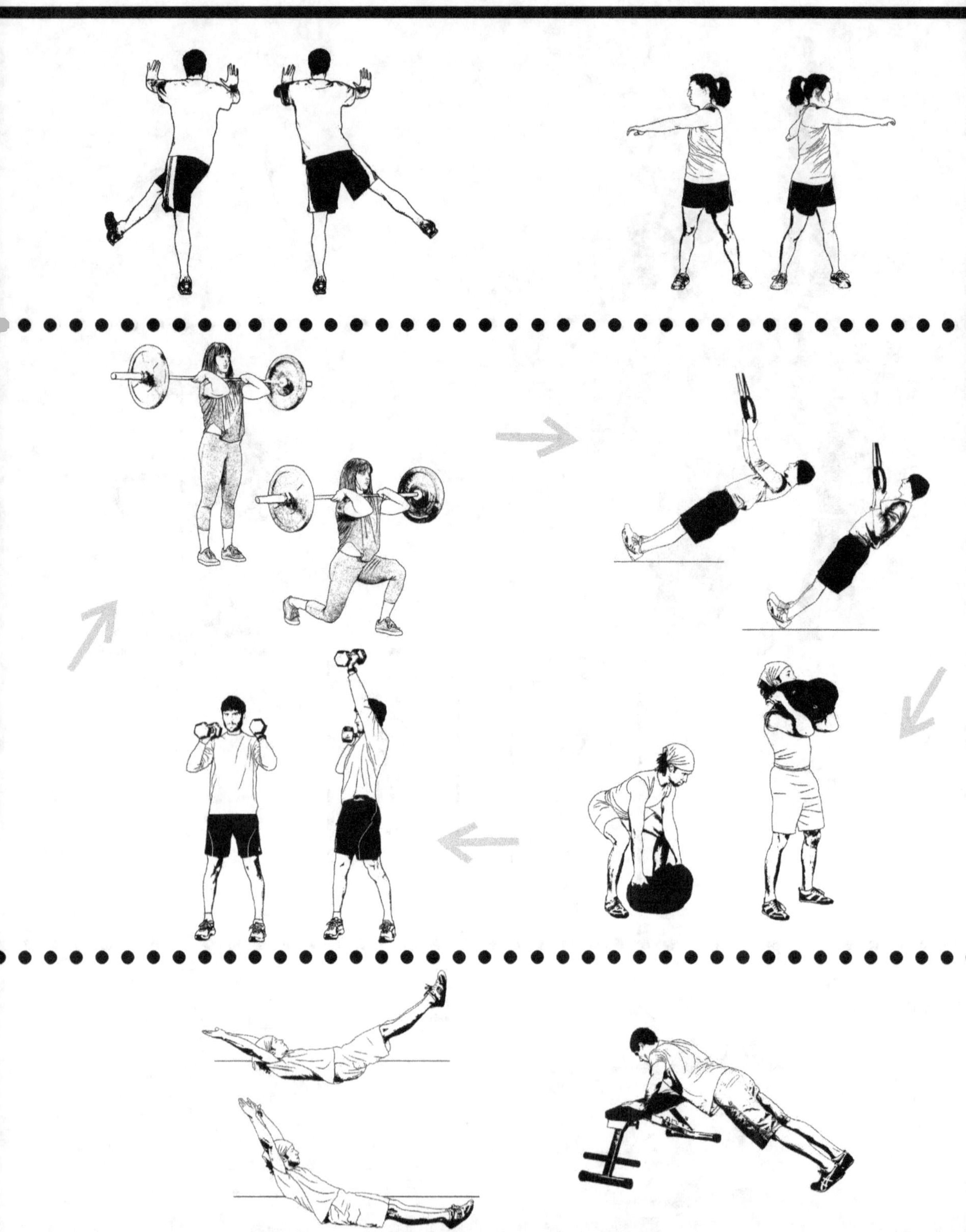

SIDE B

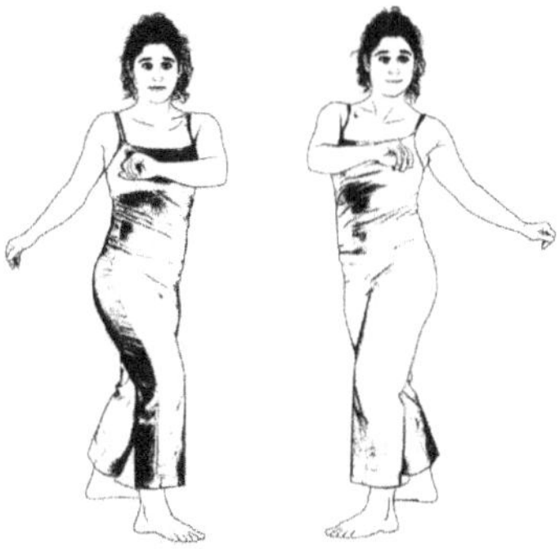

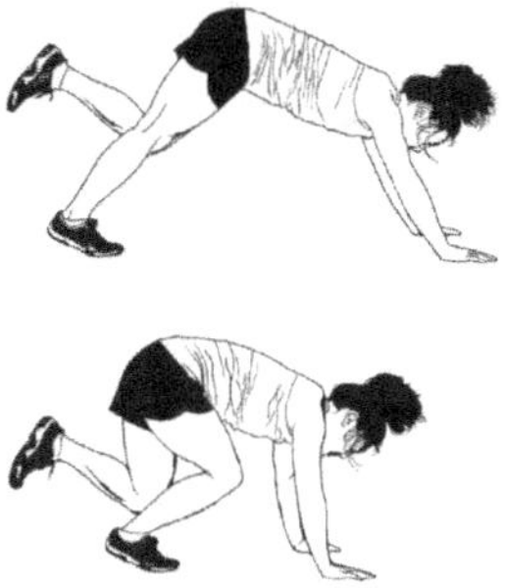

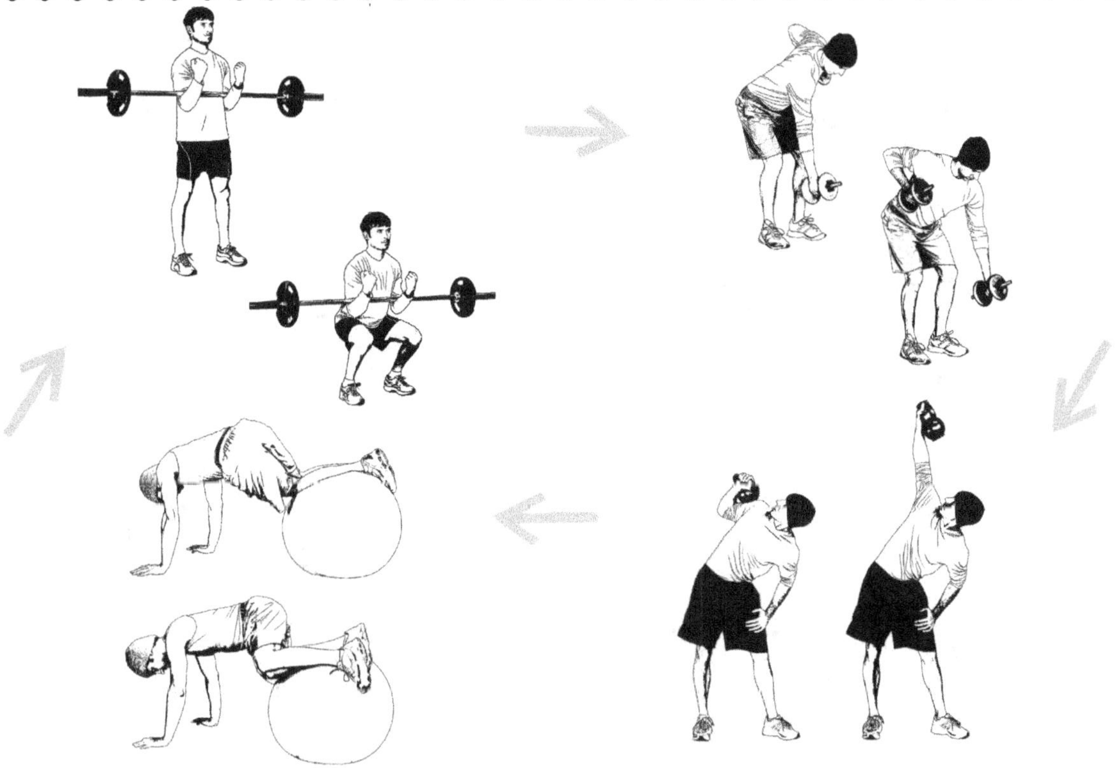

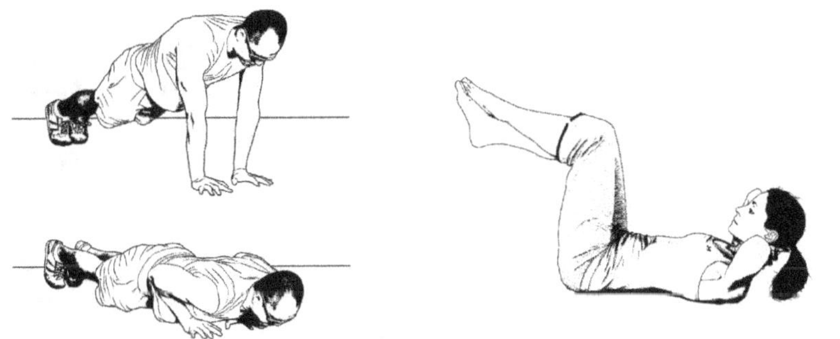

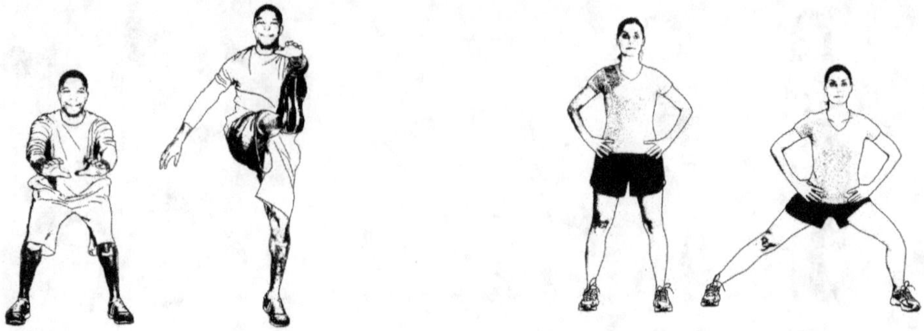

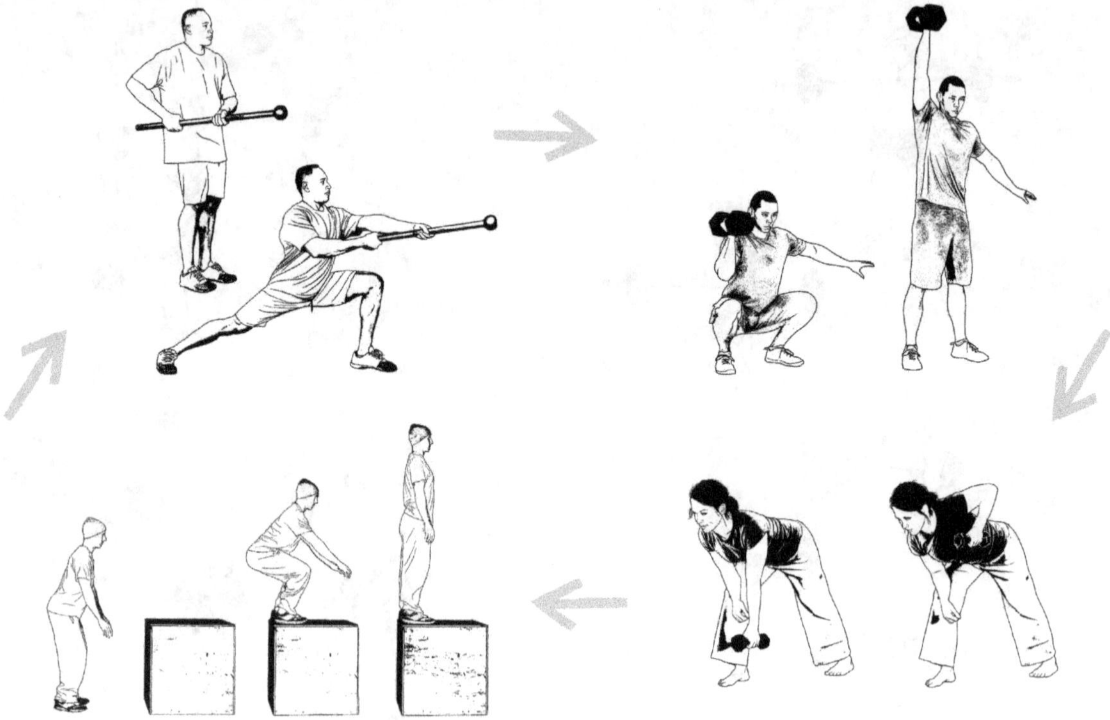

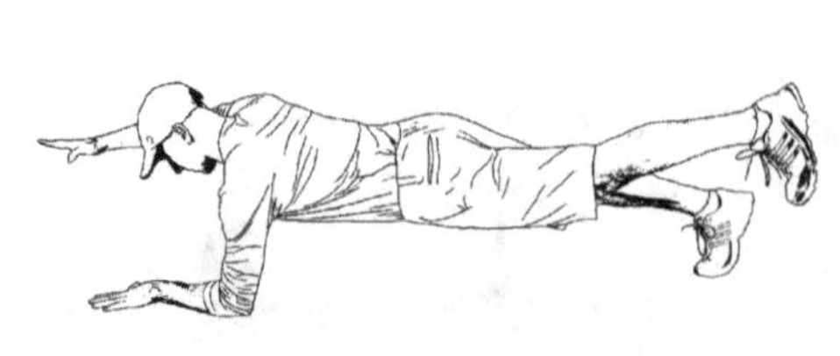
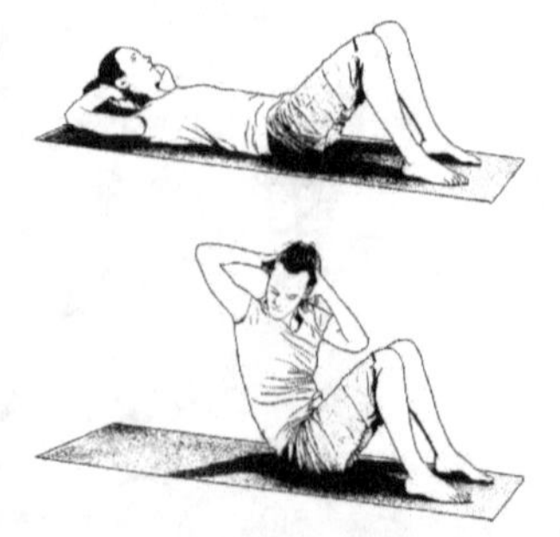

Side B

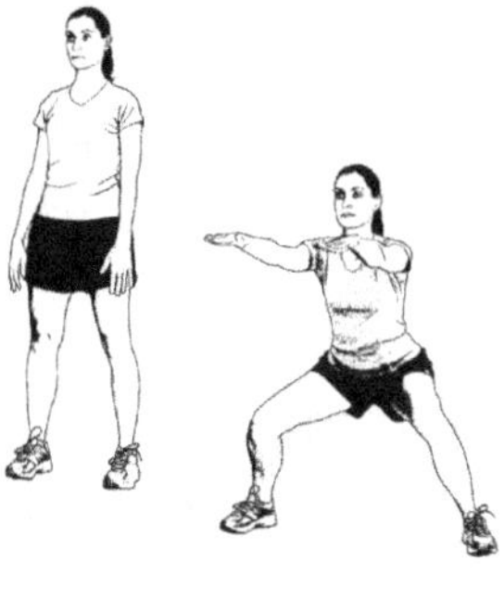

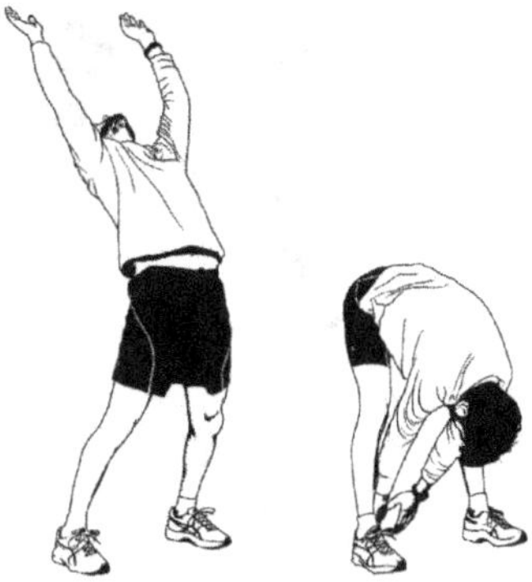

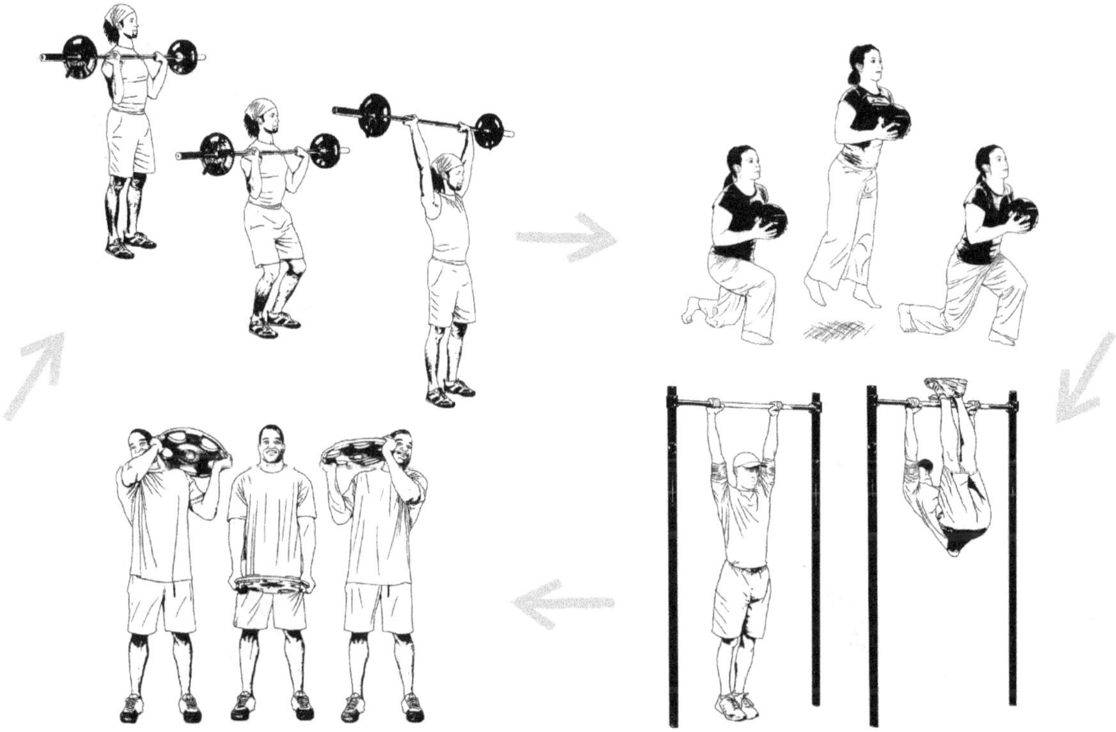

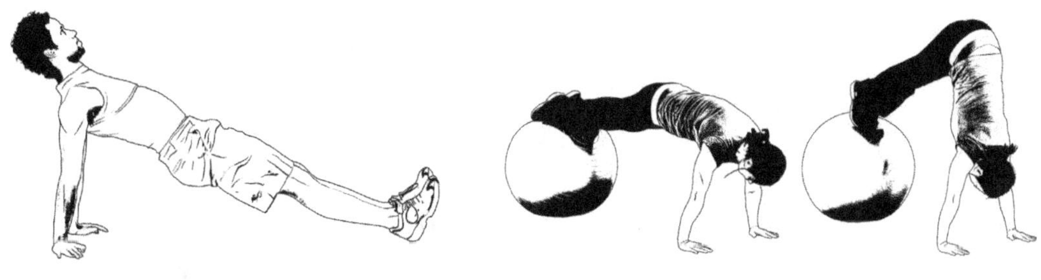

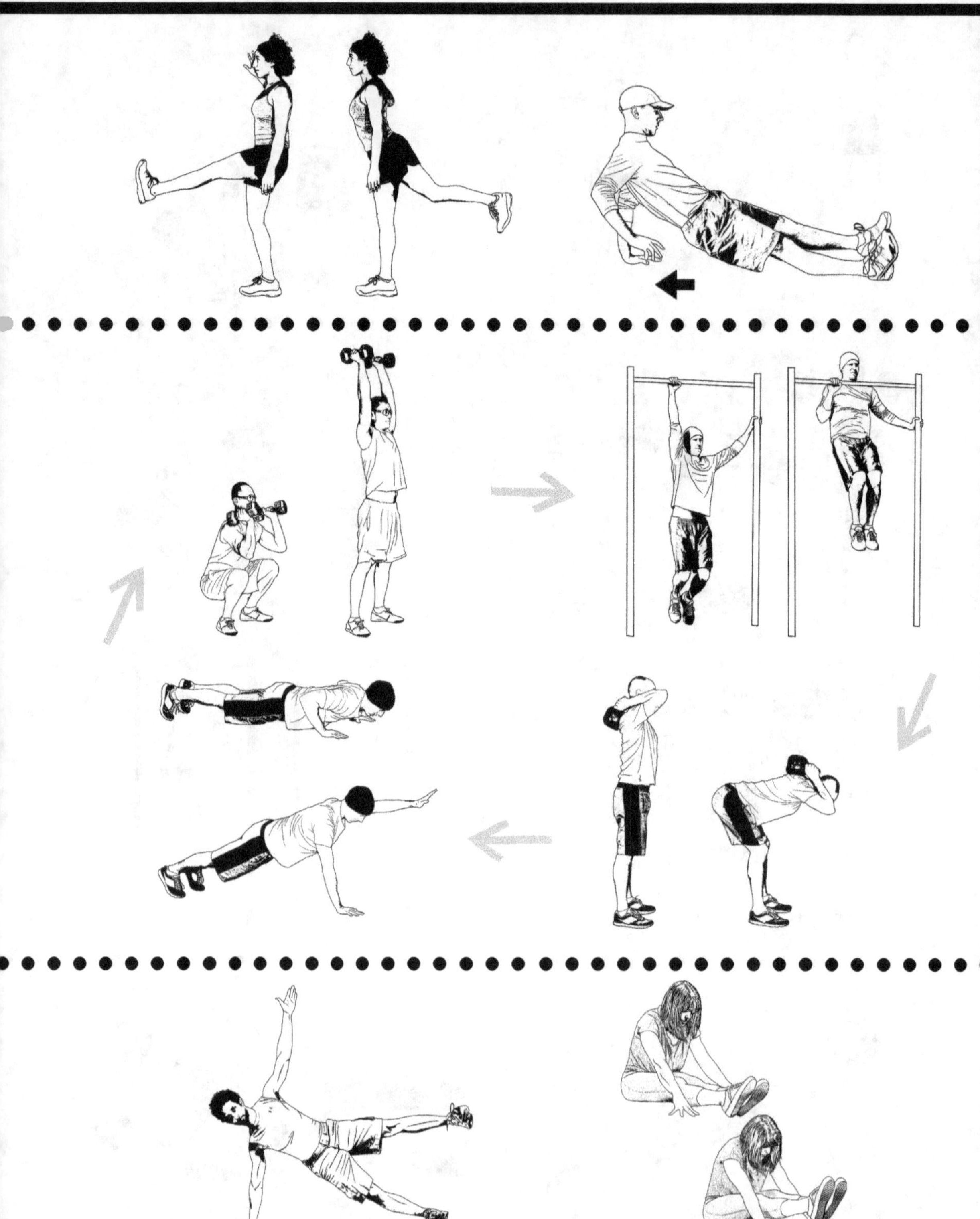

SIDE B

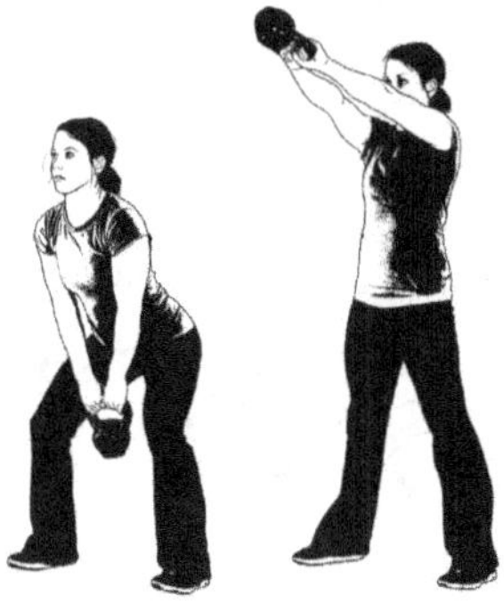

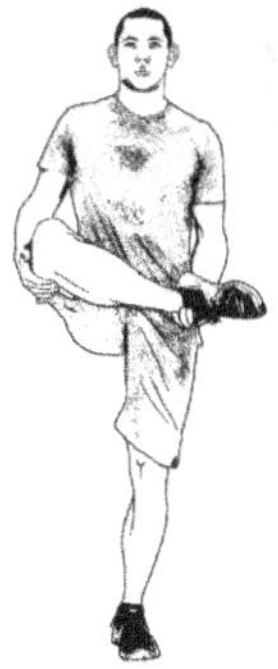

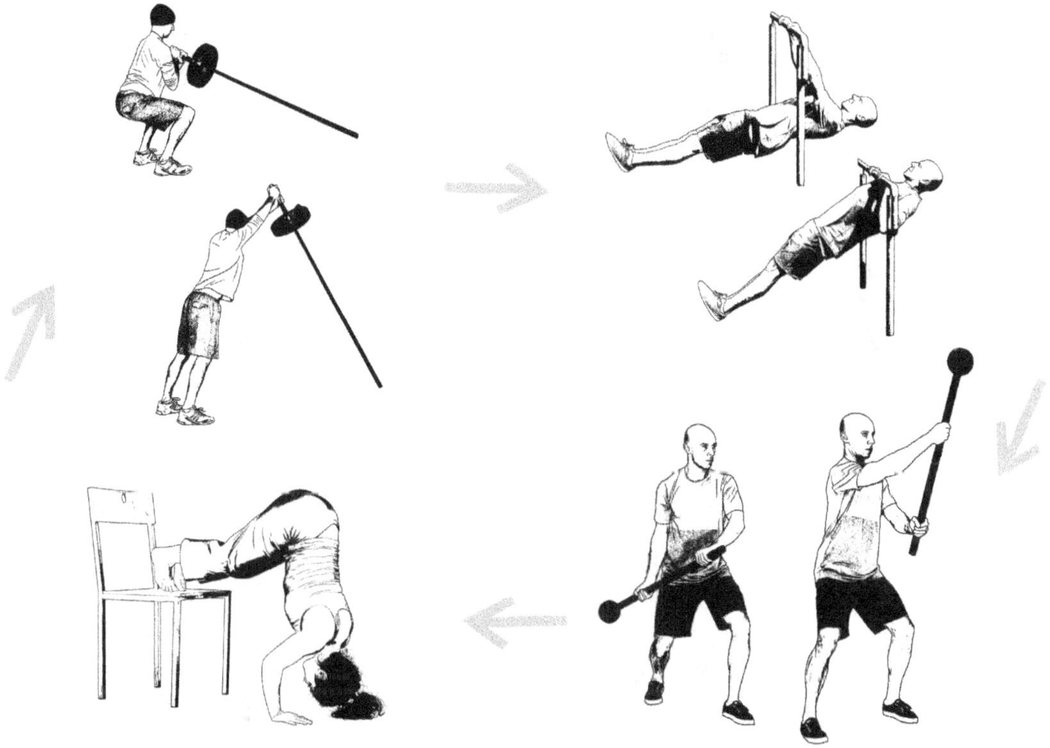

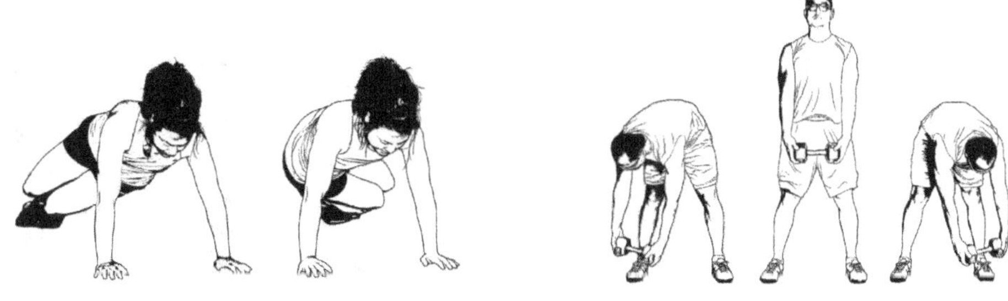

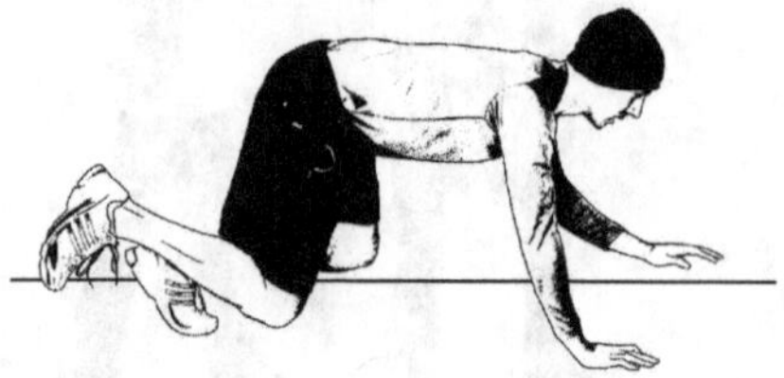

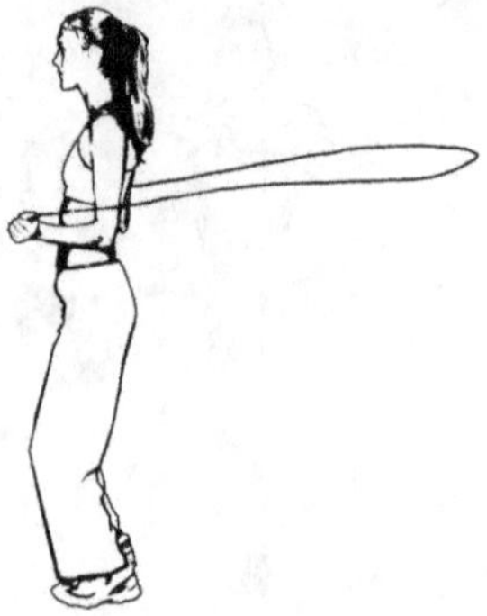

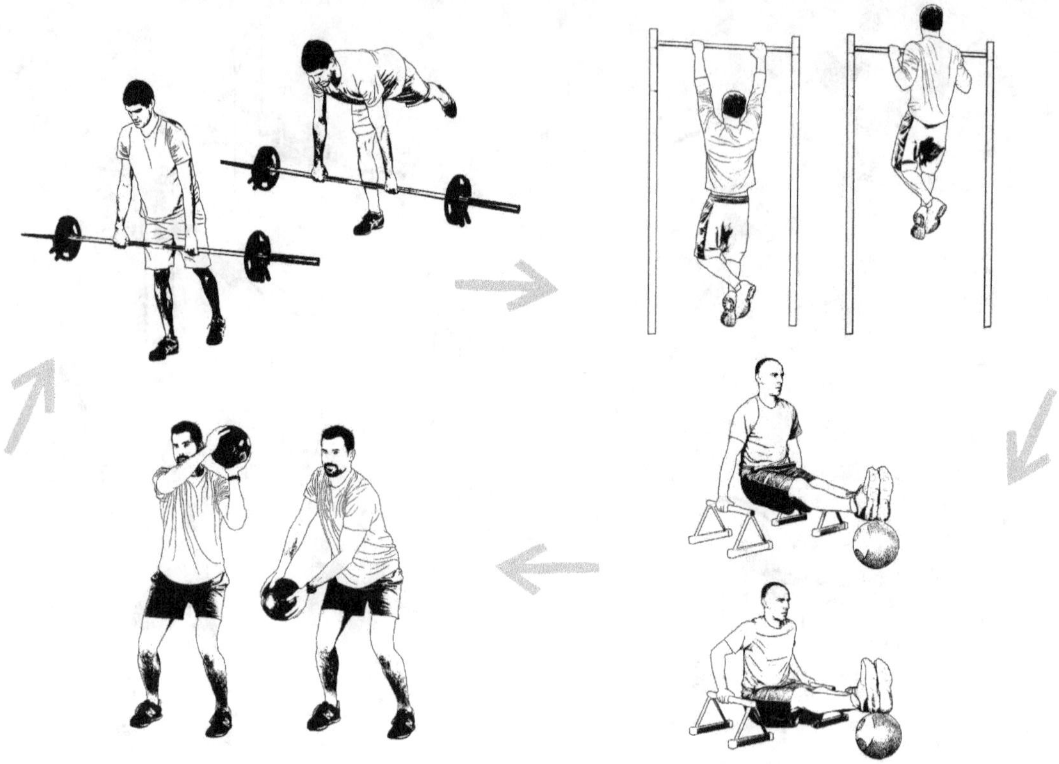

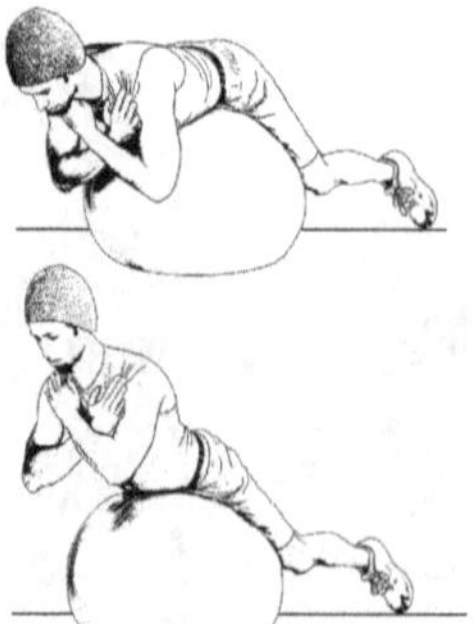

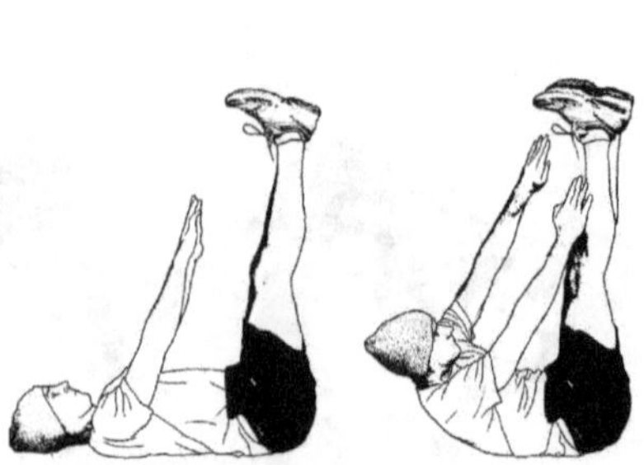

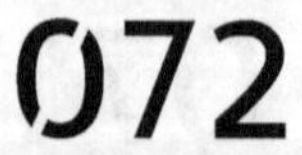

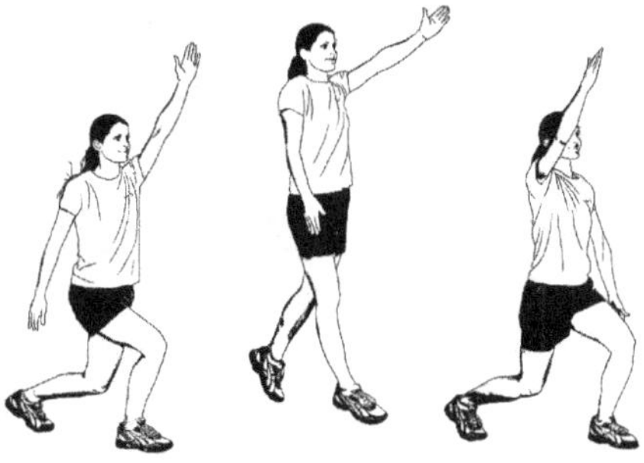

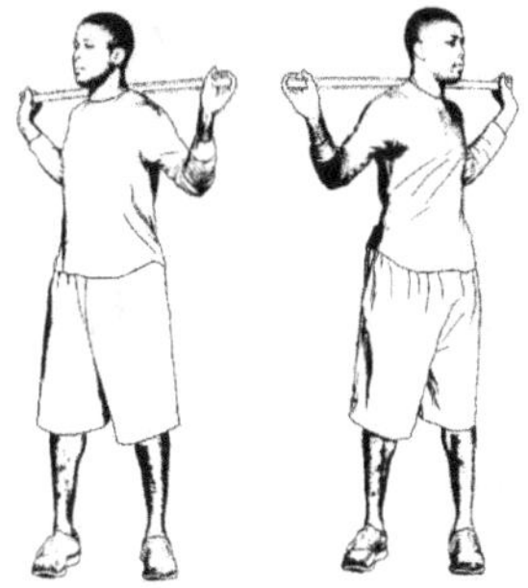

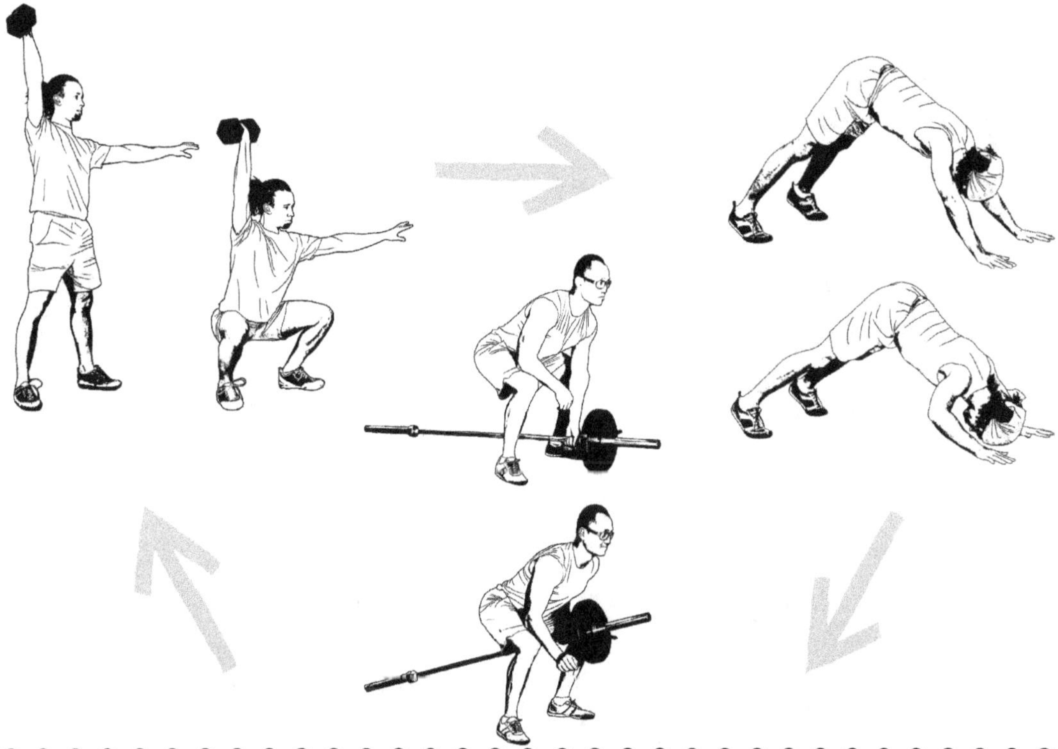

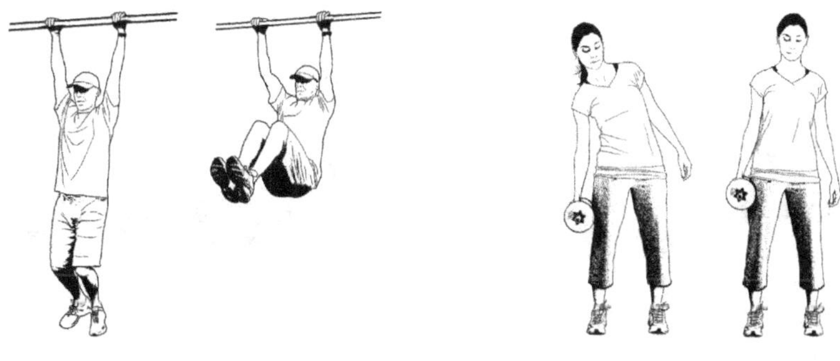

SIDE B

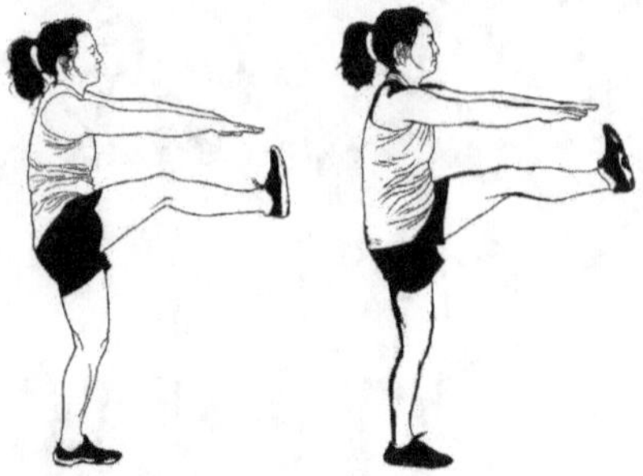

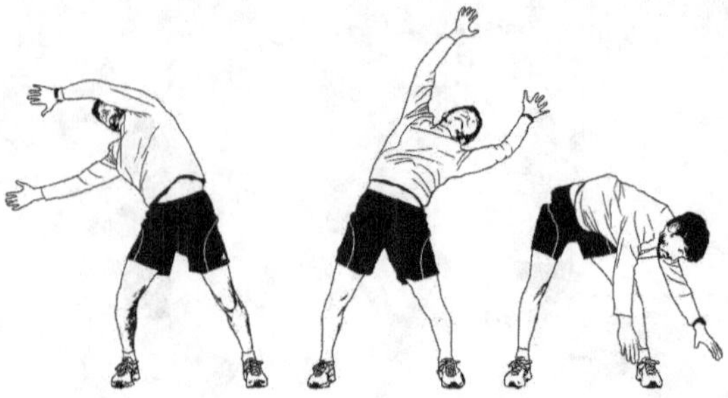

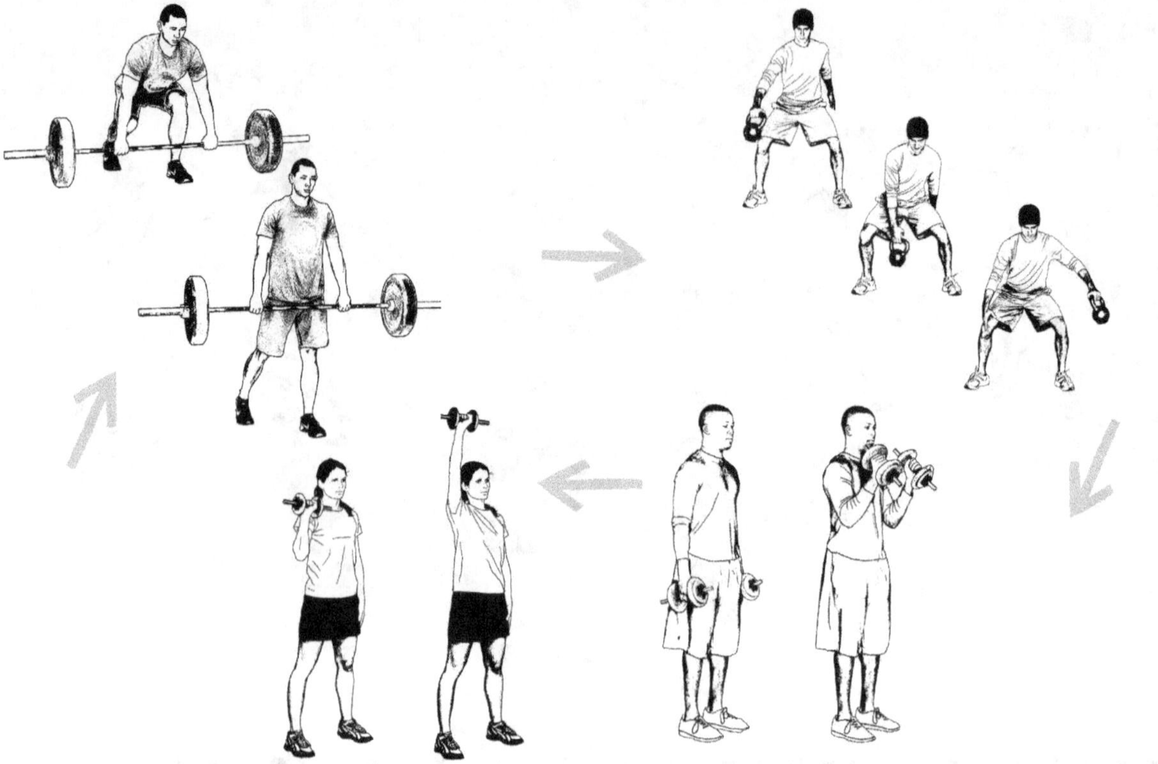

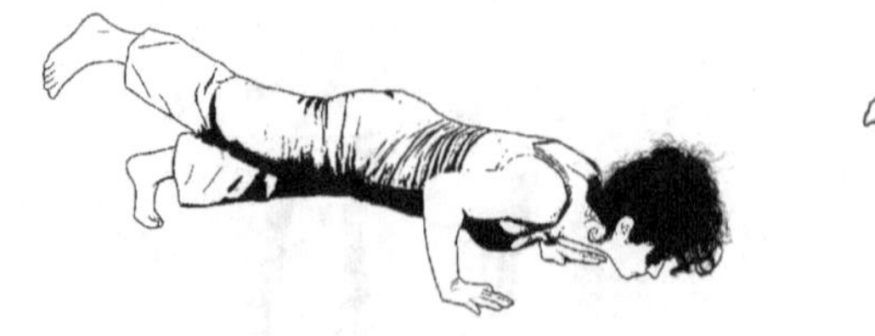

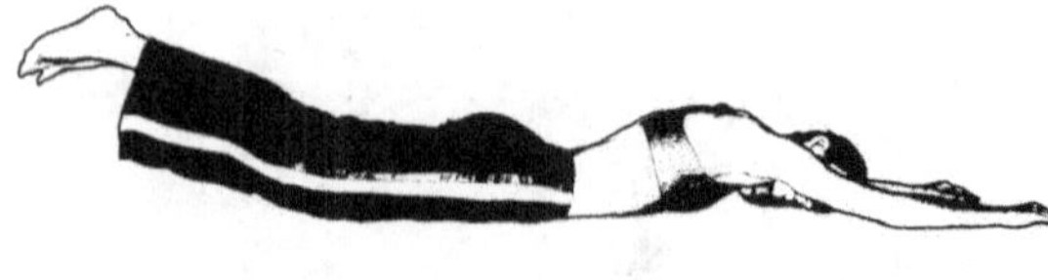

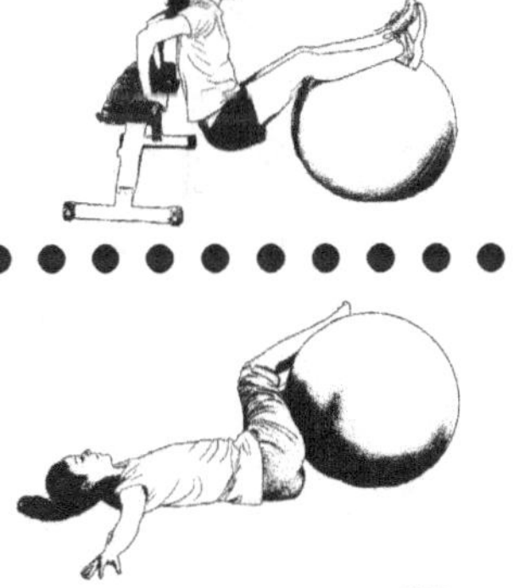

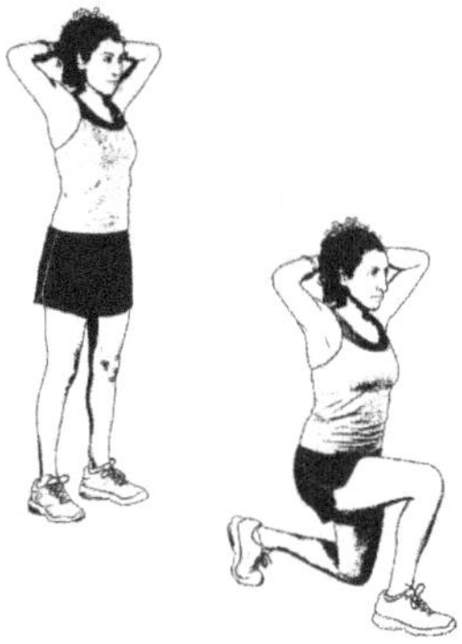

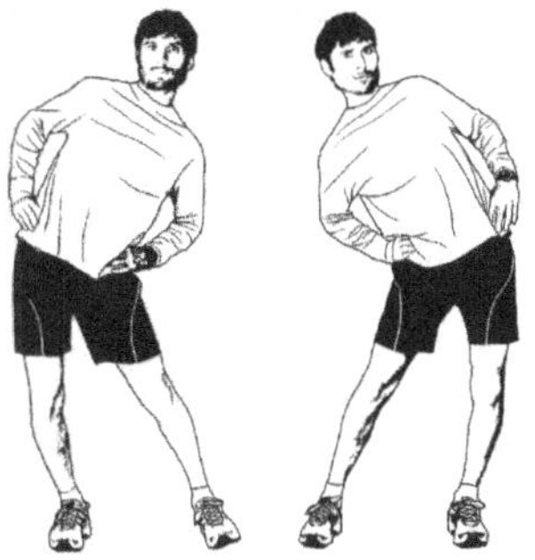

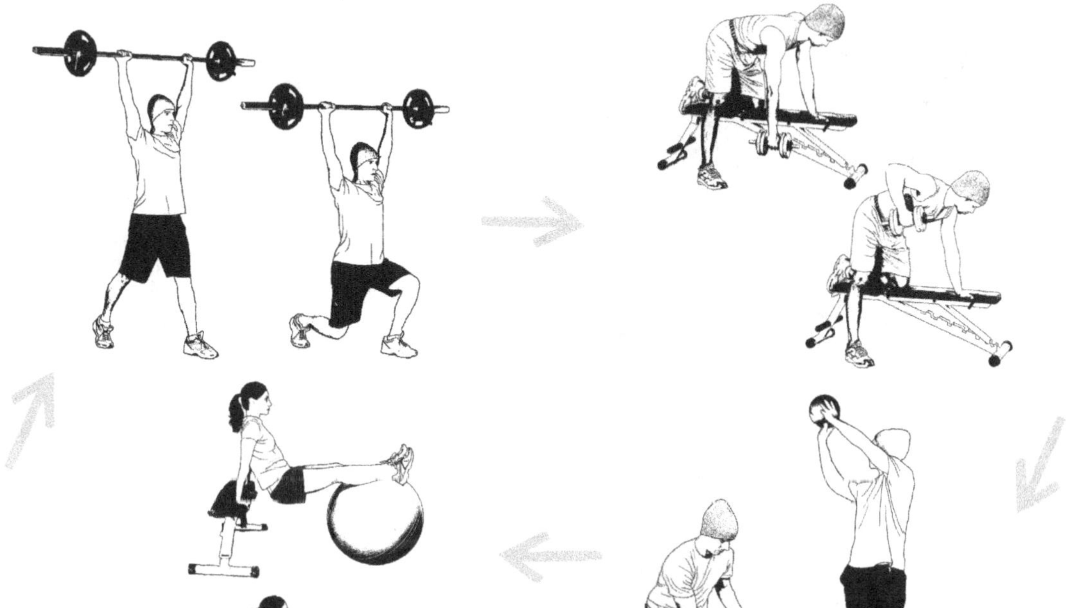

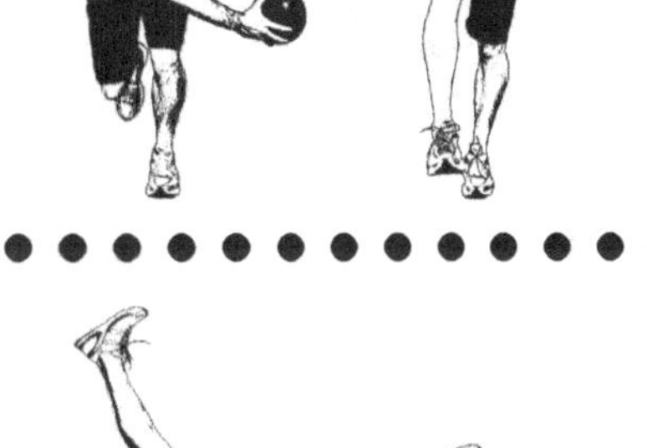

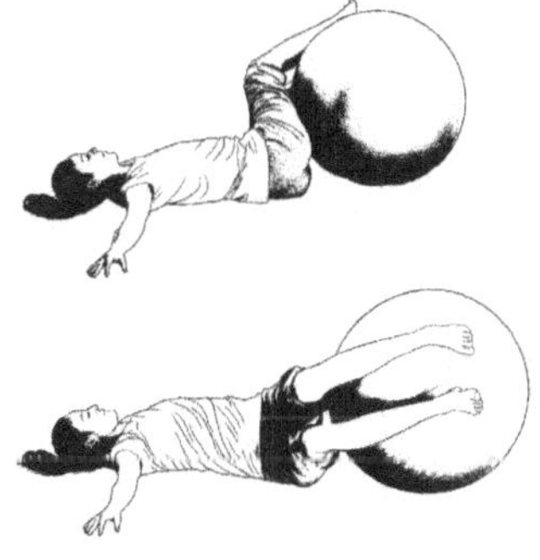

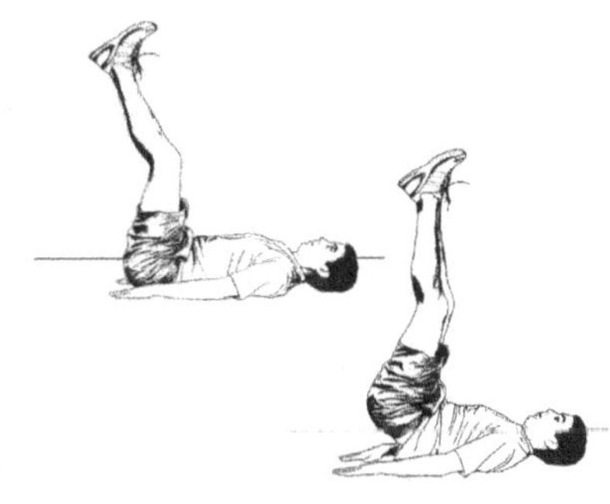

SIDE B

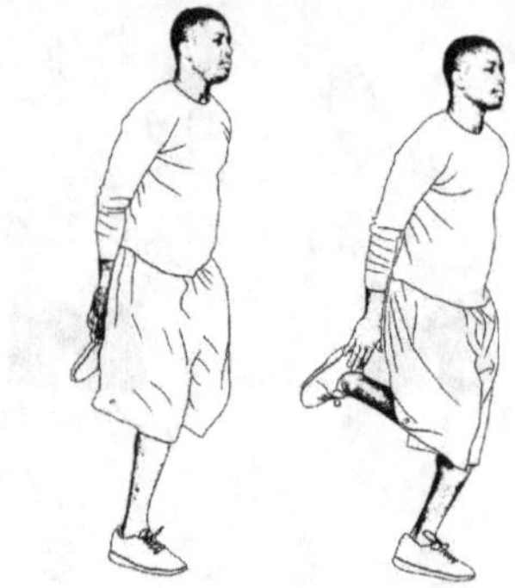

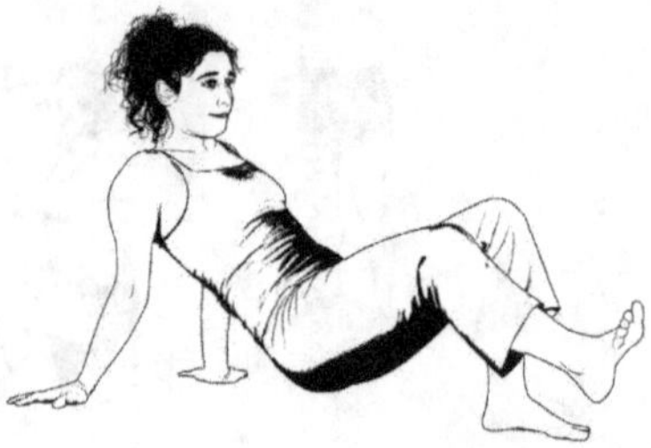

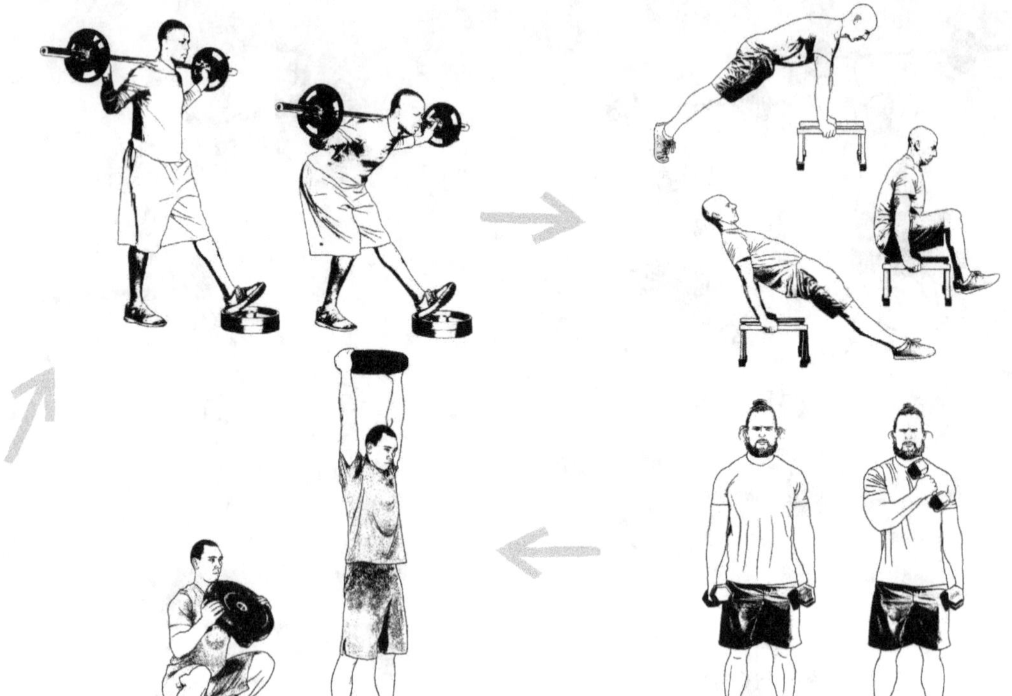

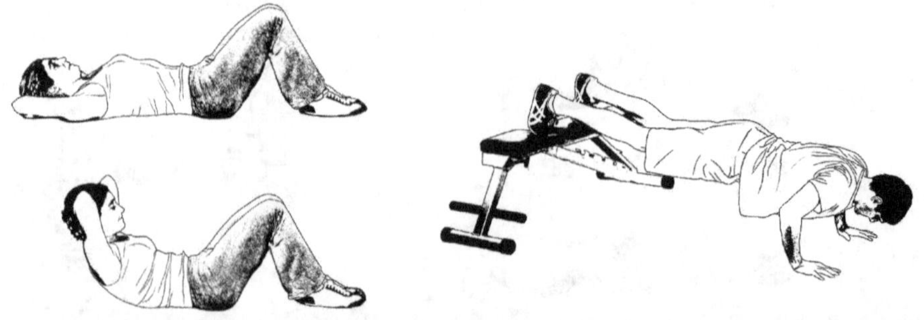

SIDE B

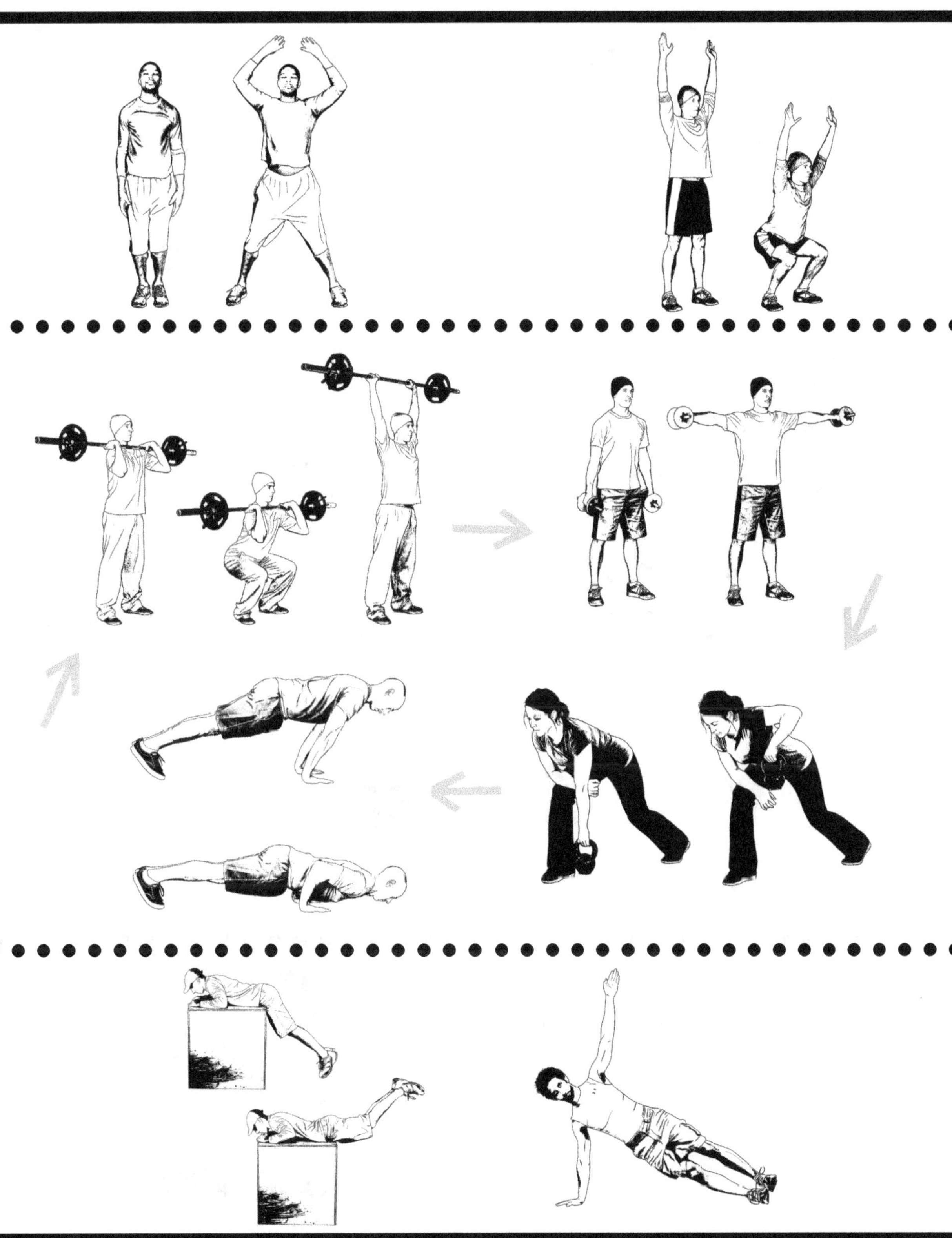

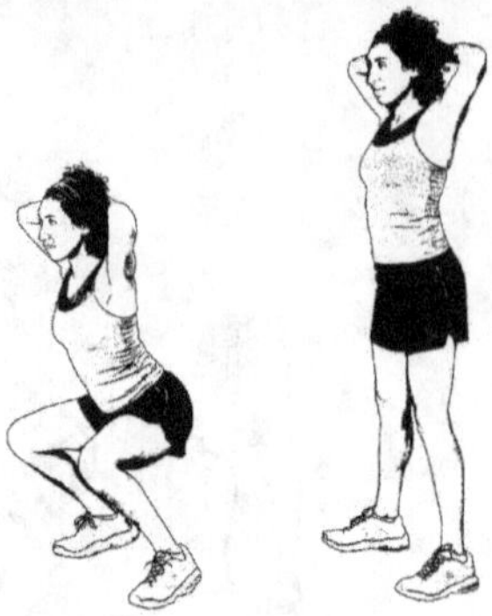

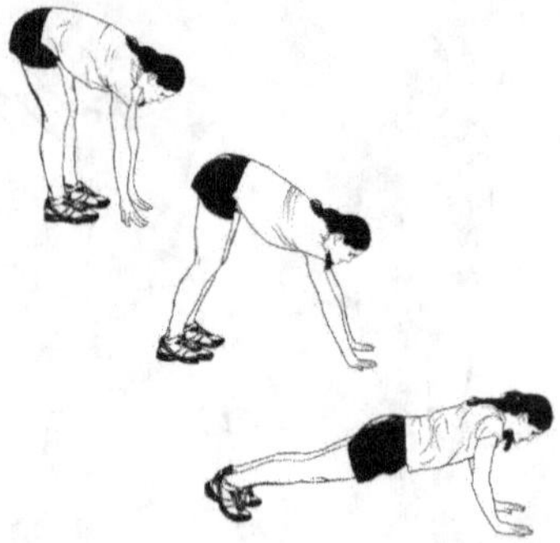

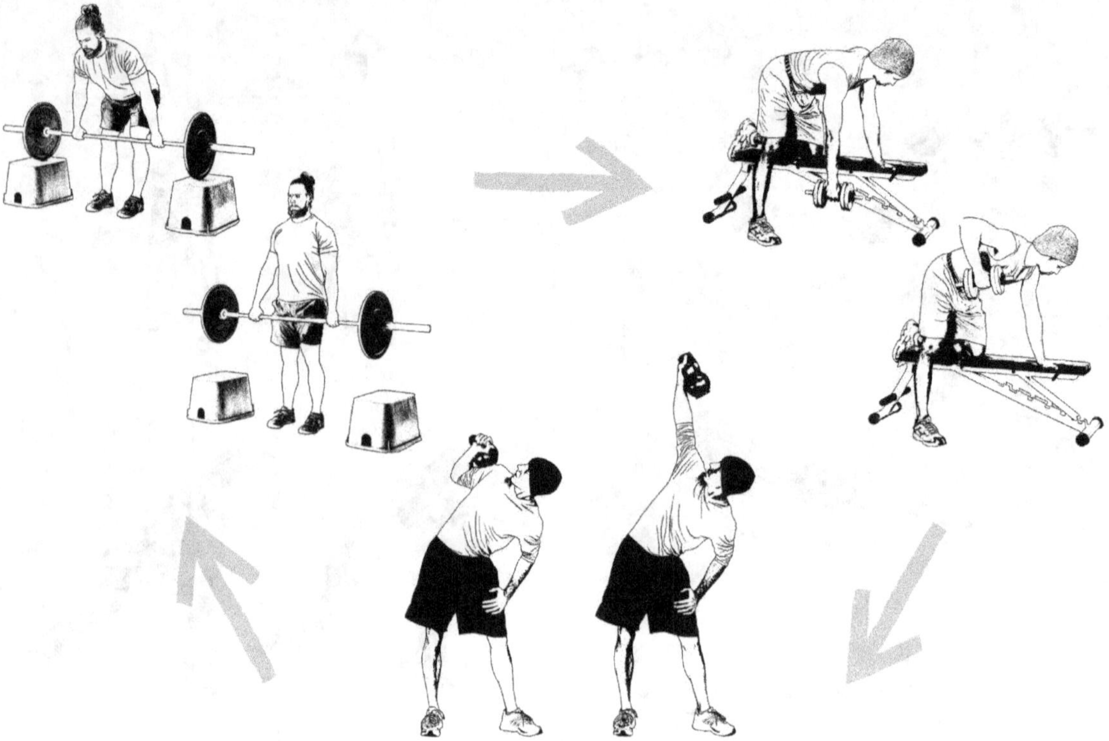

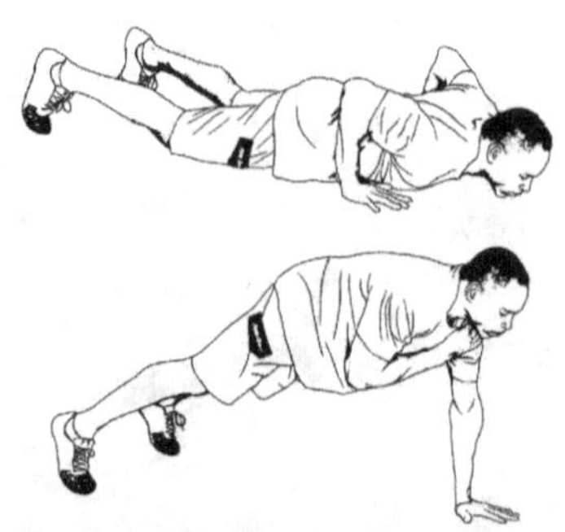
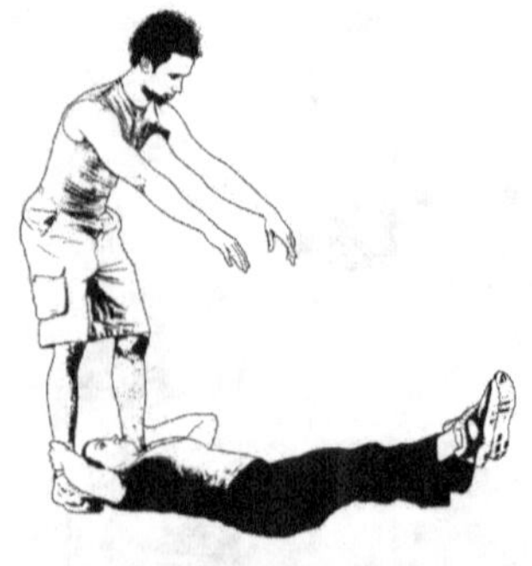

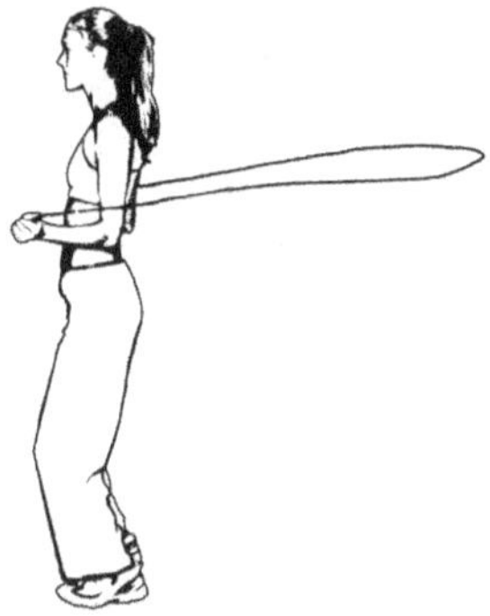

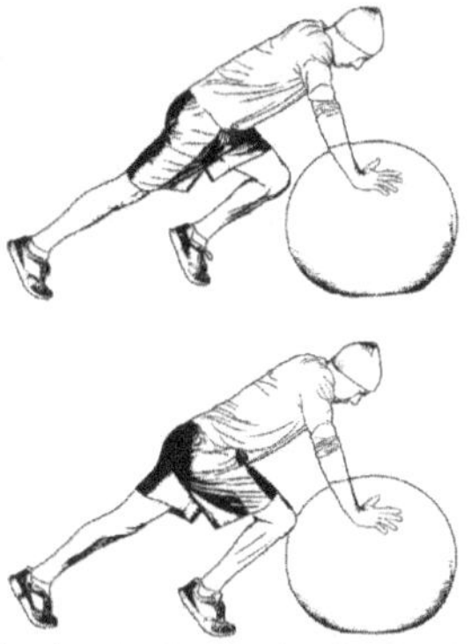

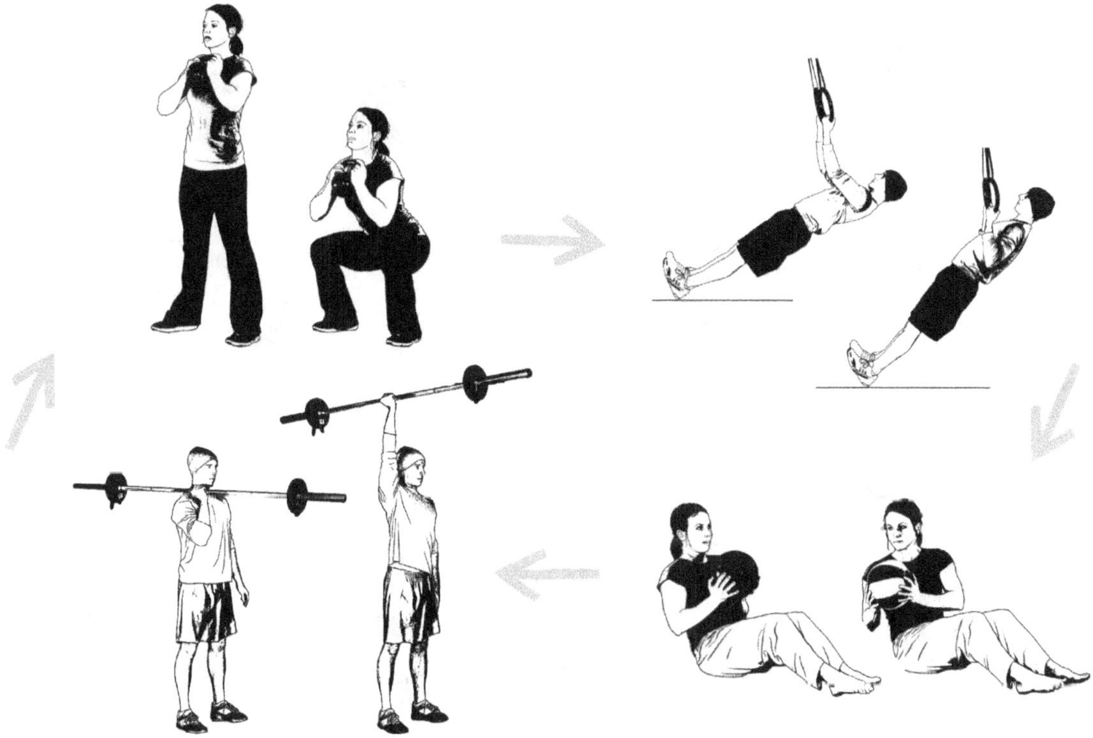

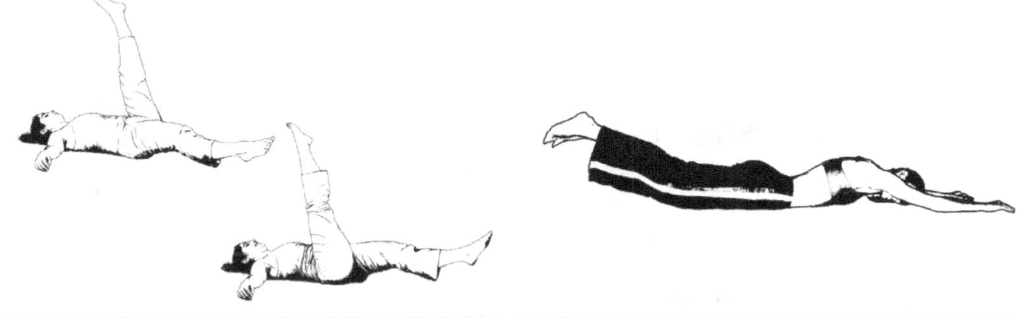

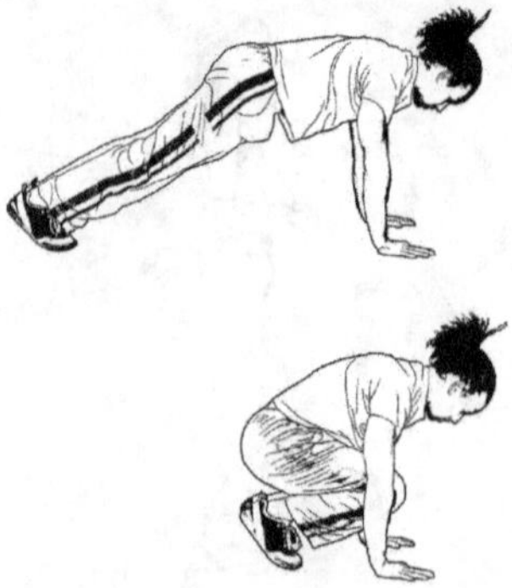

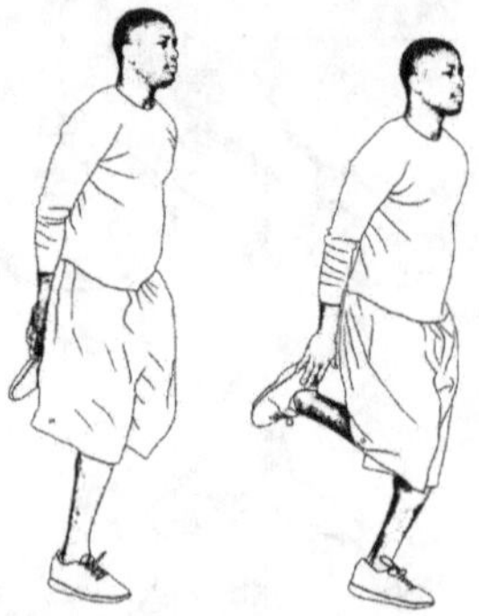

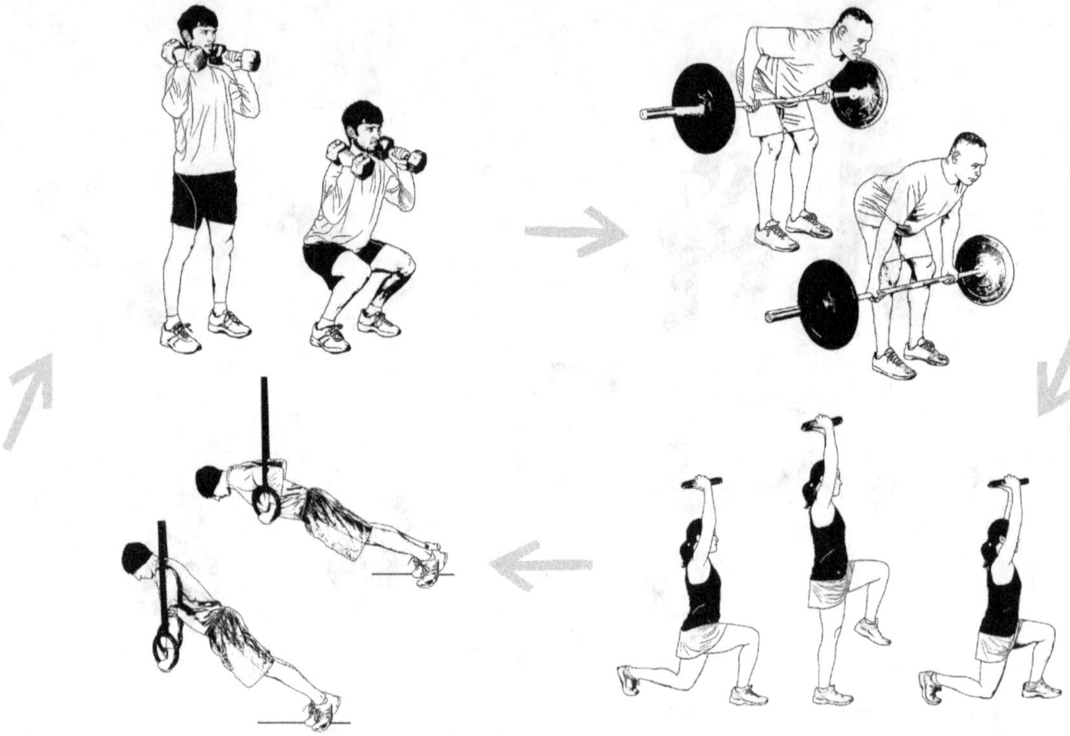

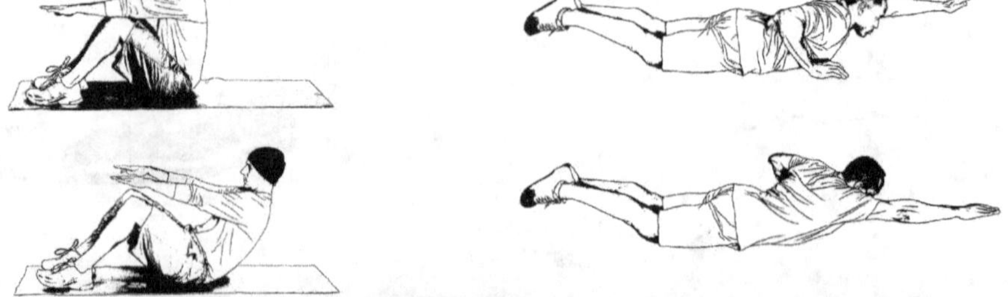

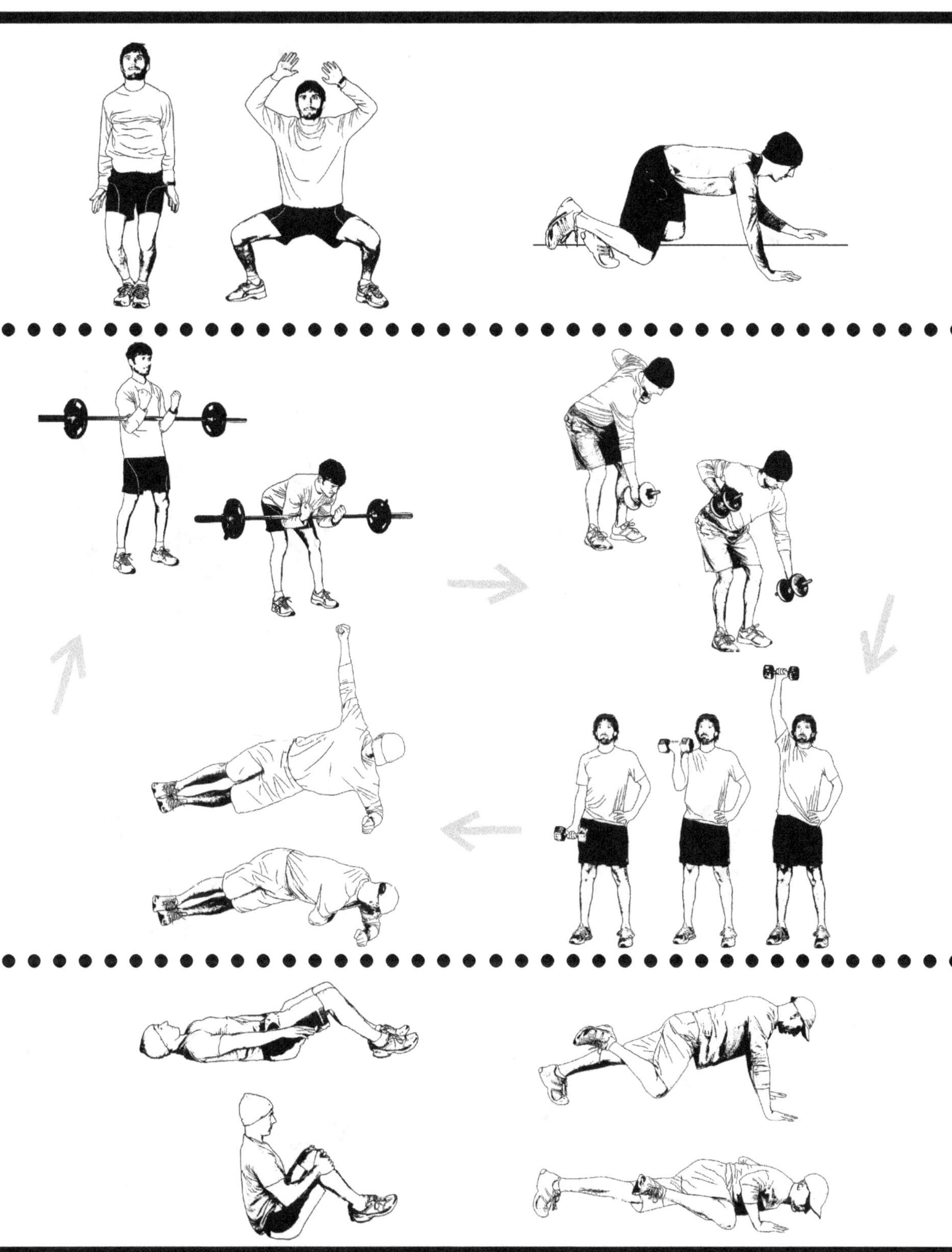

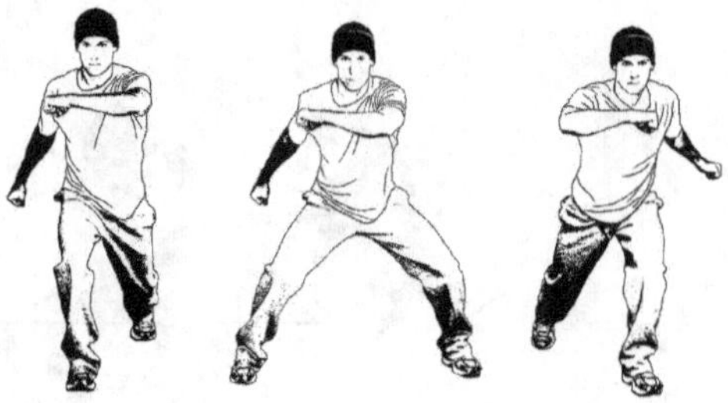

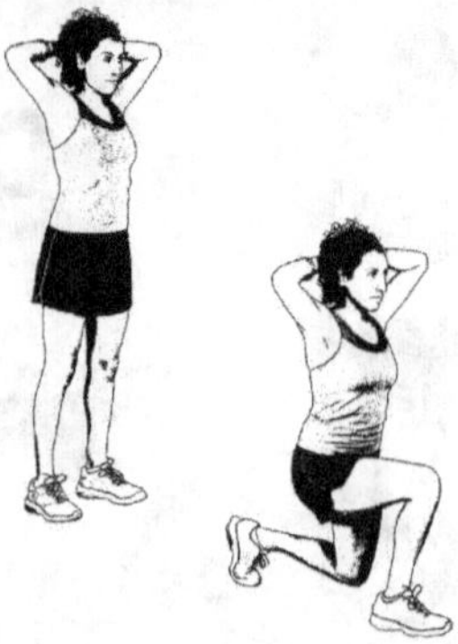

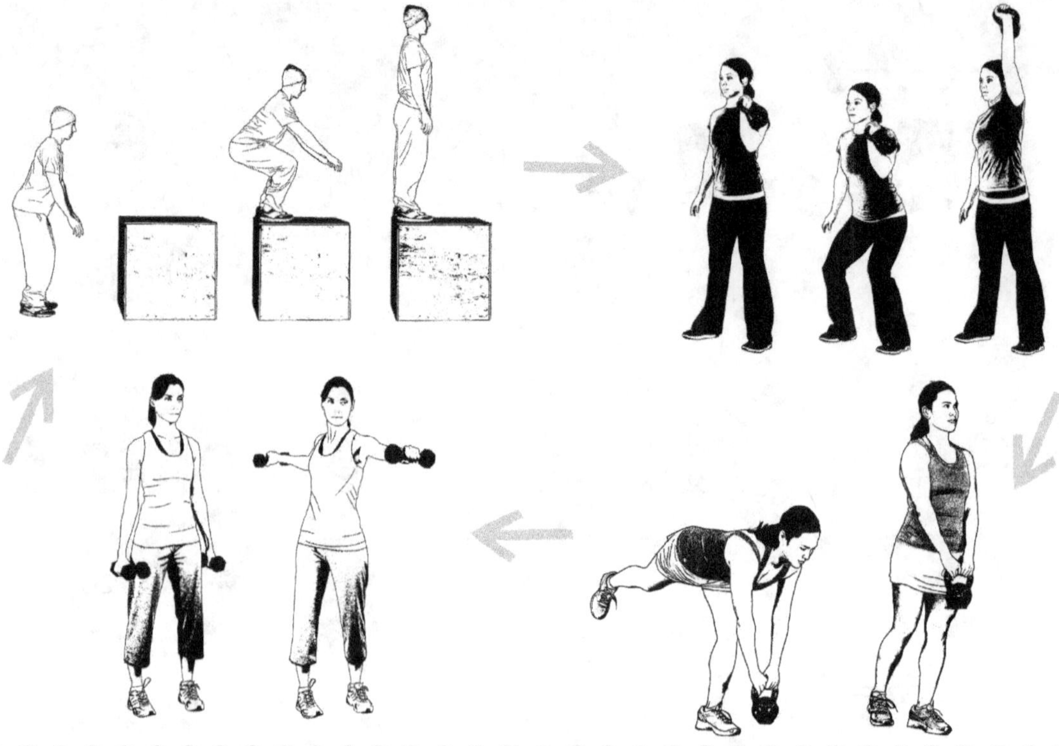

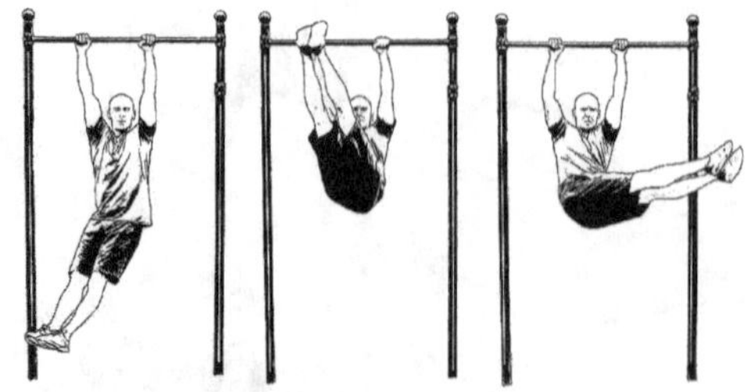

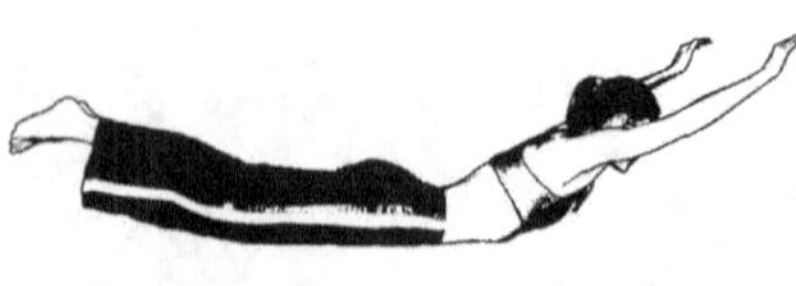

SIDE B

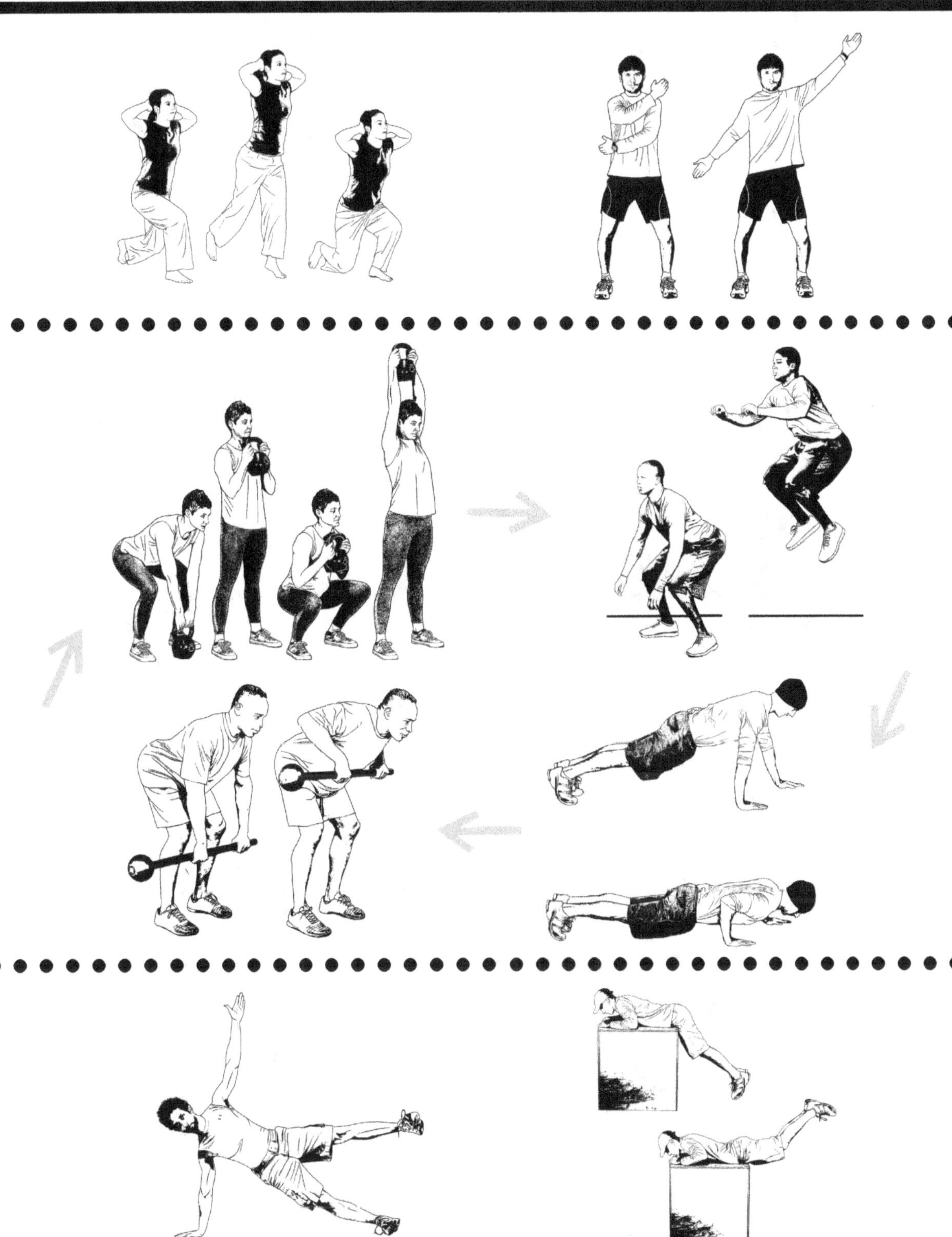

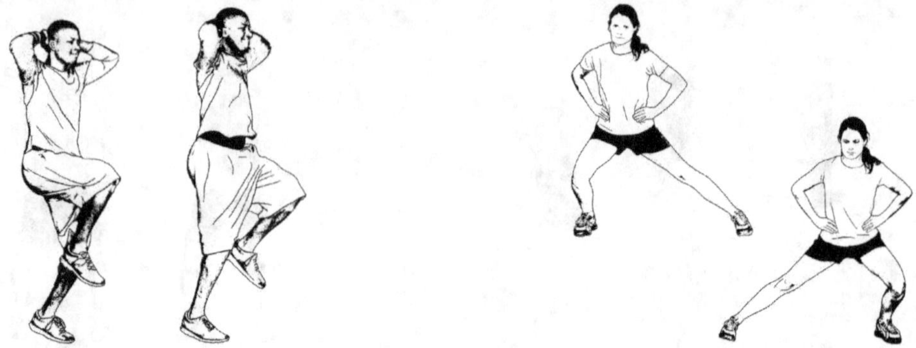

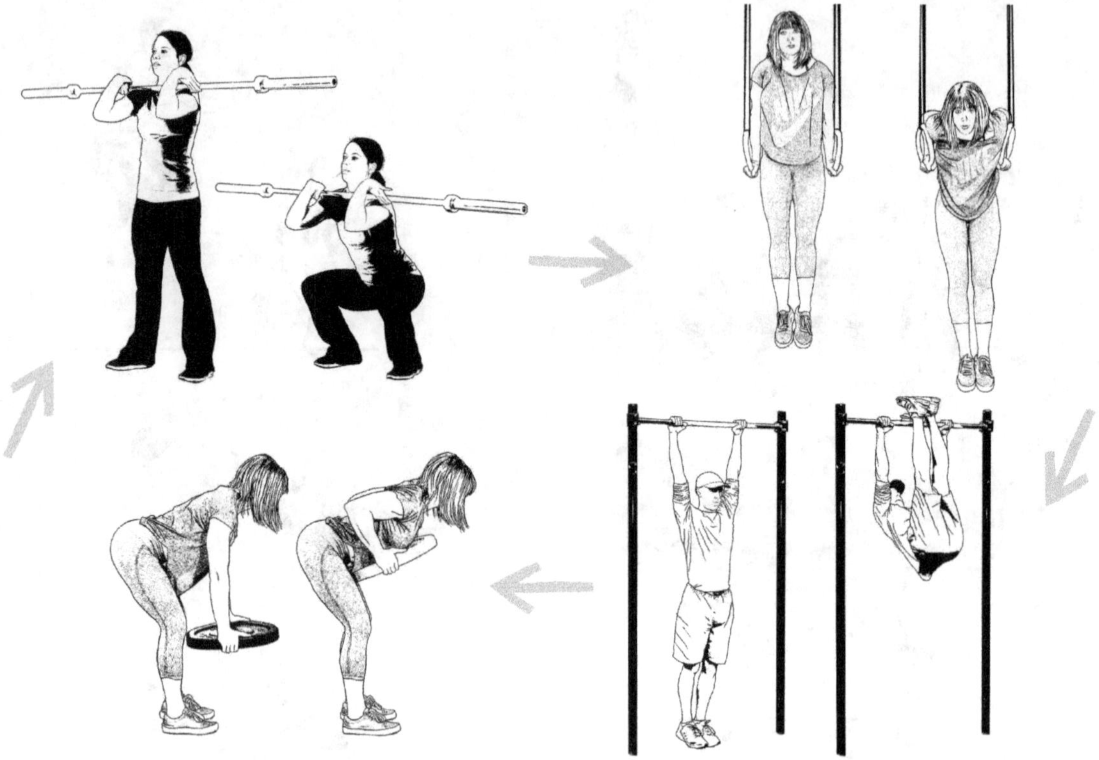

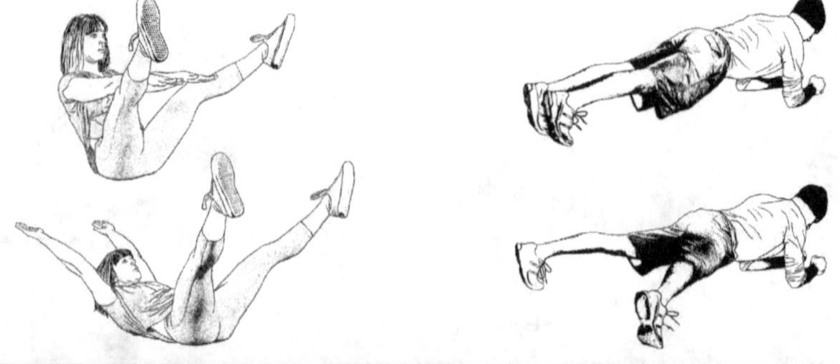

Side B

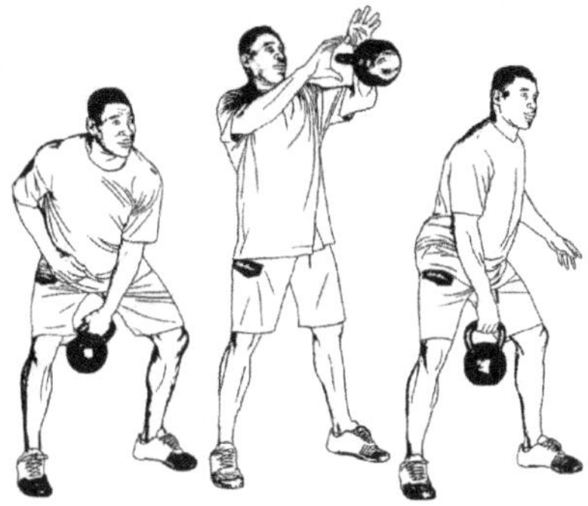

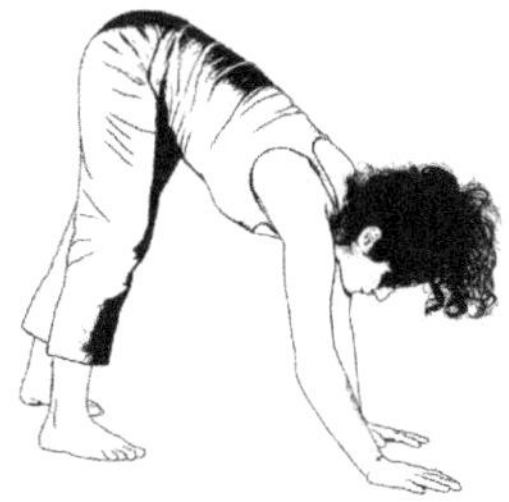

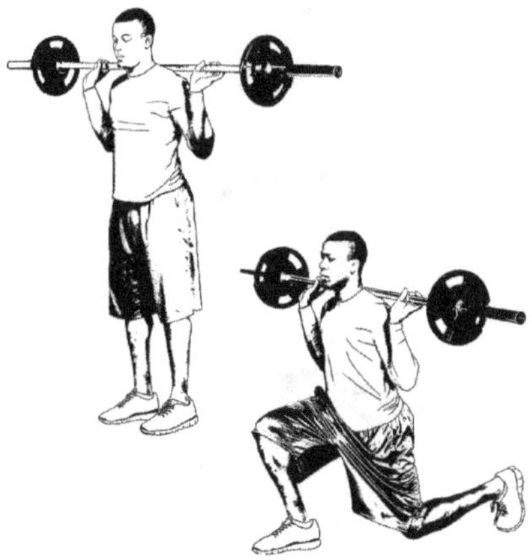

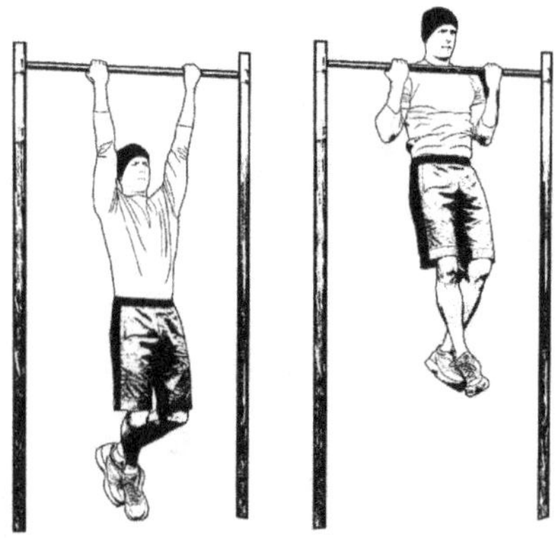

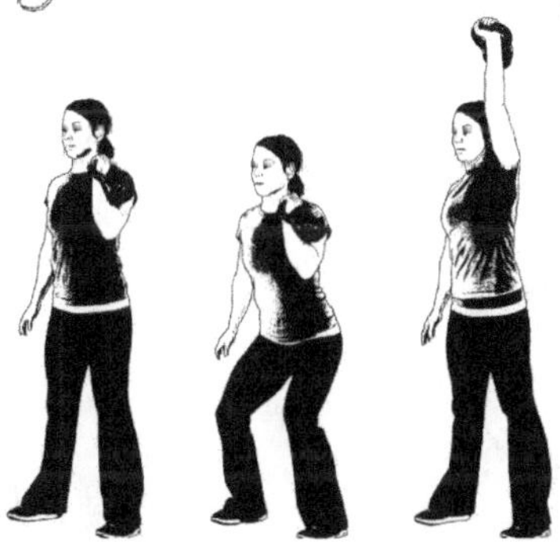

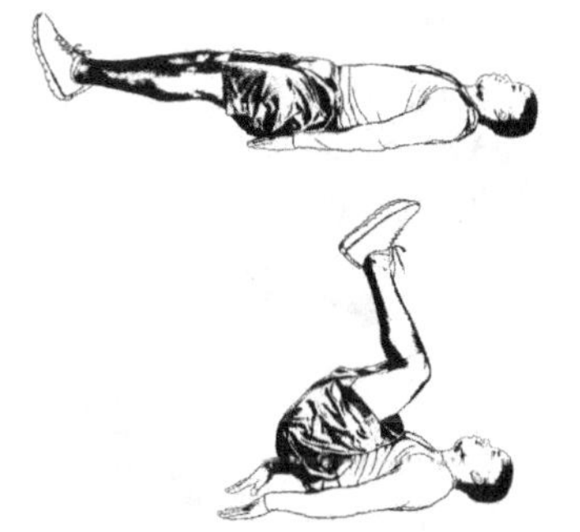

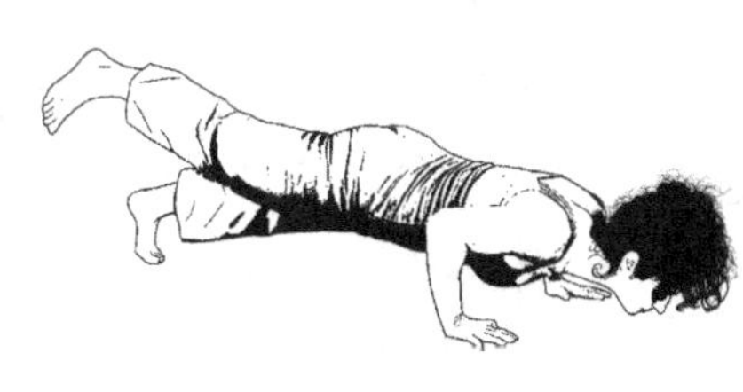

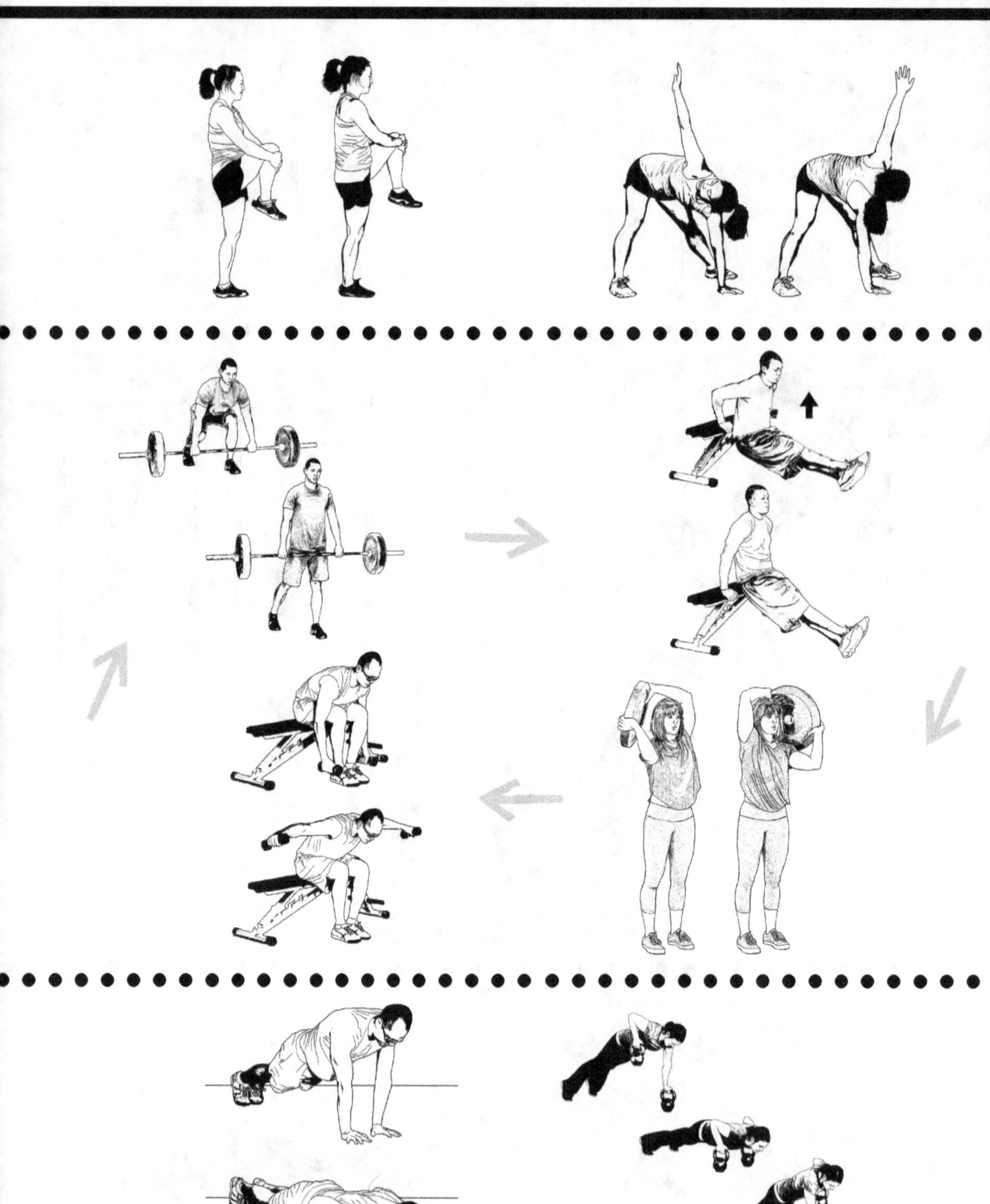

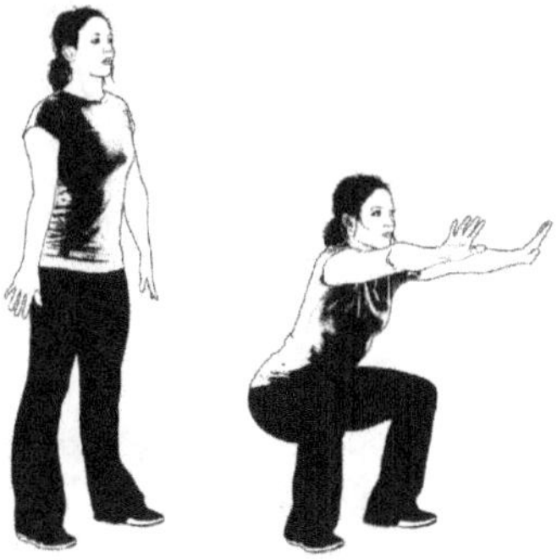

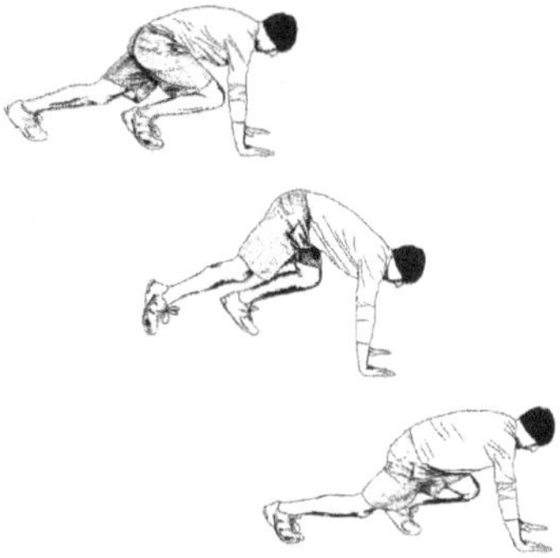

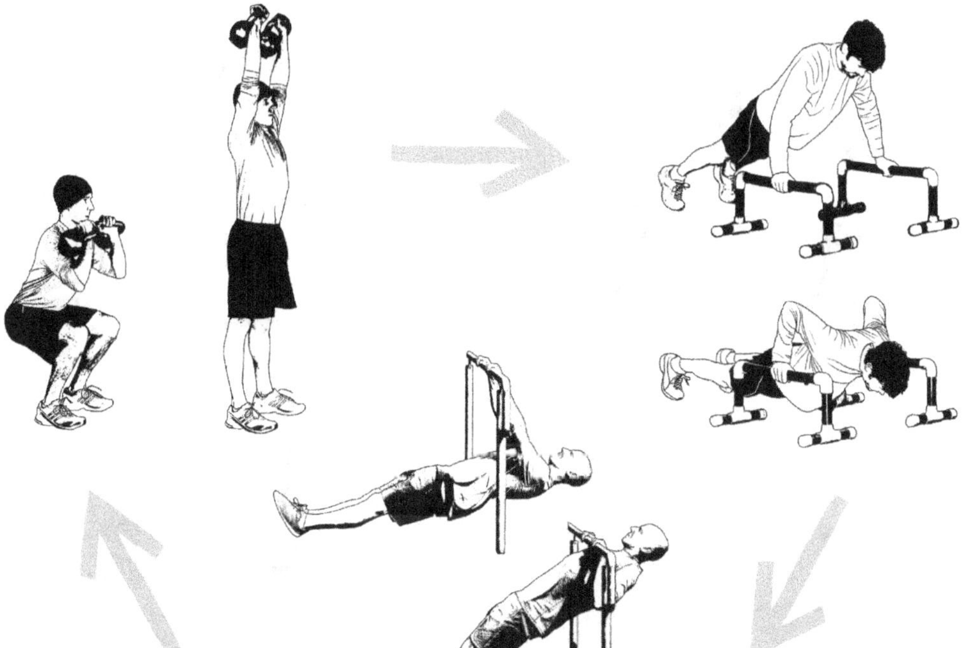

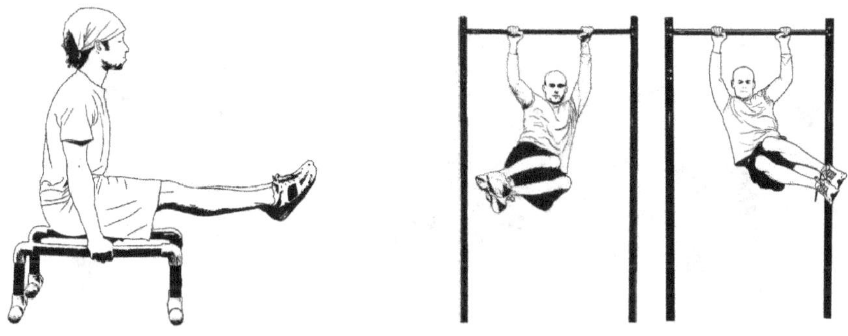

Side B

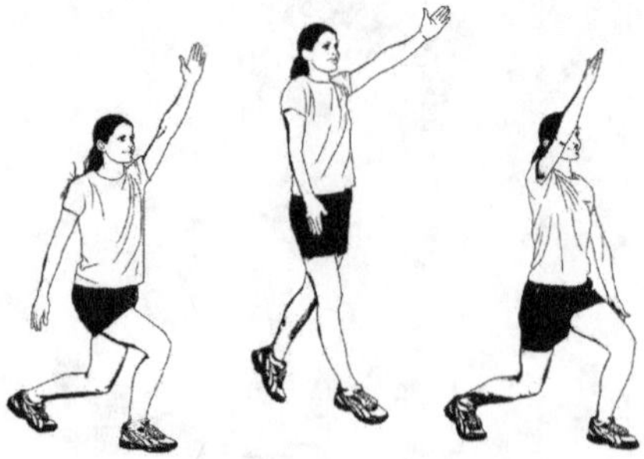

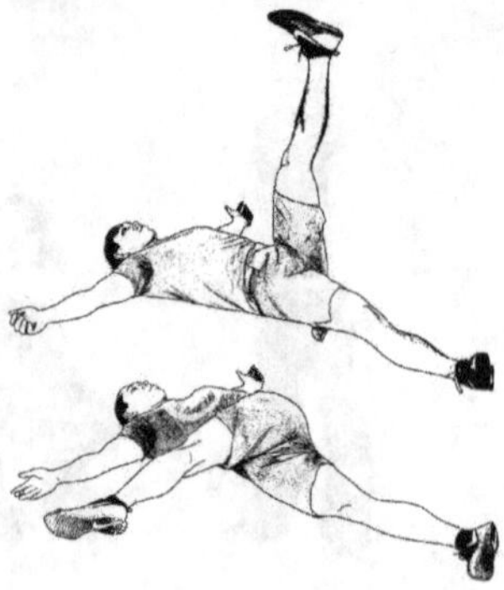

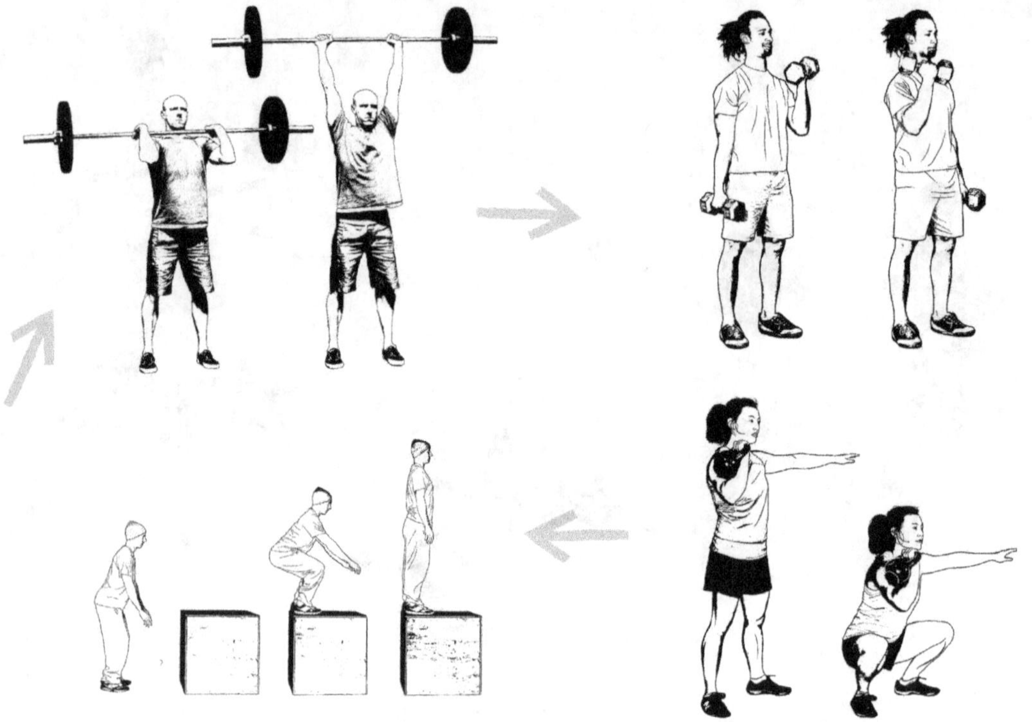

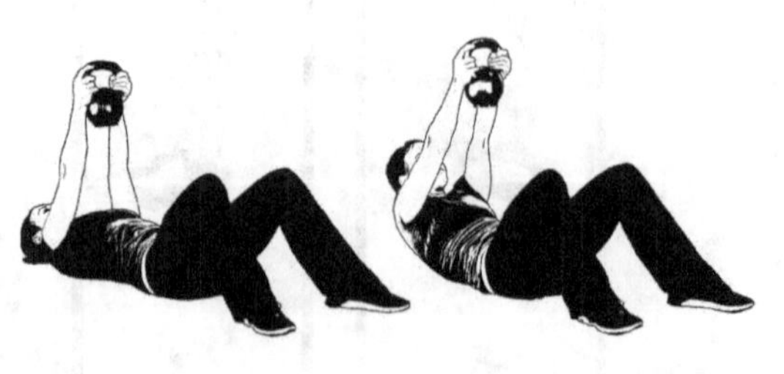

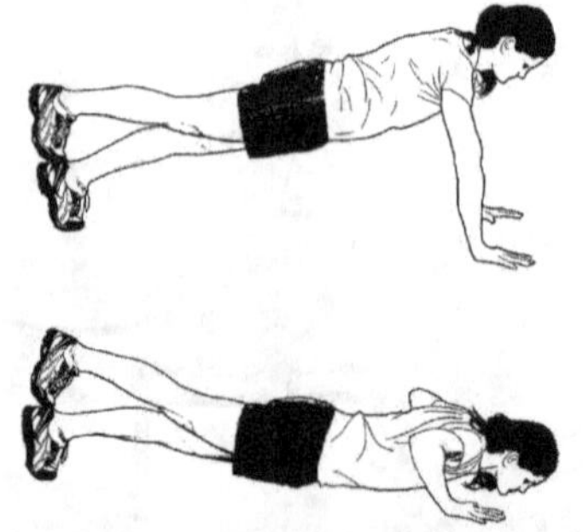

Side B

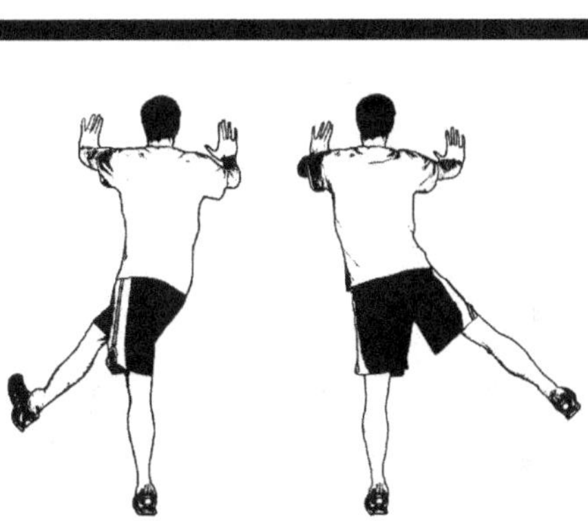

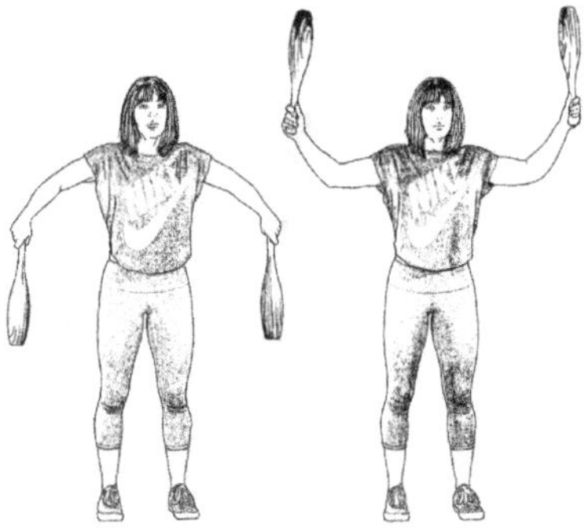

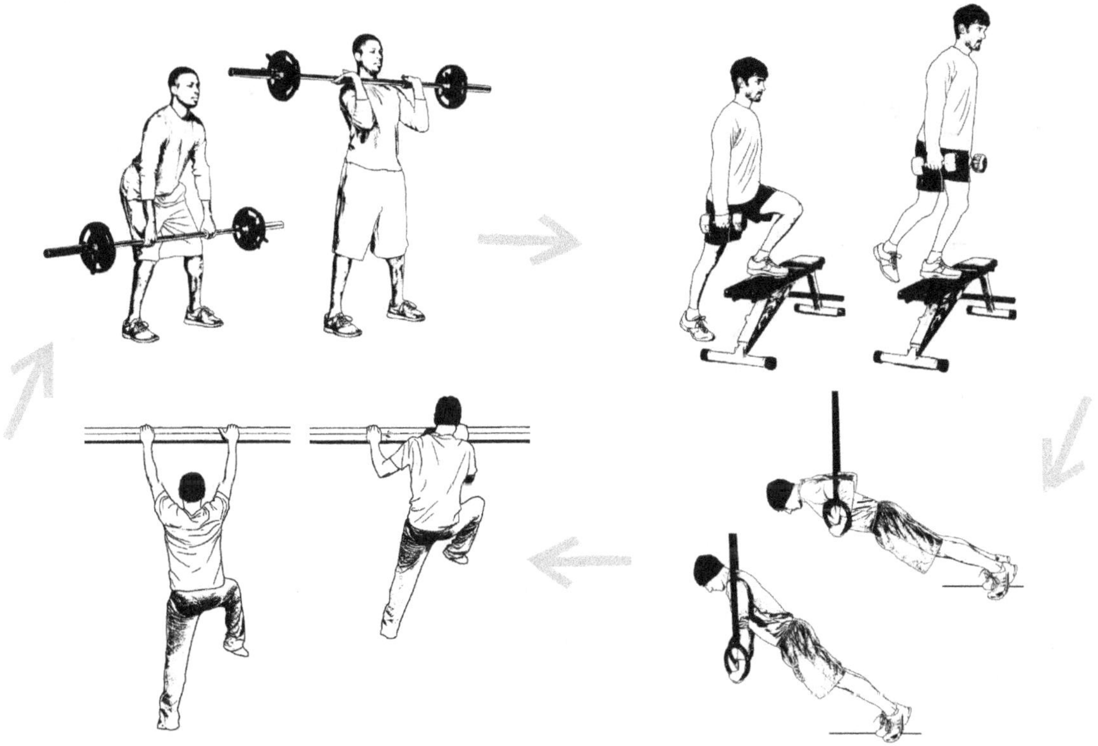

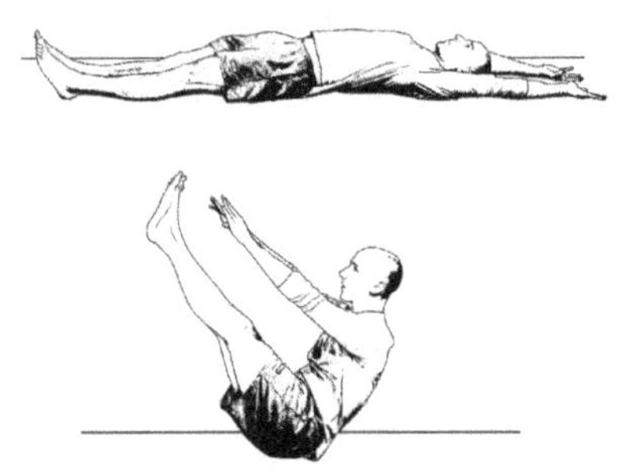

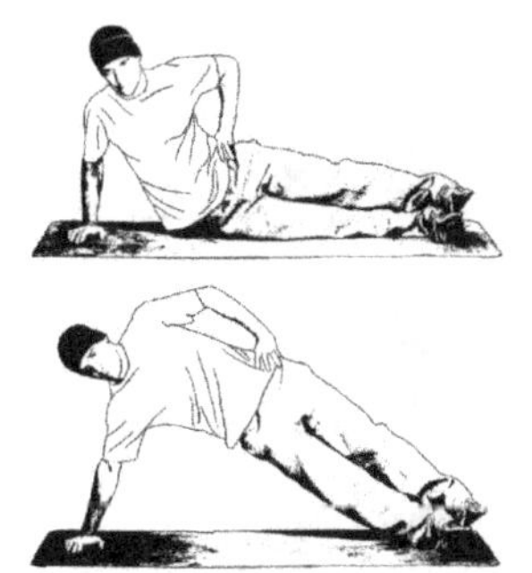

SIDE B

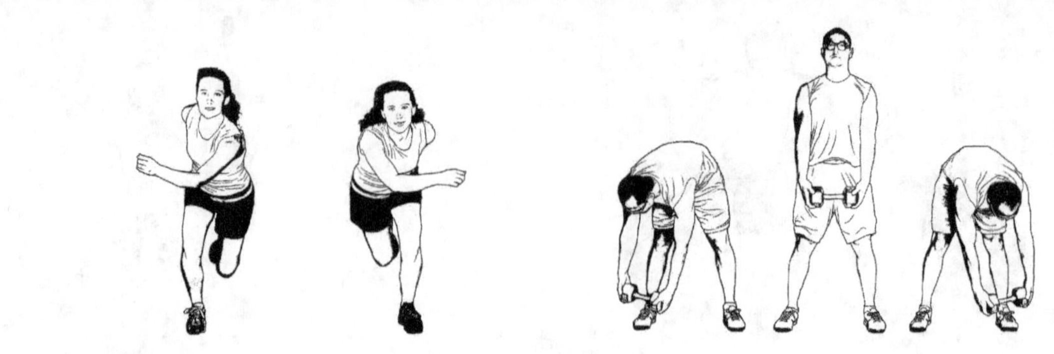

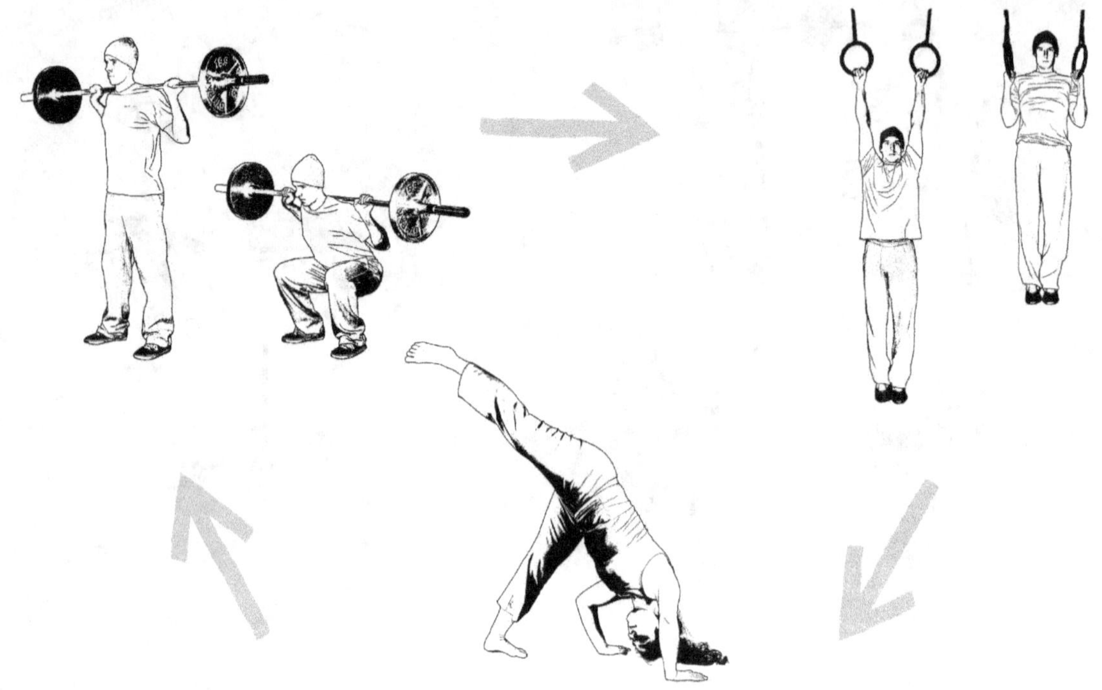

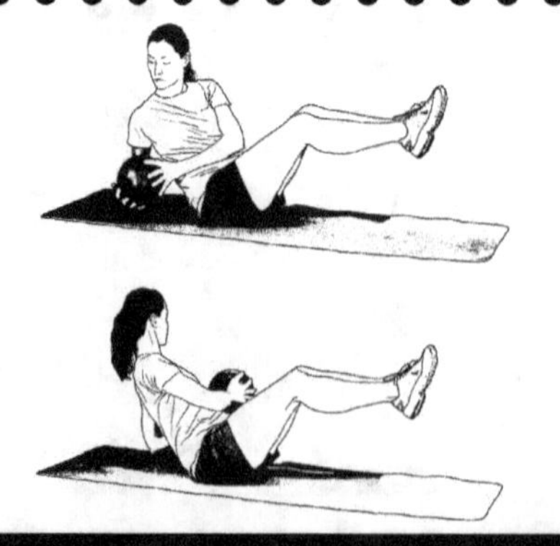

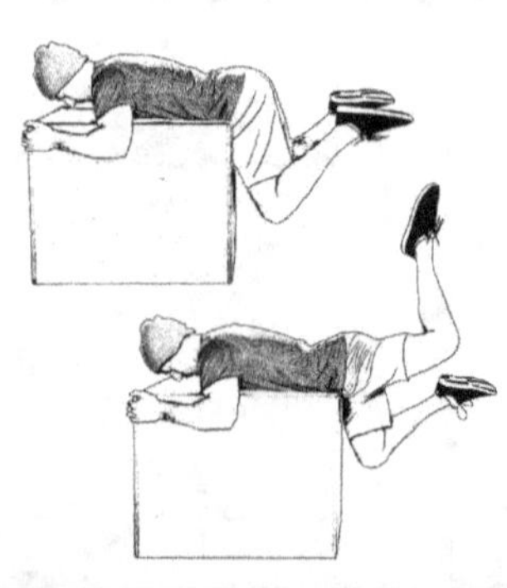

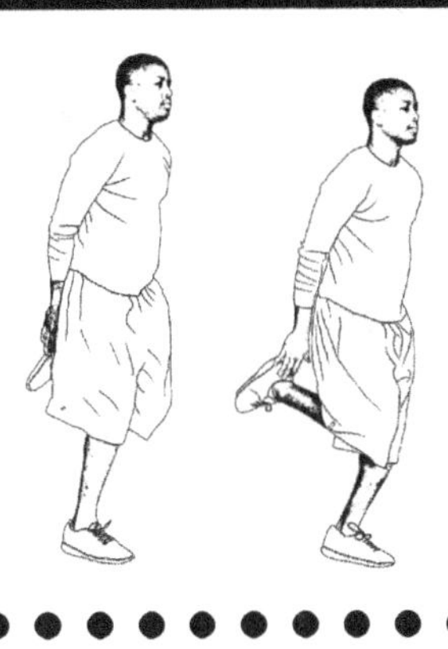
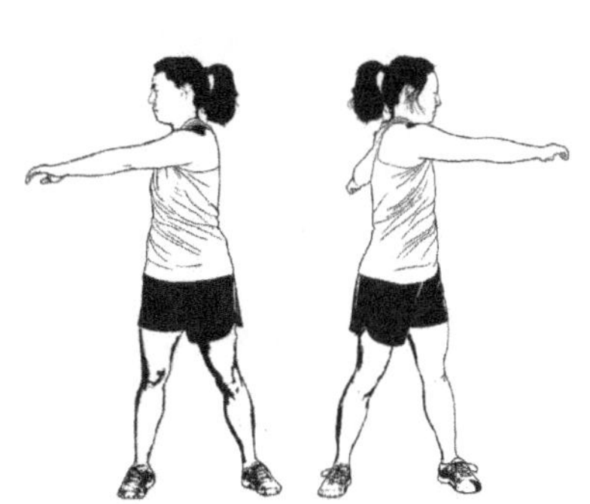
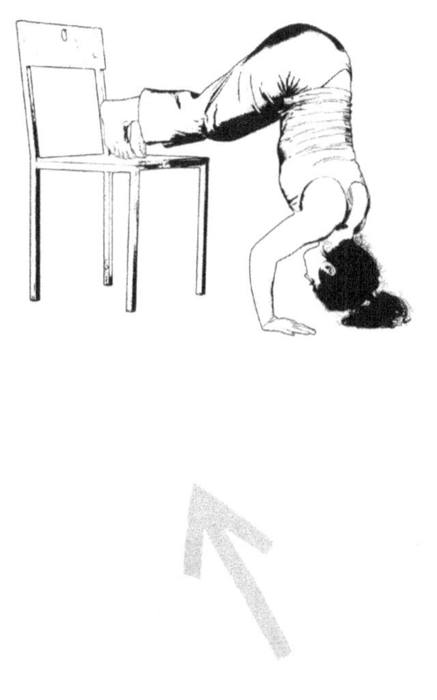
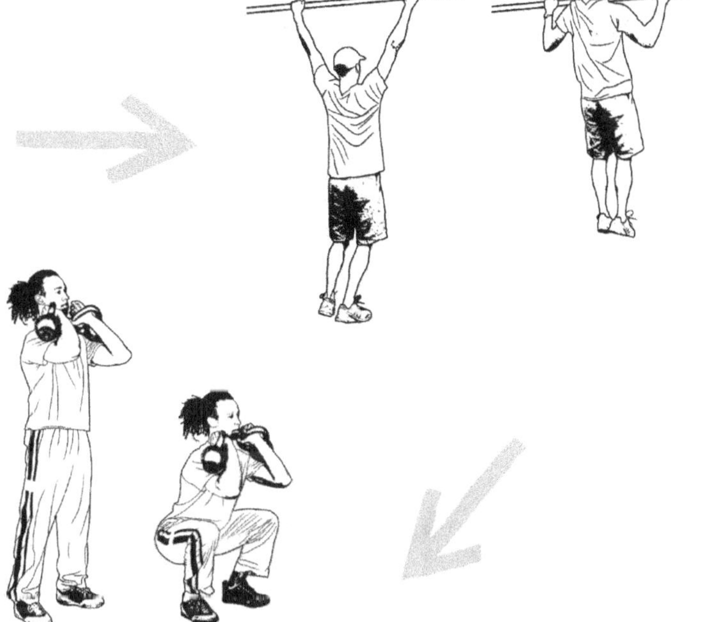
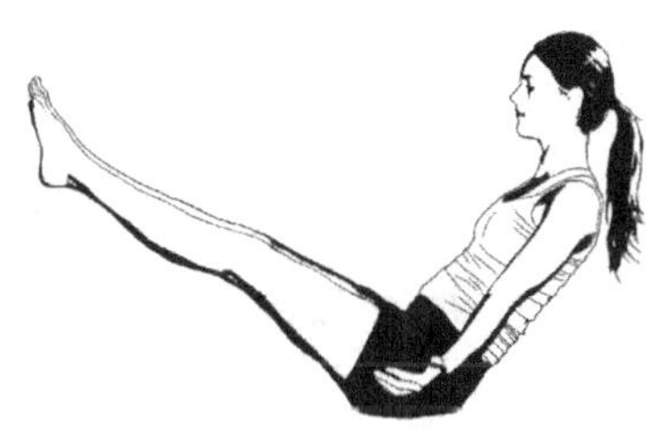
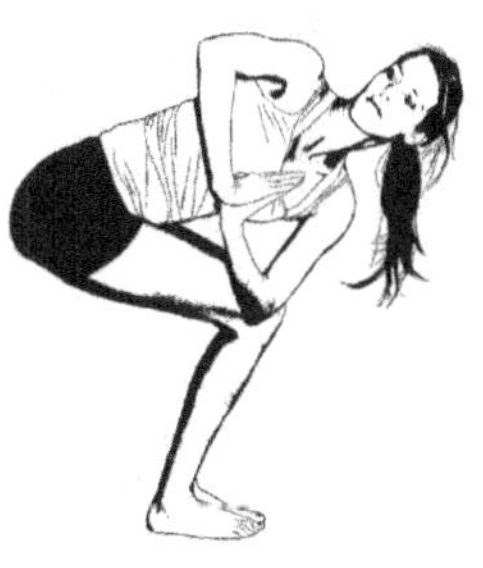

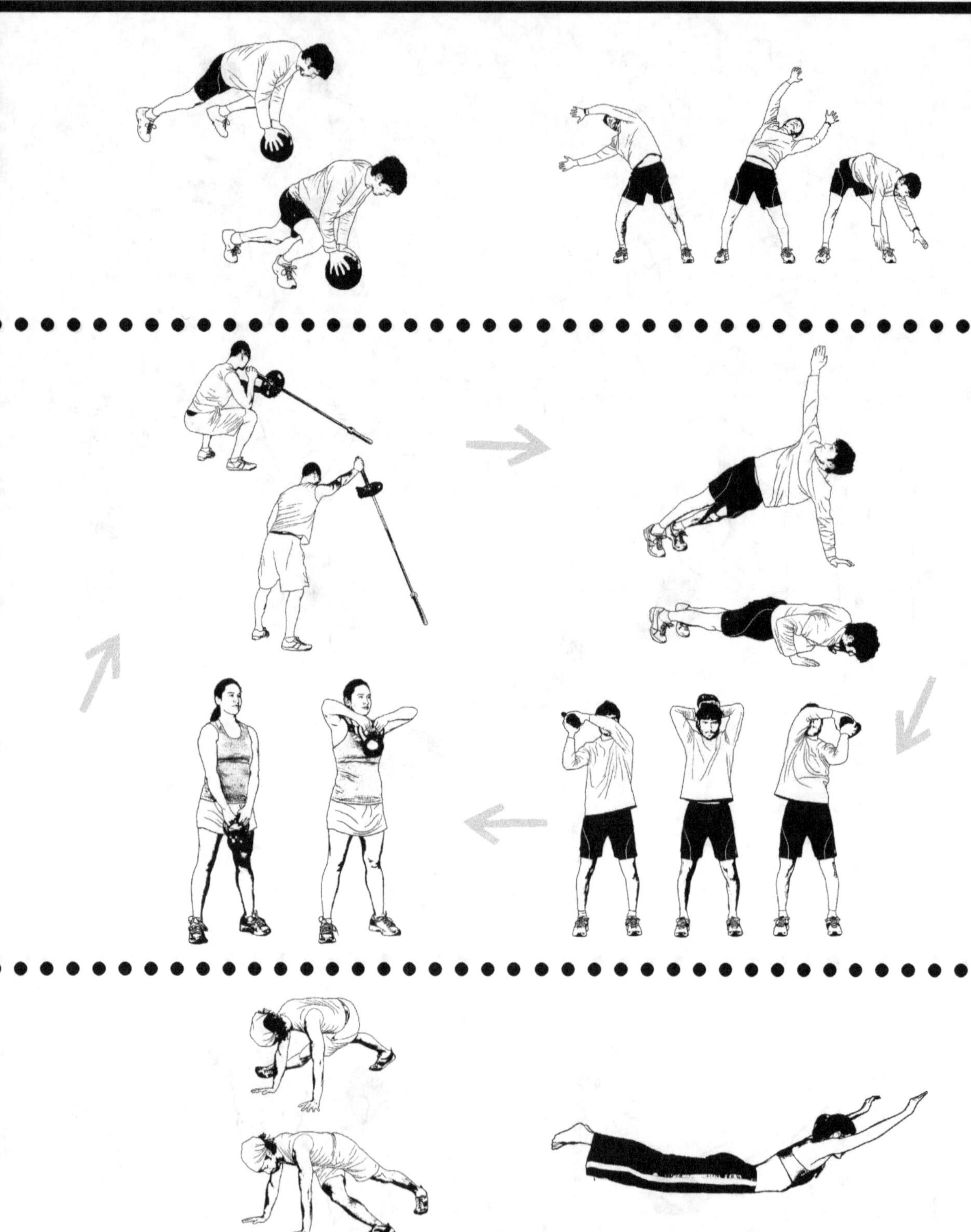

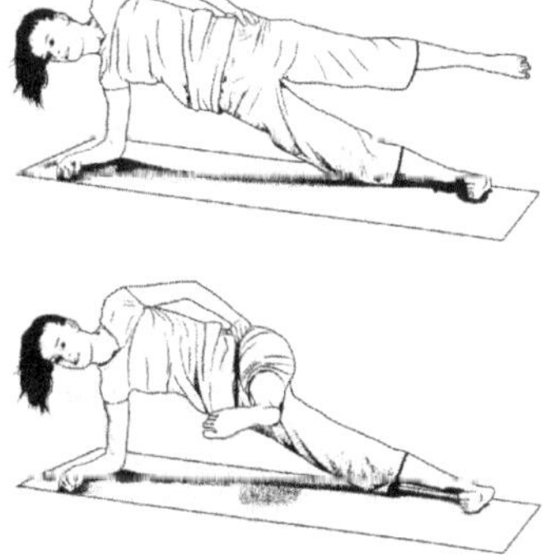

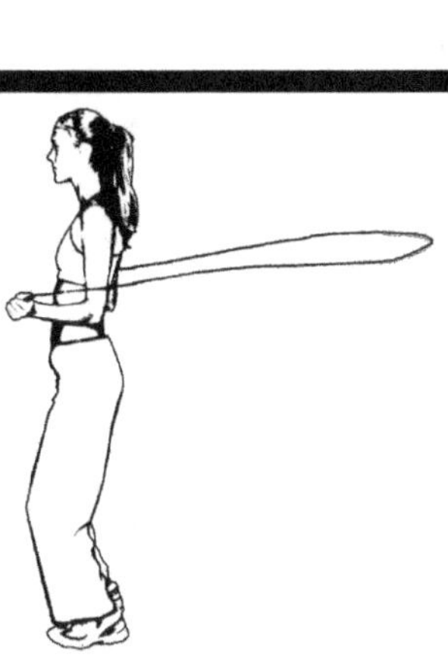

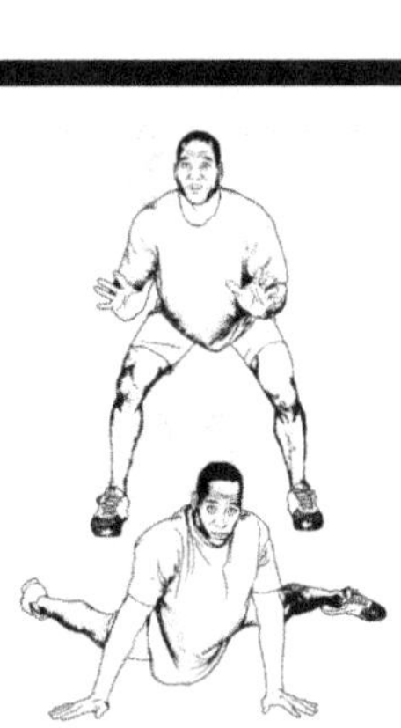

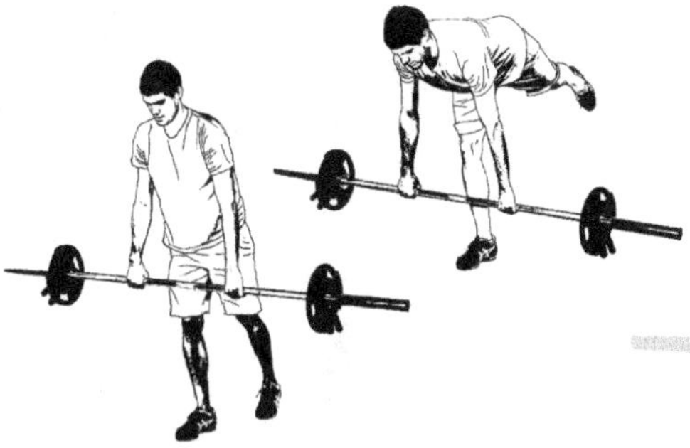

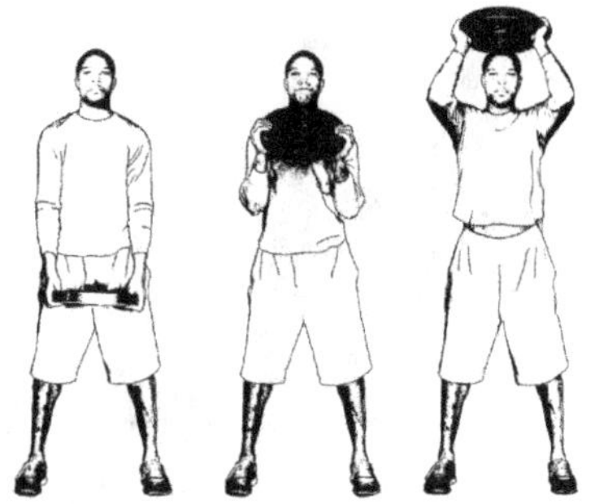

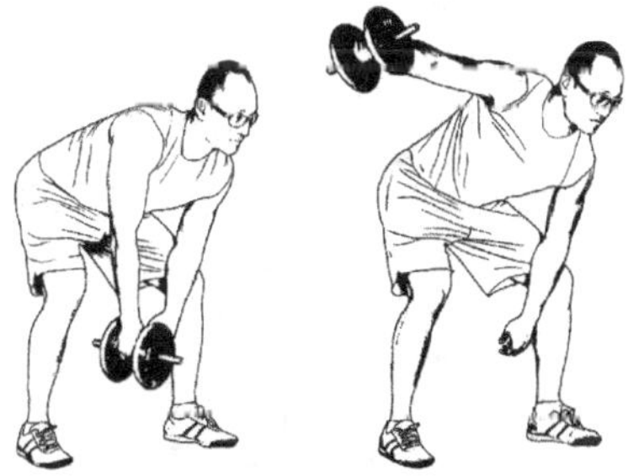

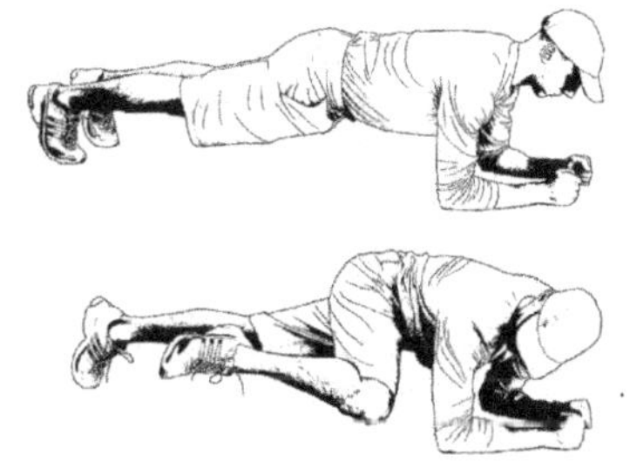
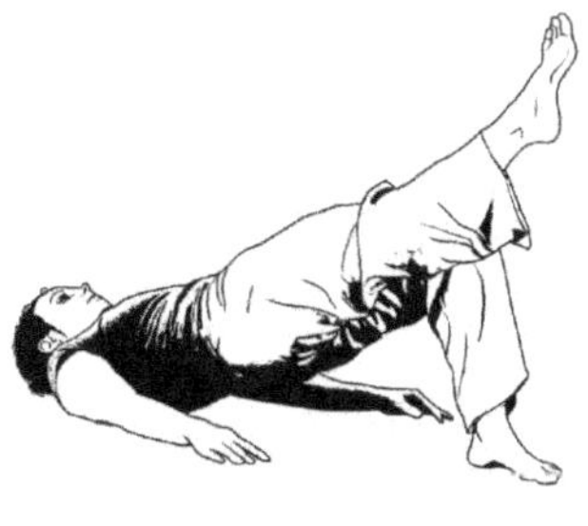

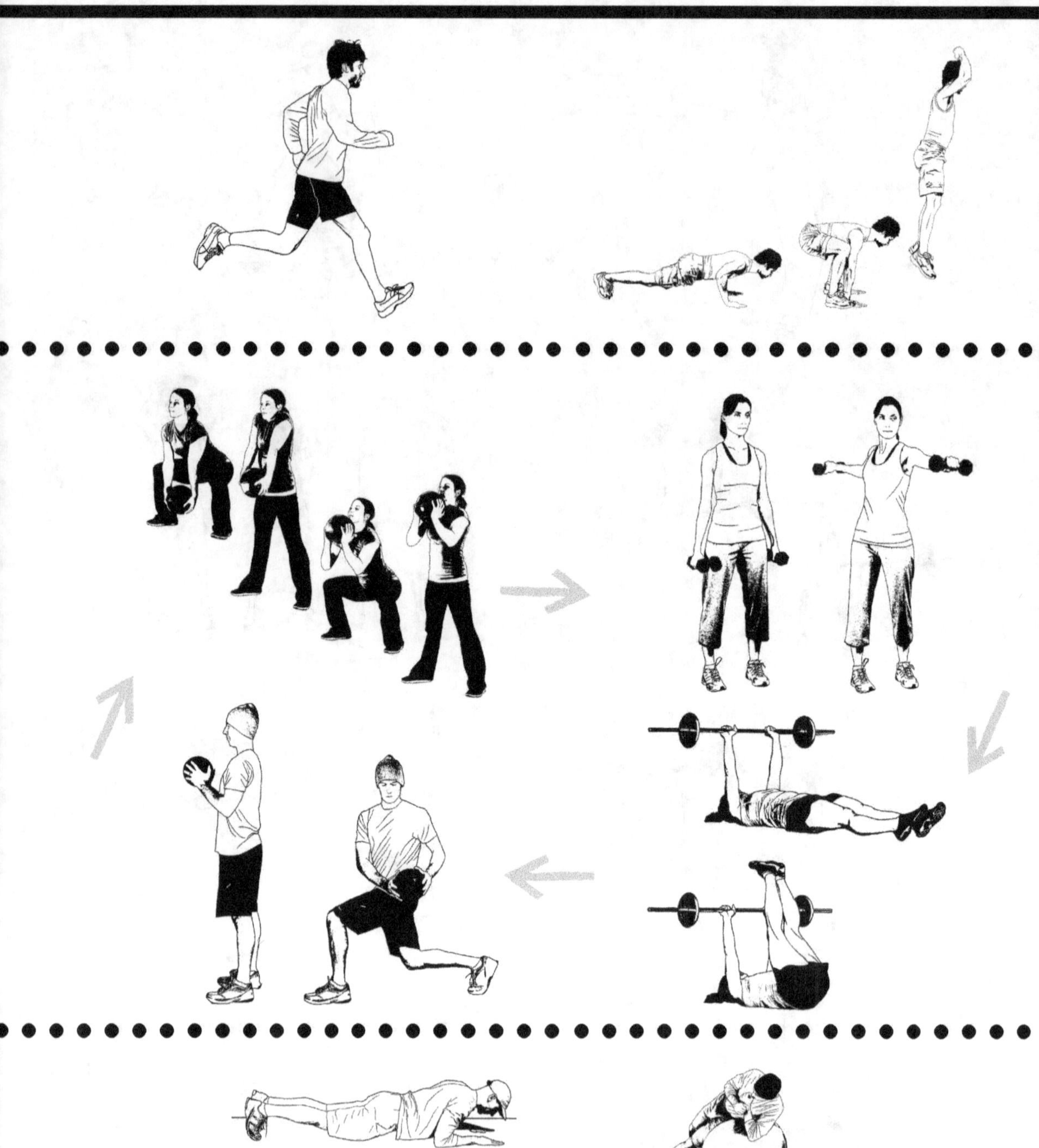

SIDE B

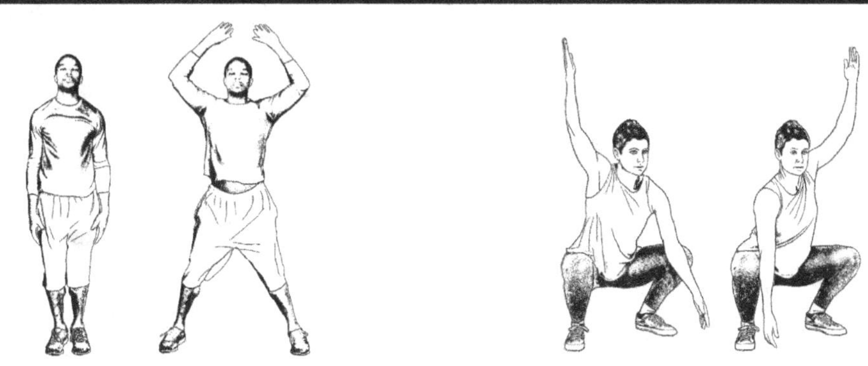

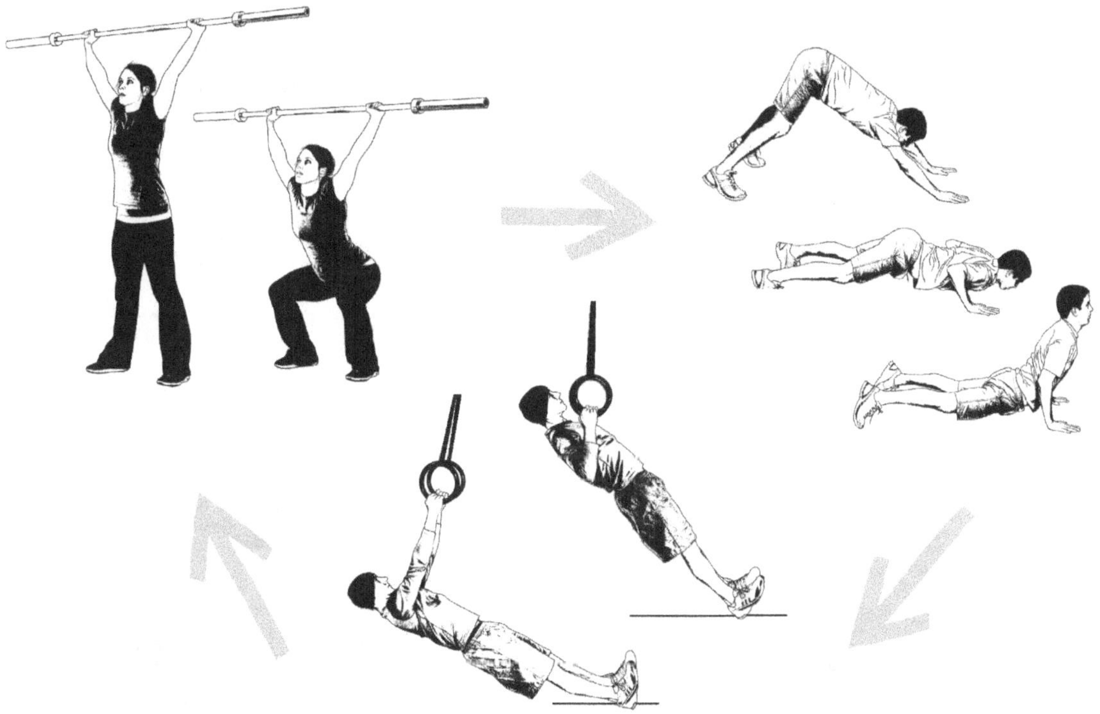

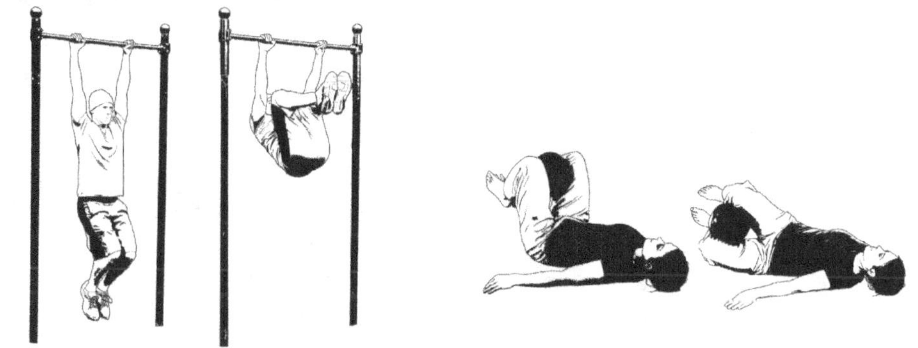

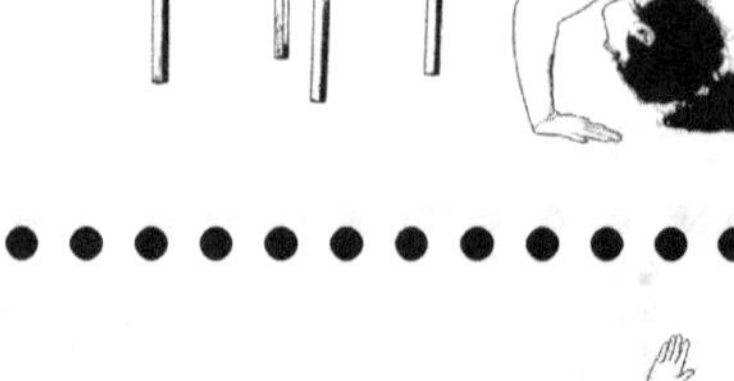

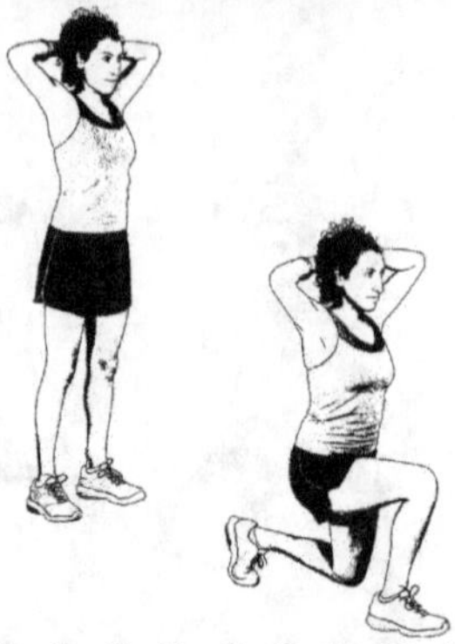

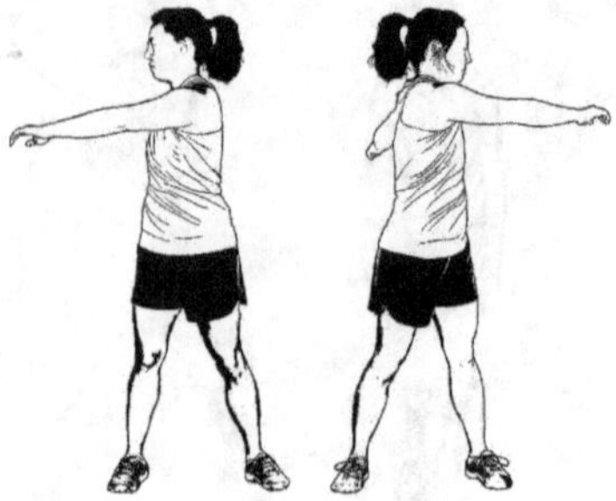

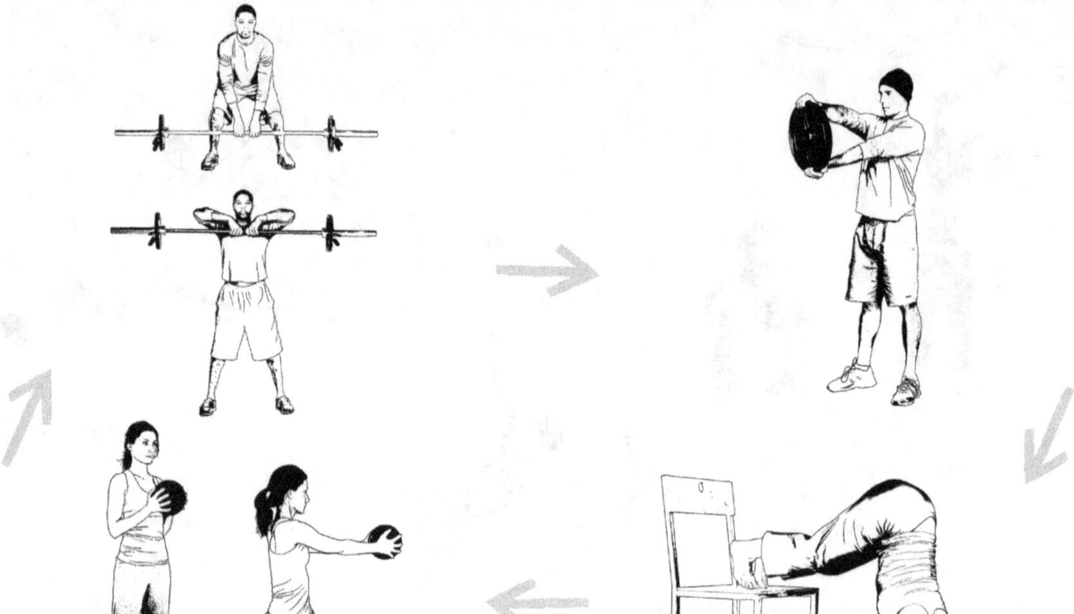

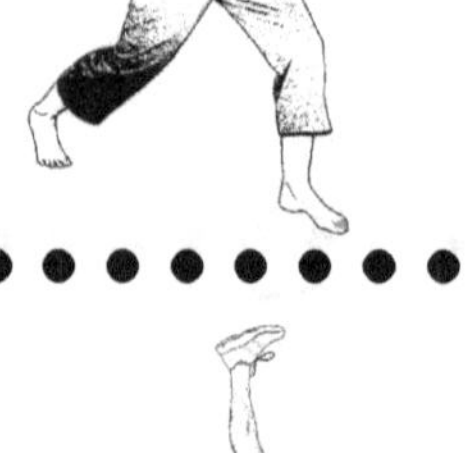

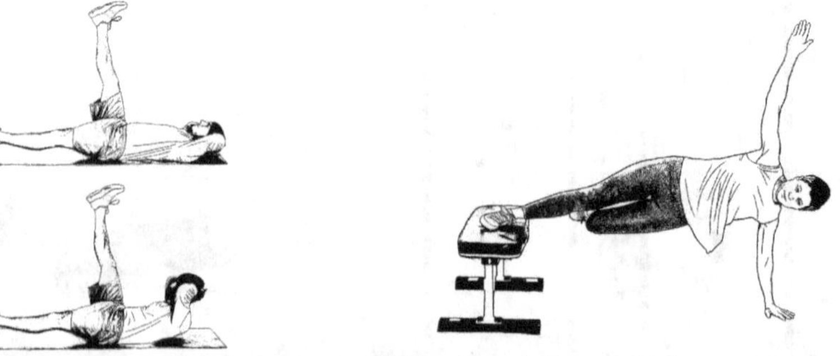

SIDE B

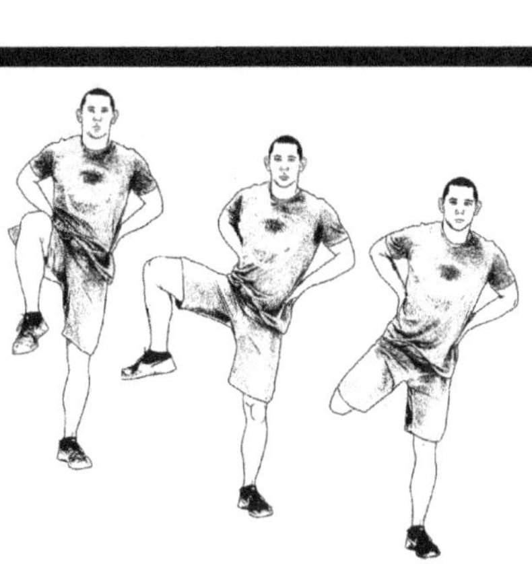

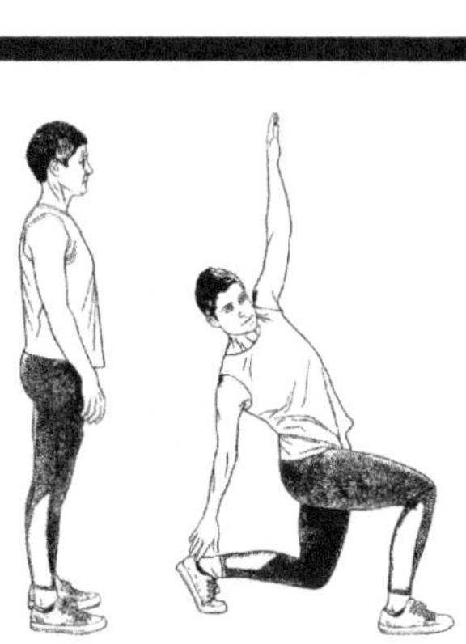

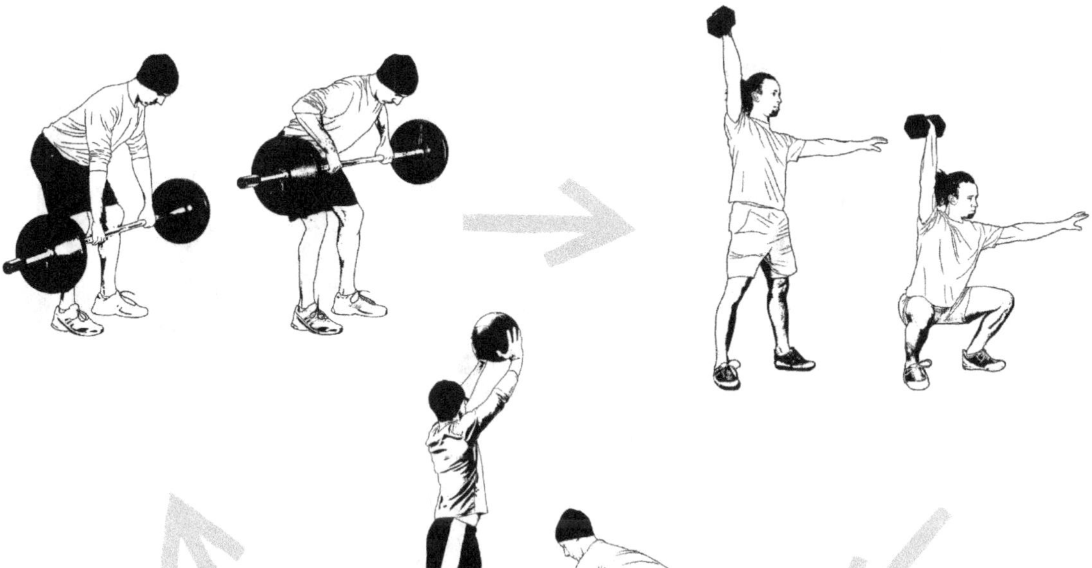

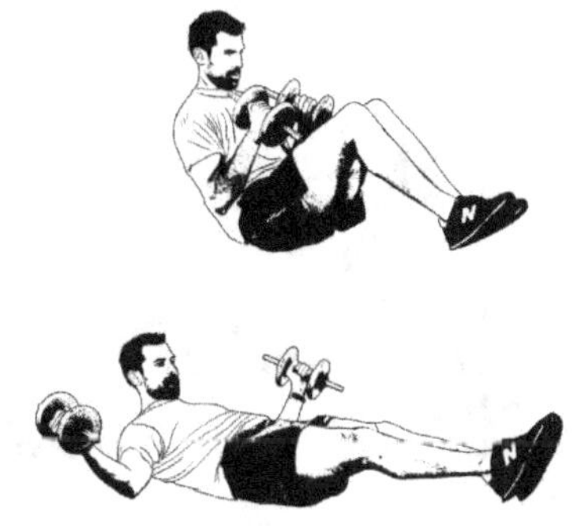

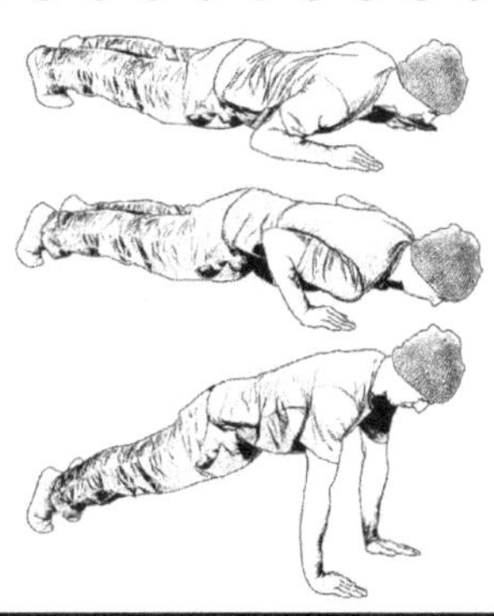

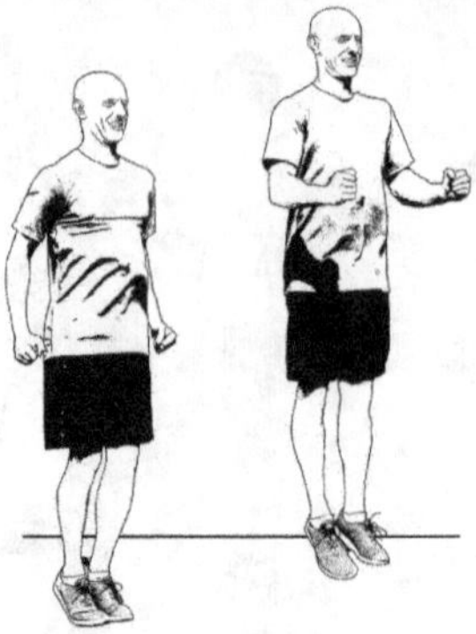

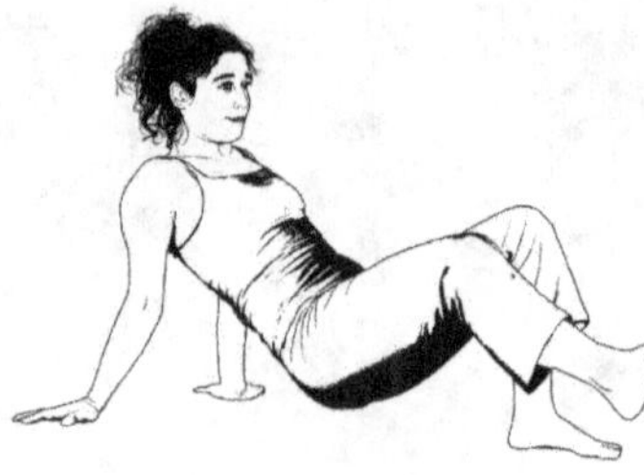

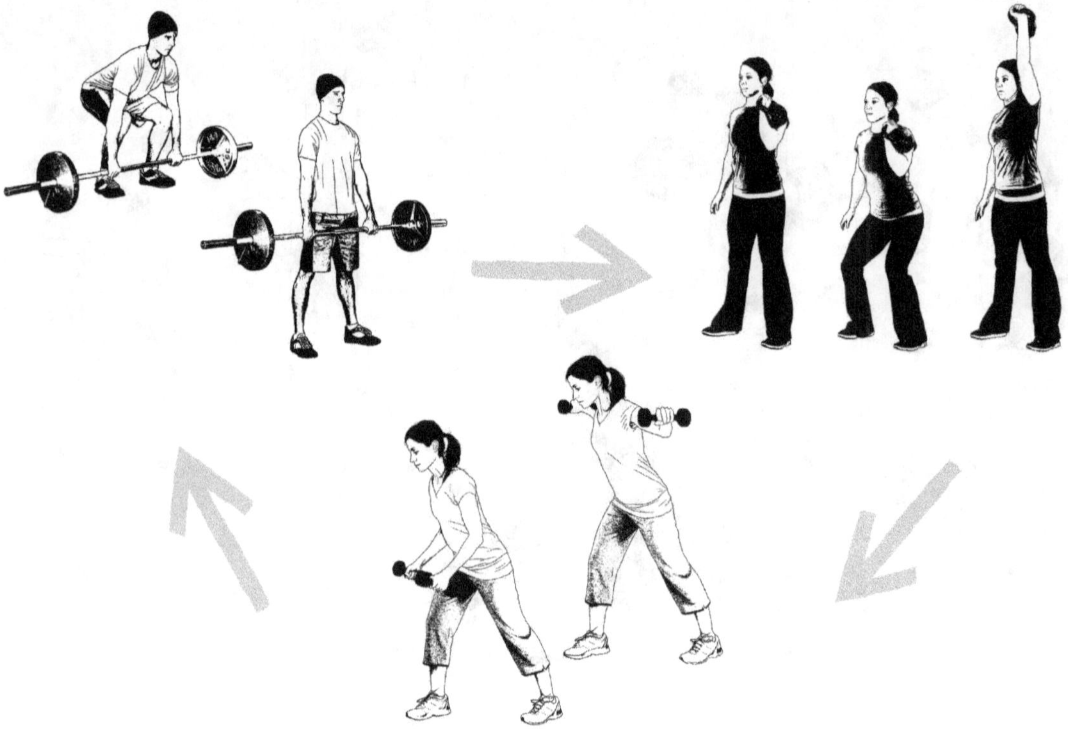

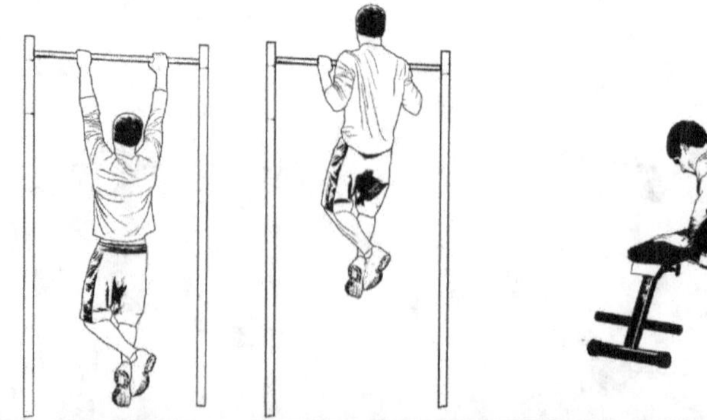

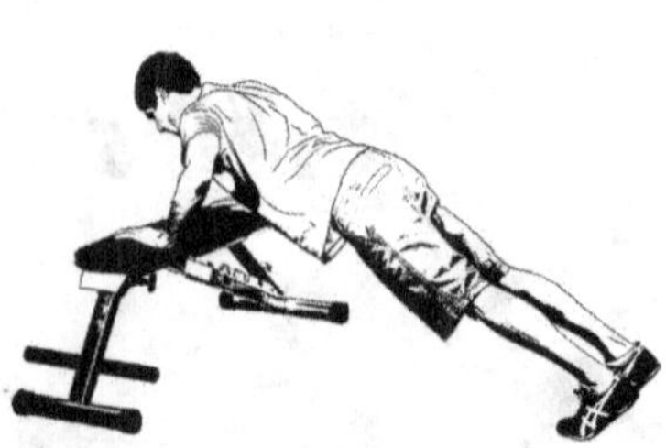

SIDE B

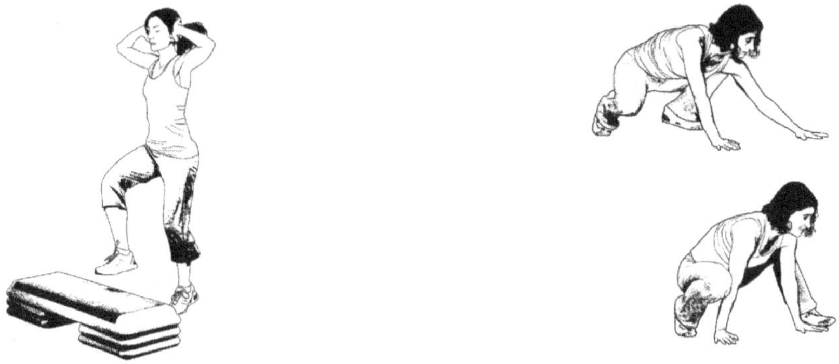

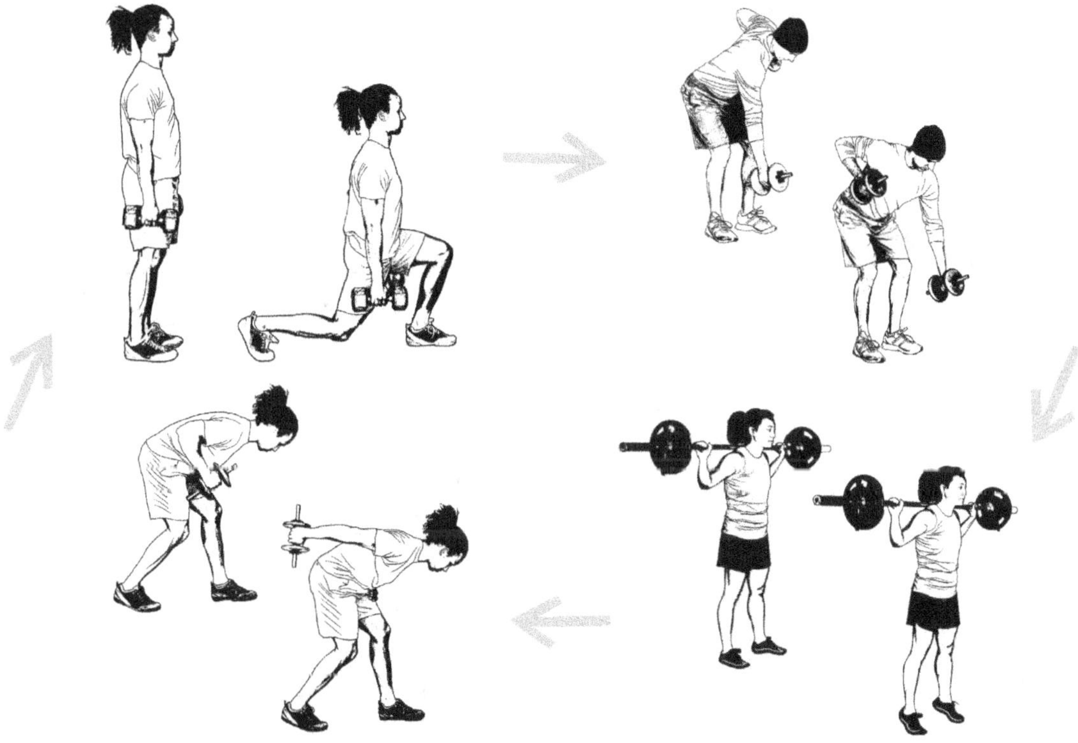

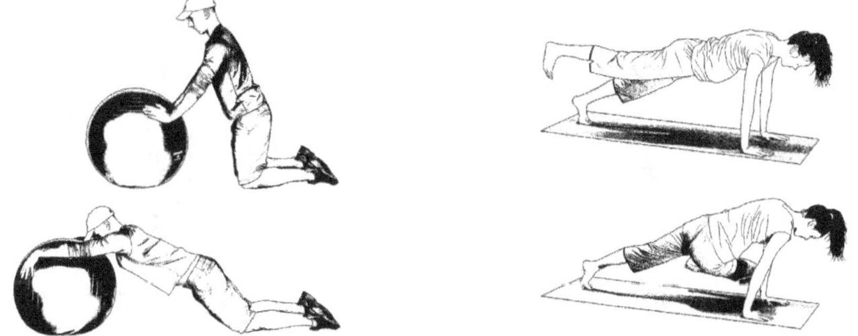

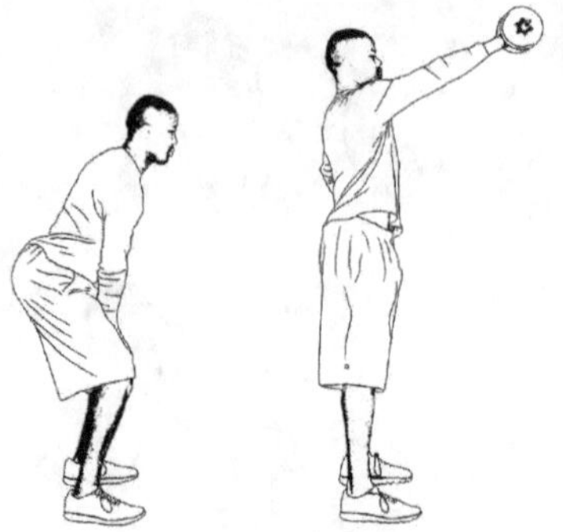

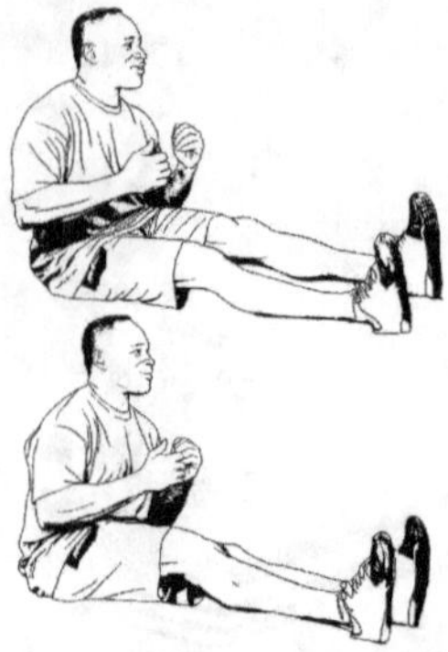

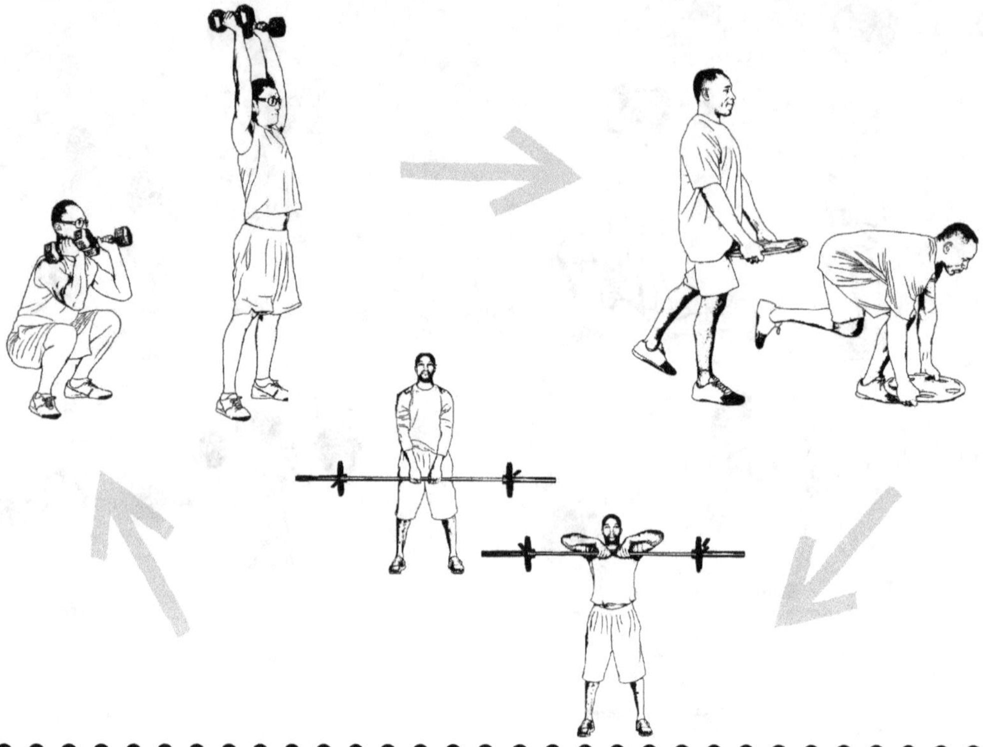

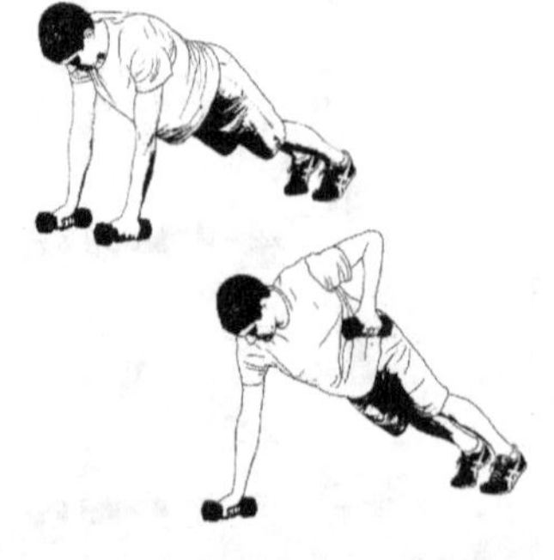

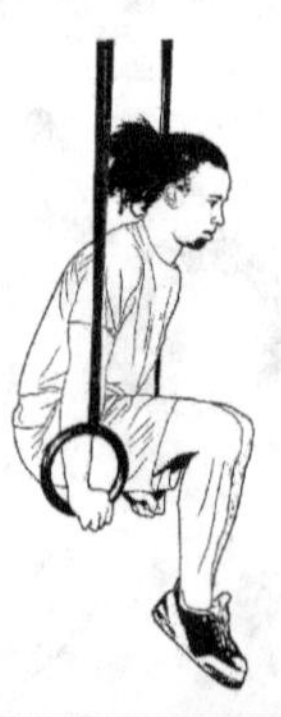

SIDE B

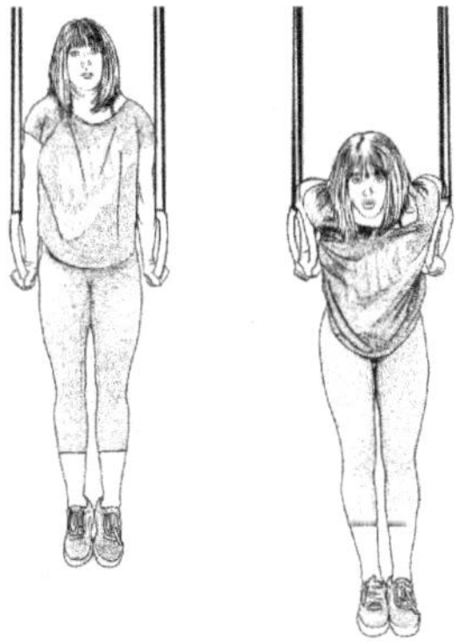

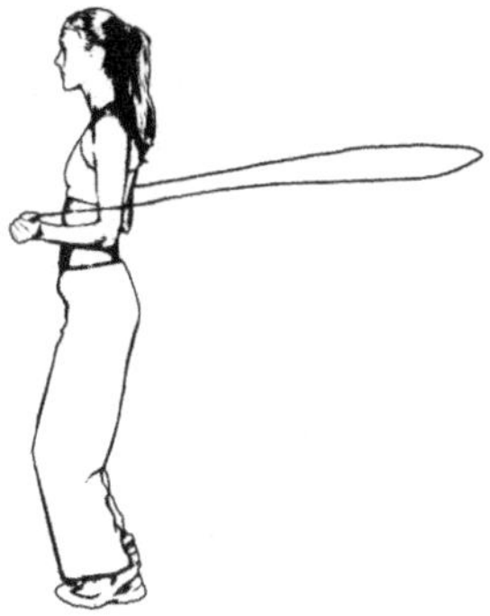

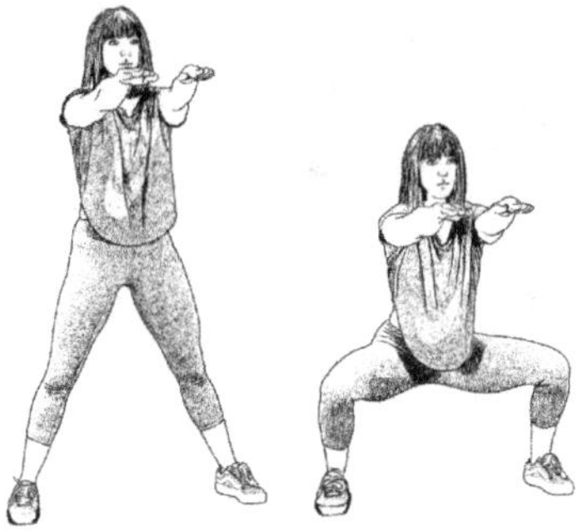

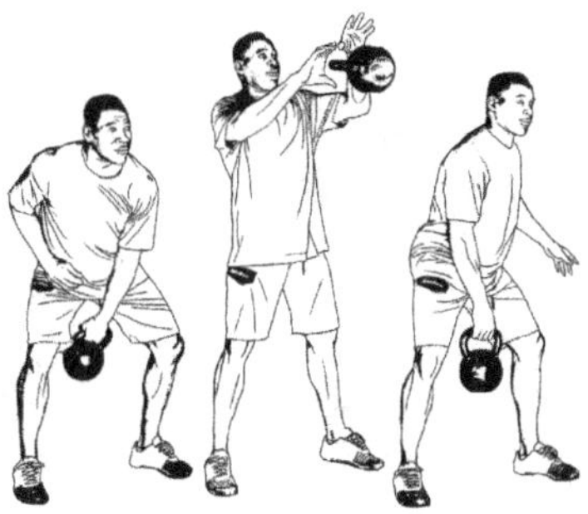

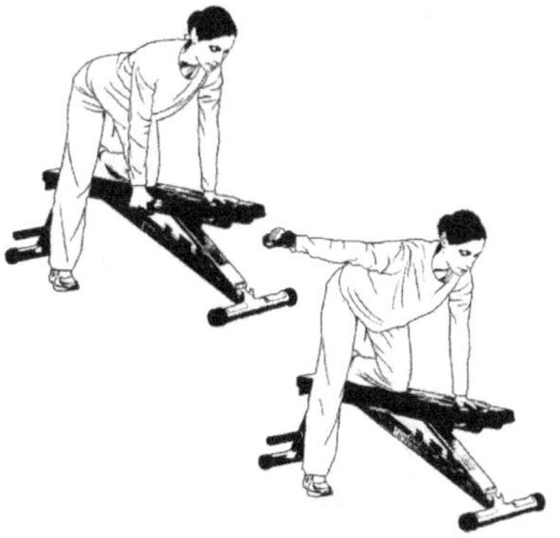

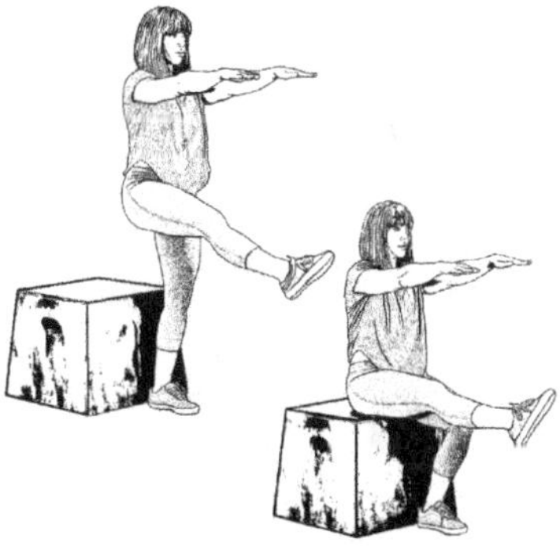

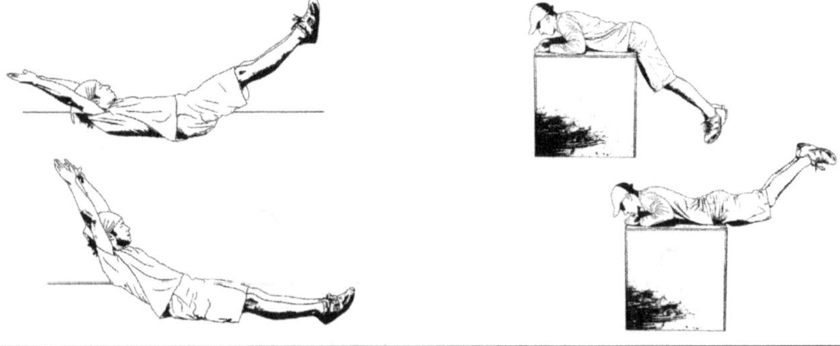

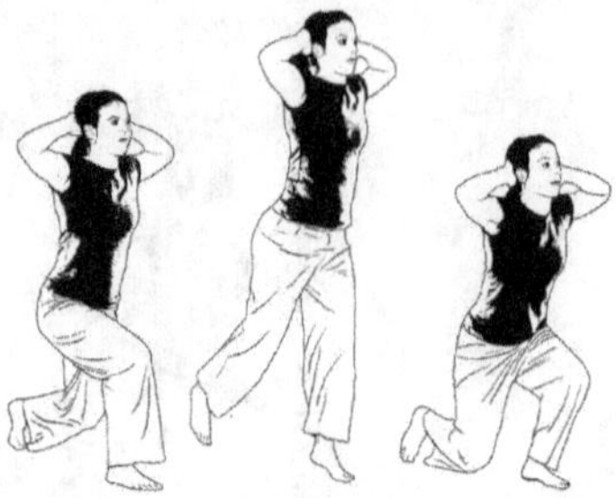

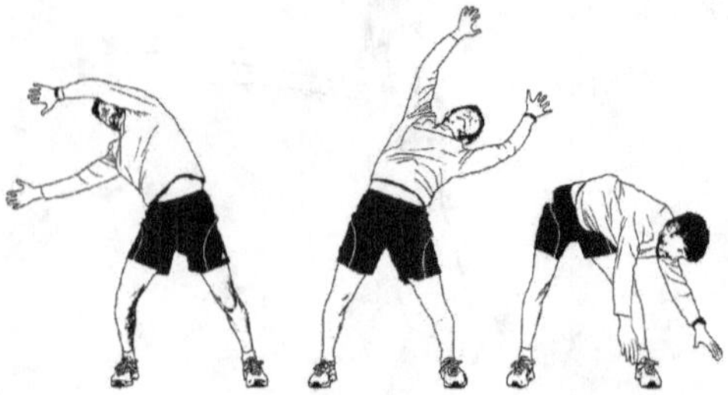

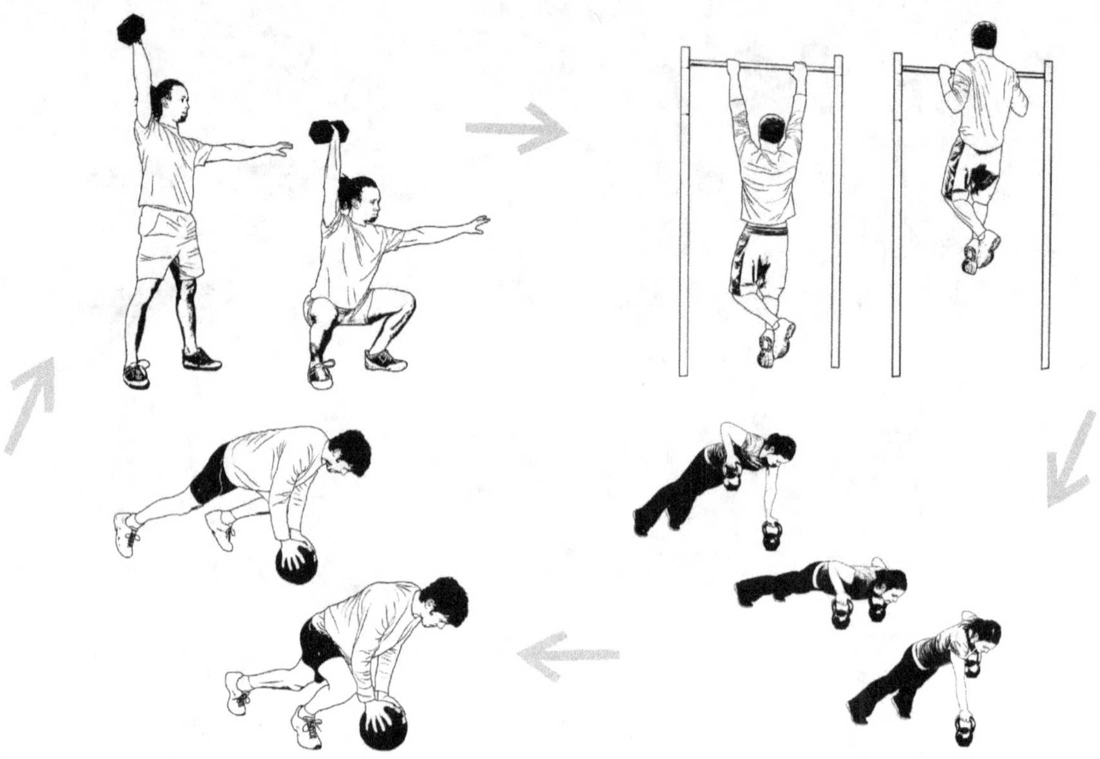

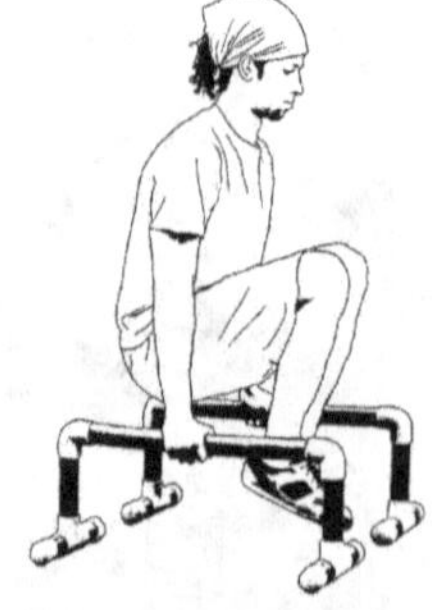

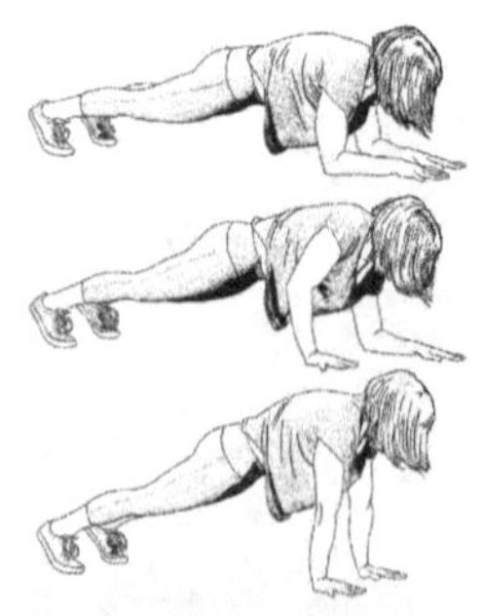

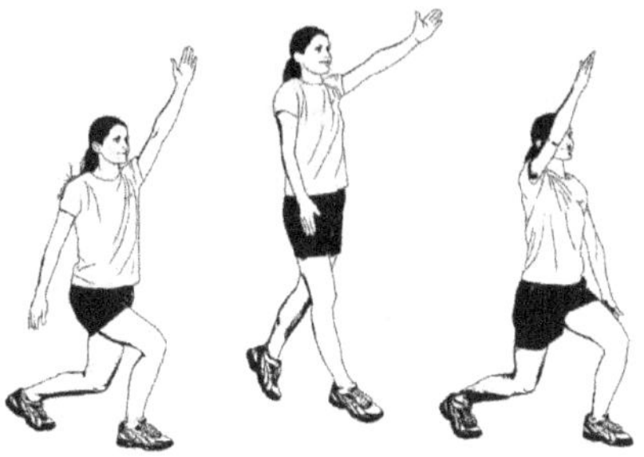

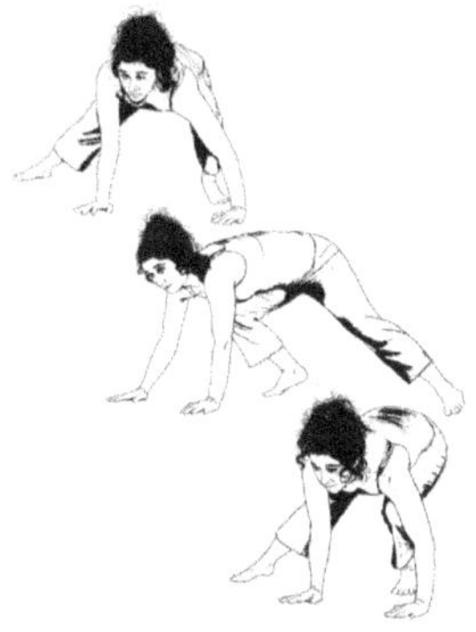

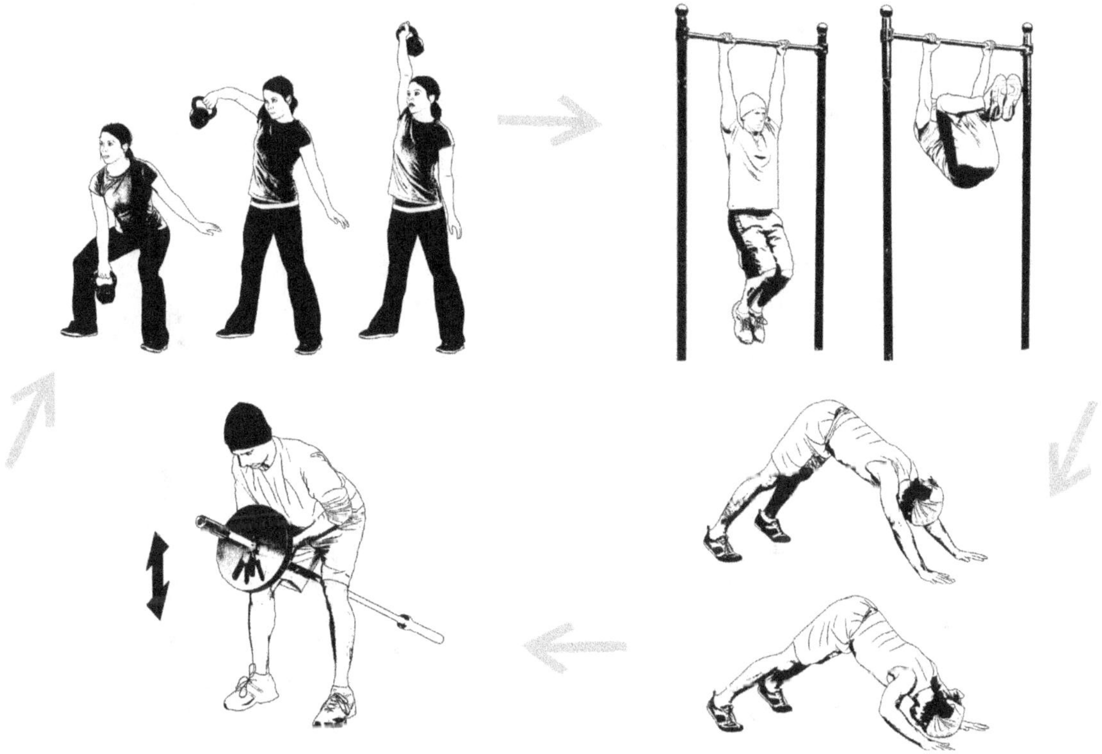

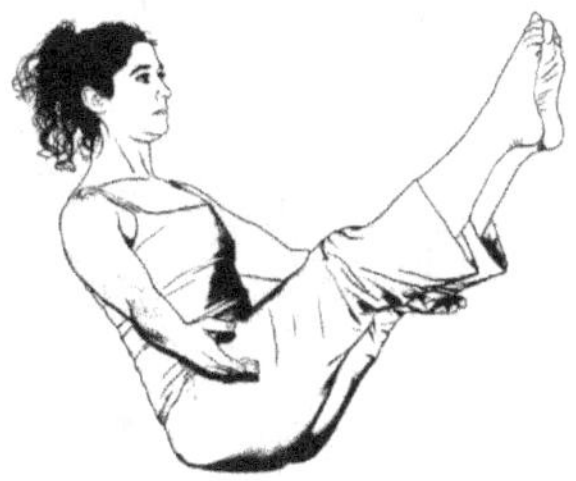

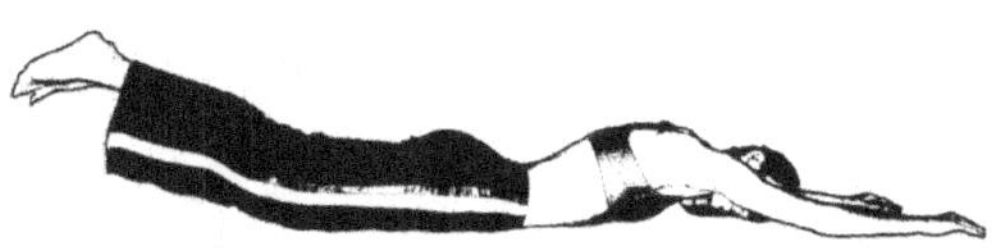

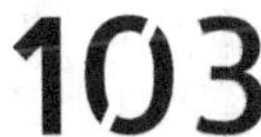

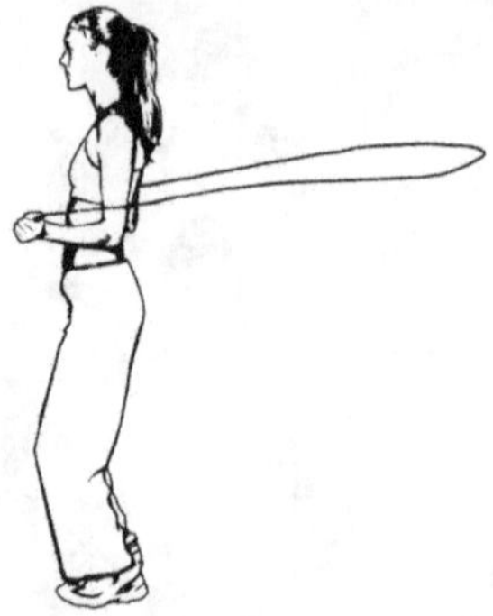

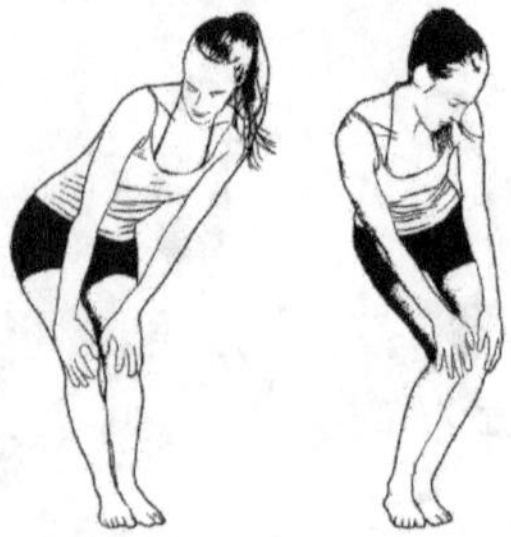

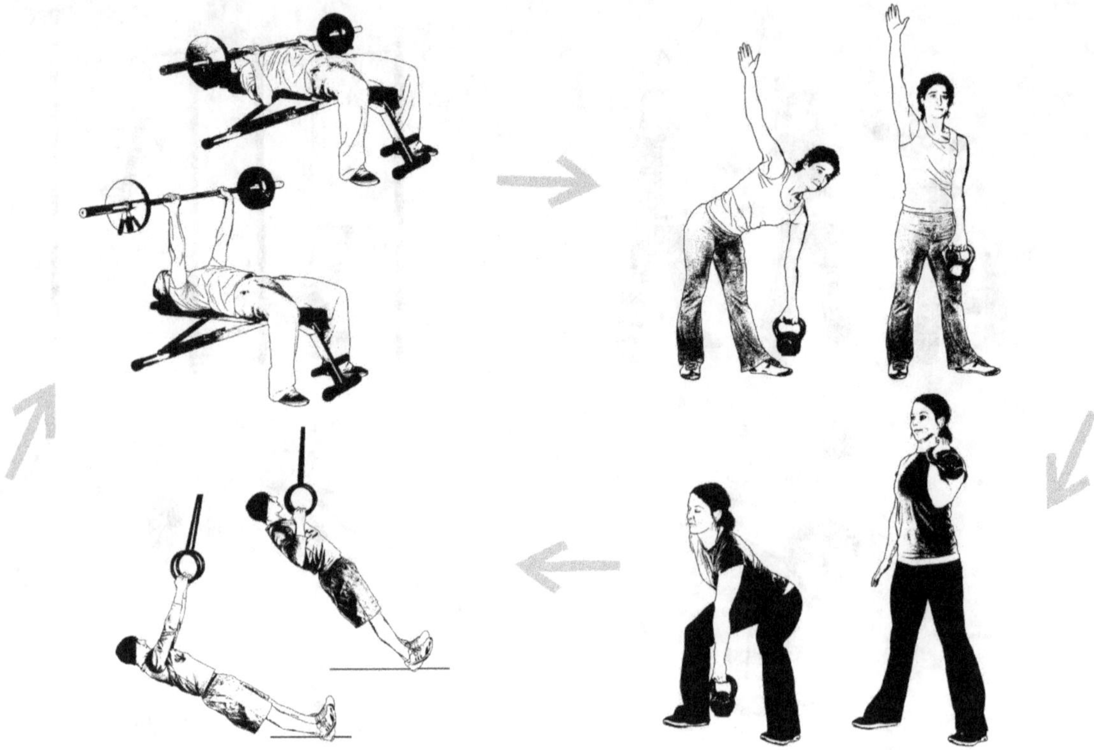

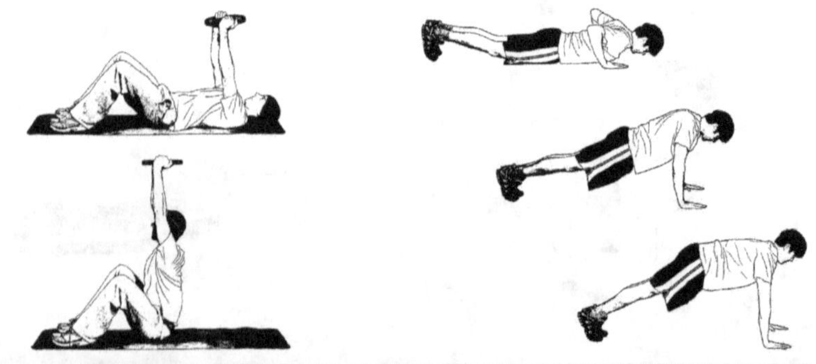

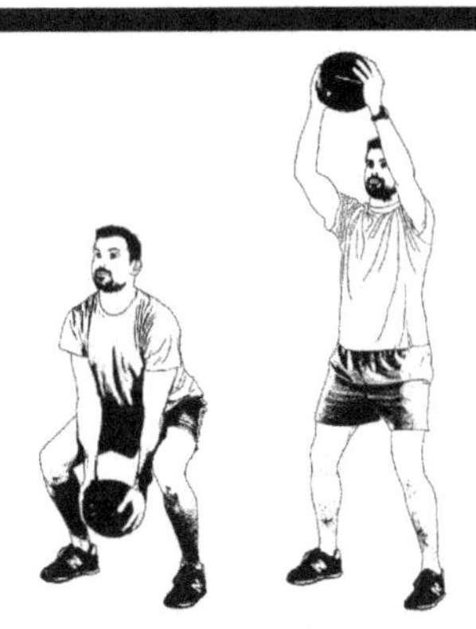

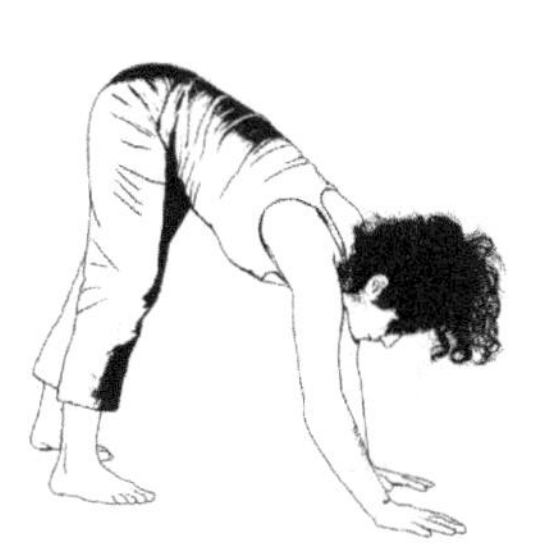

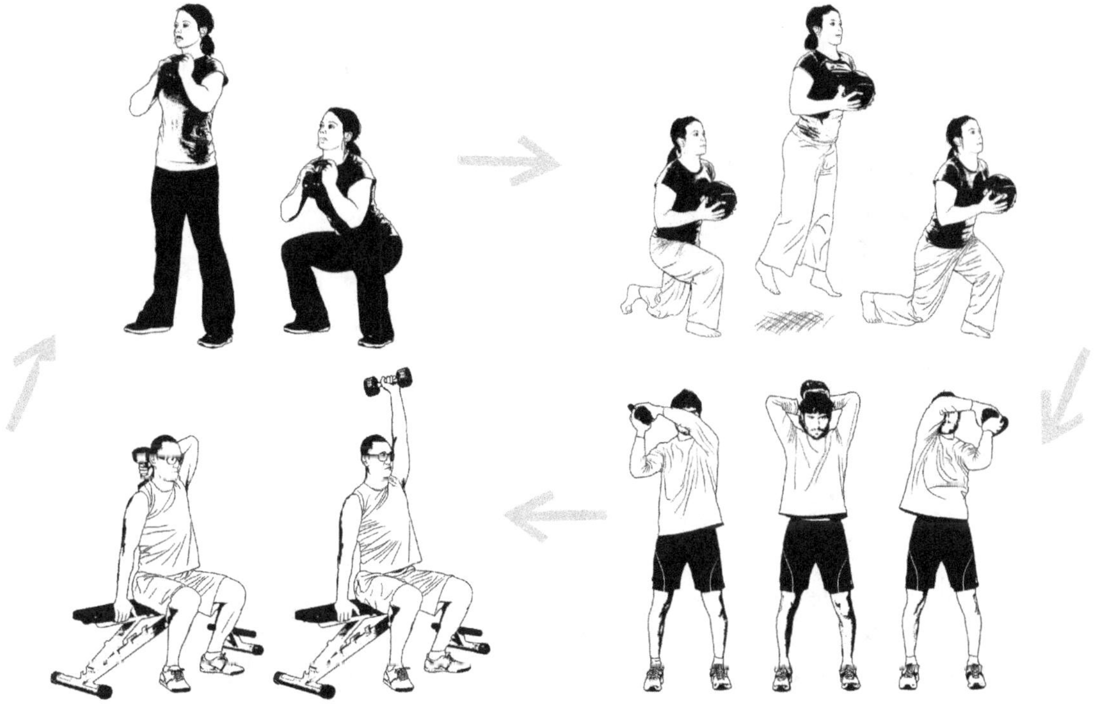

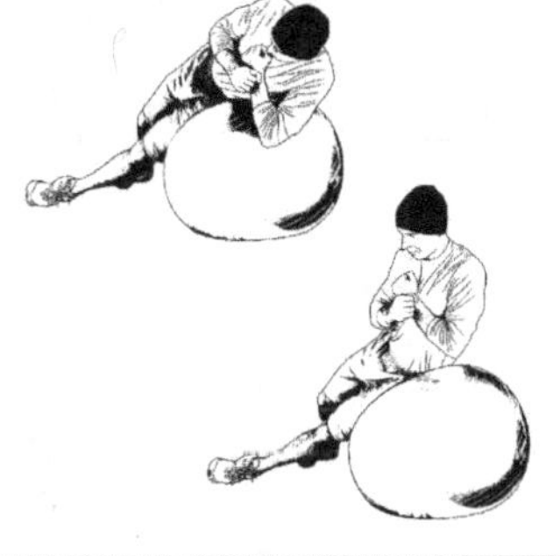

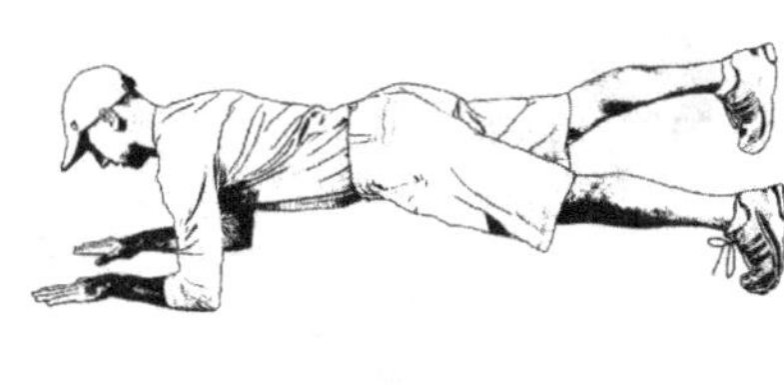

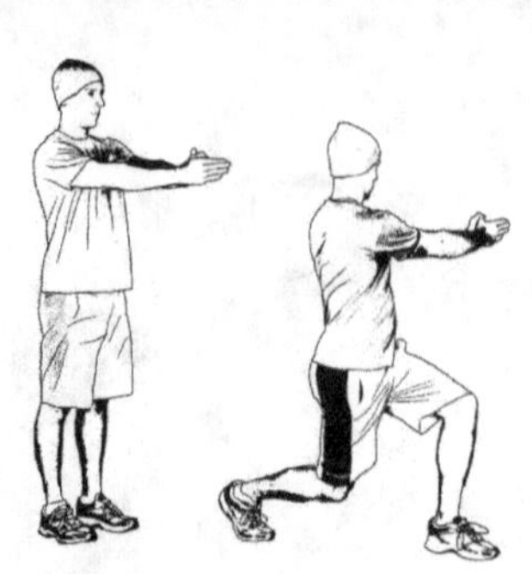

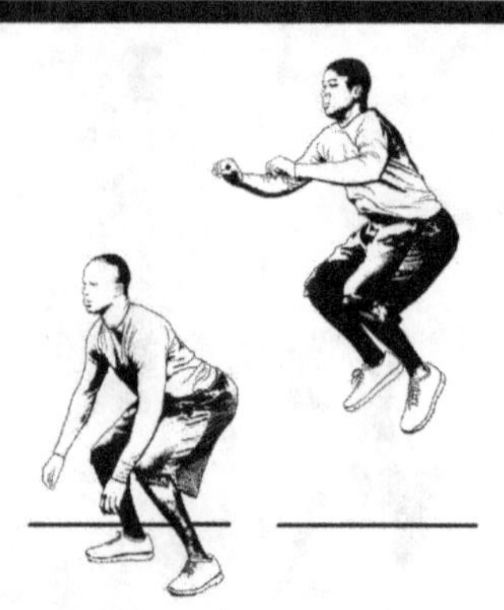

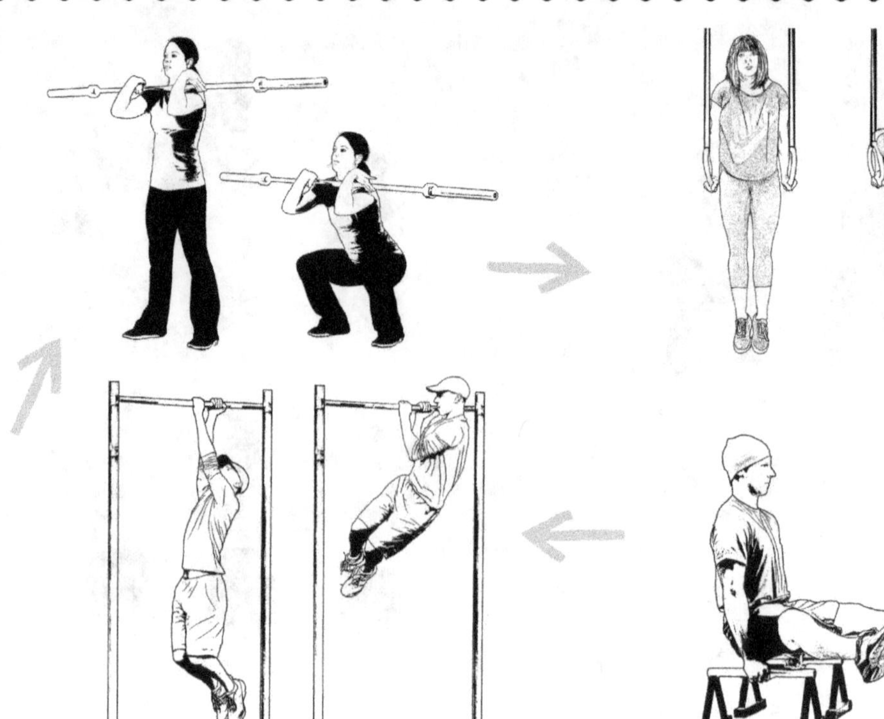

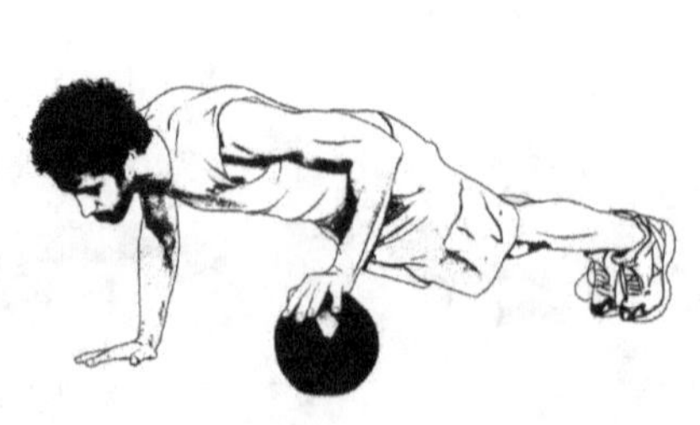

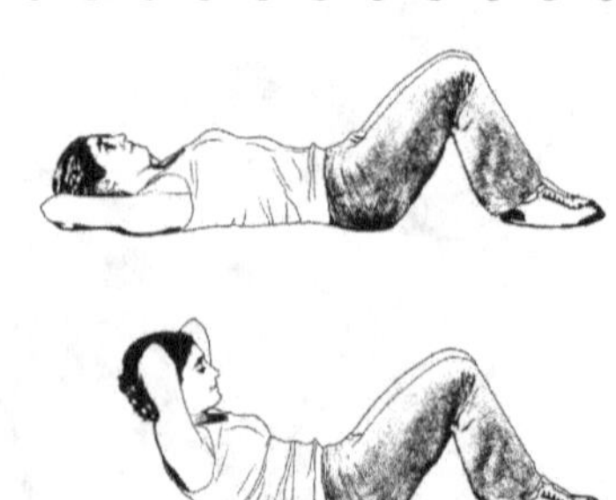

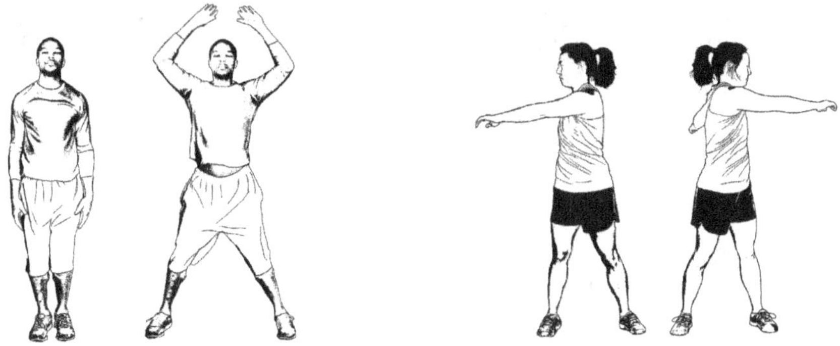

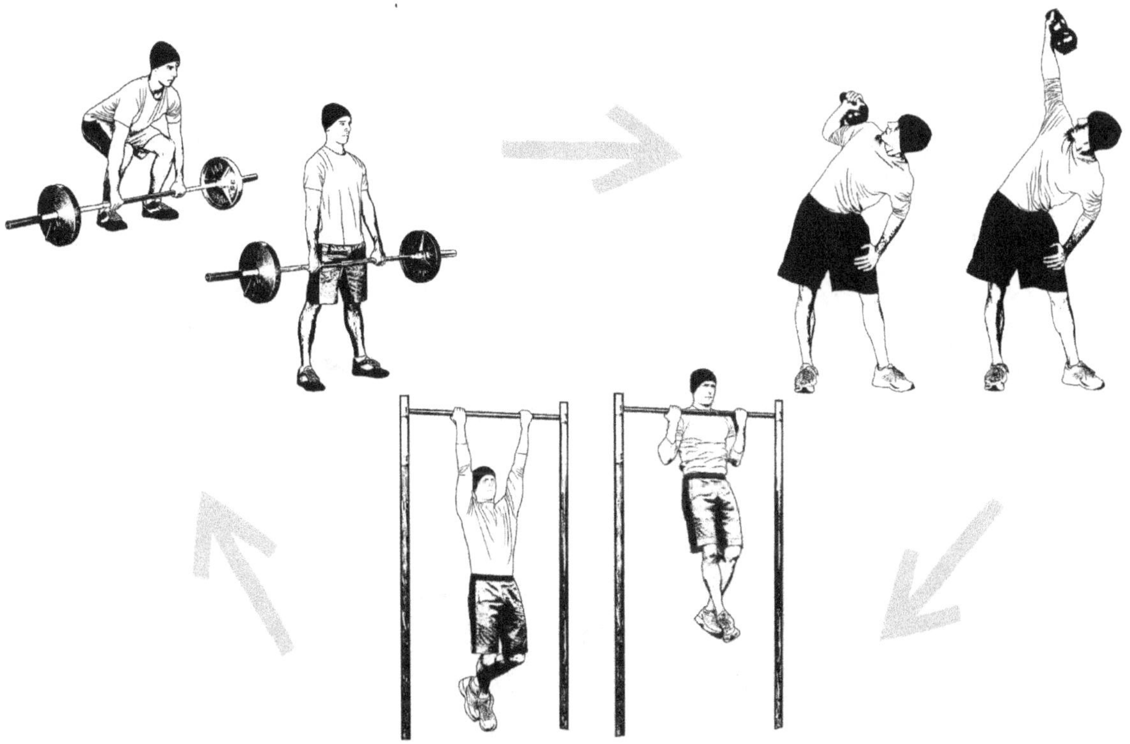

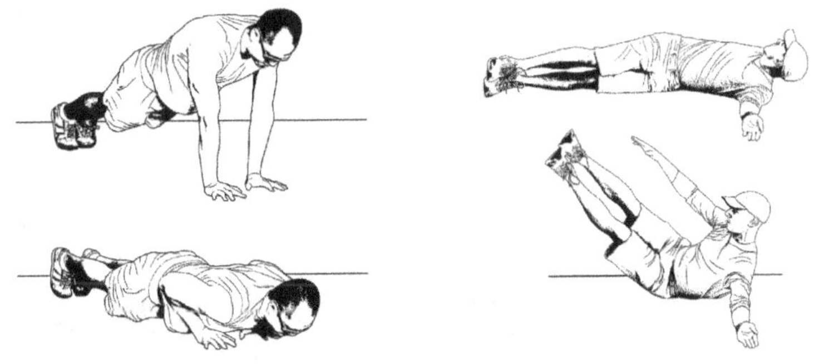

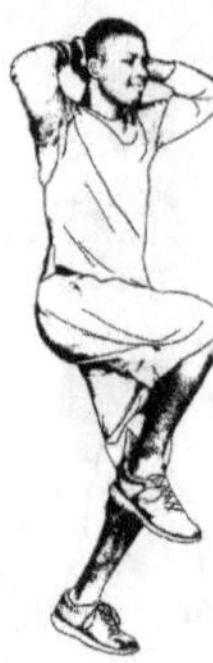

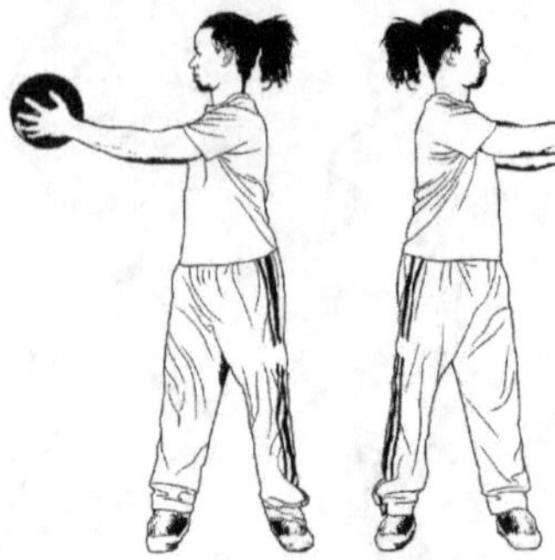

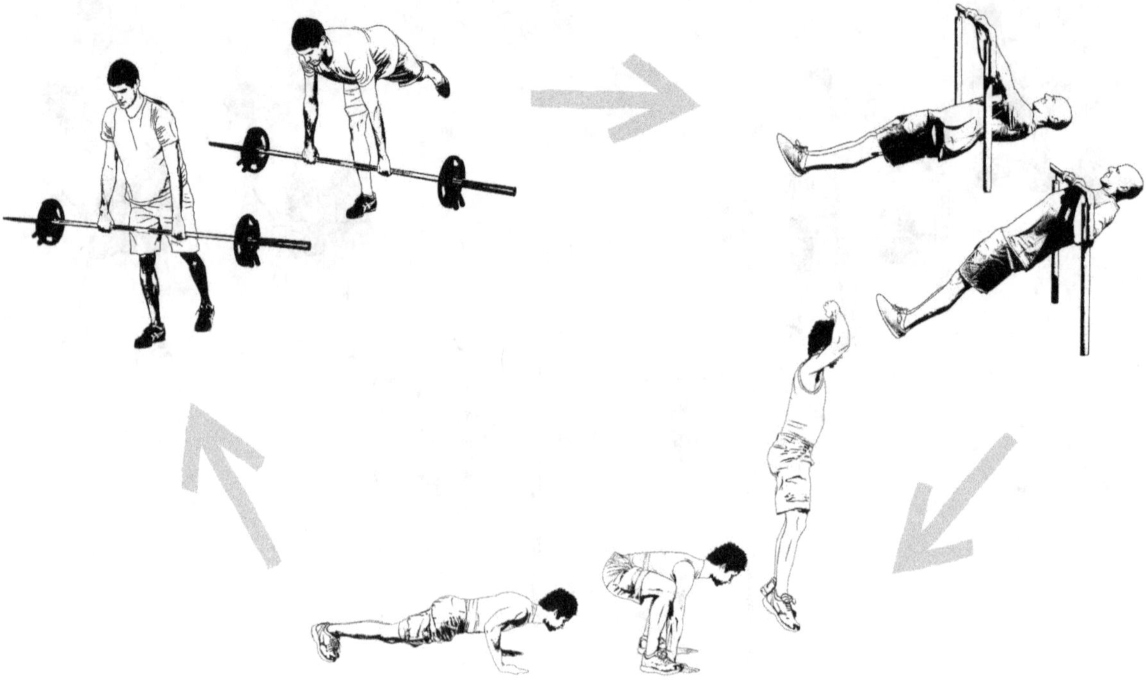

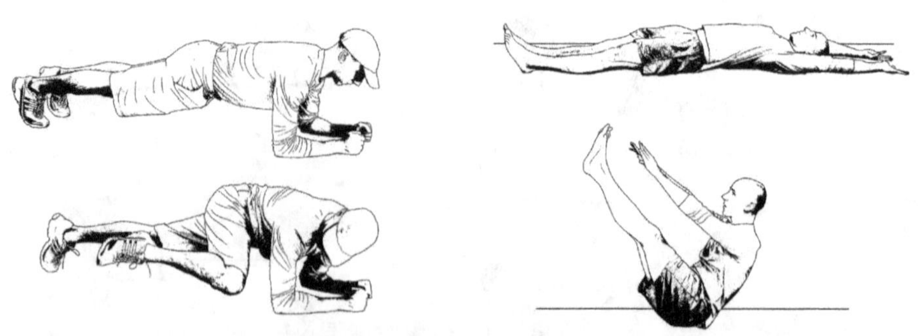

Side B

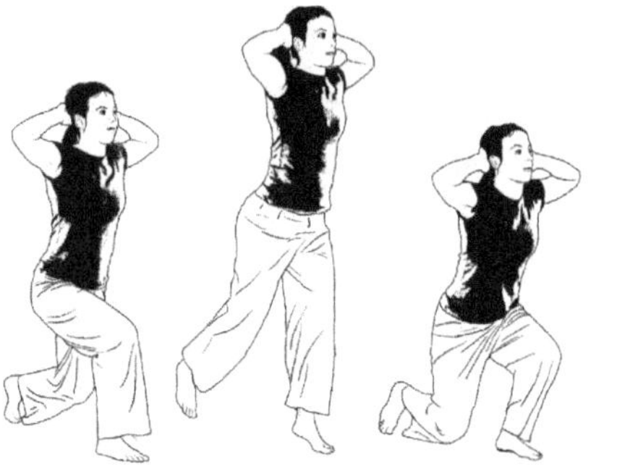

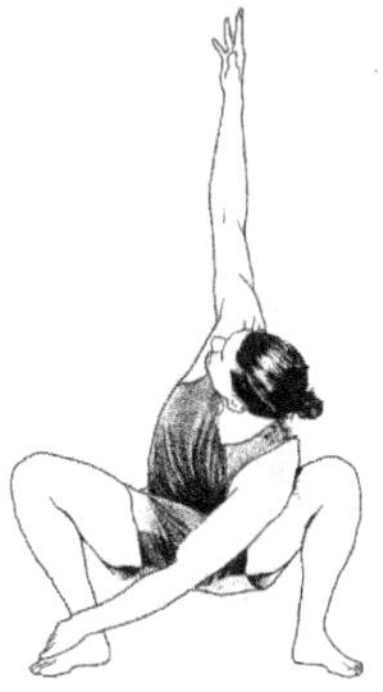

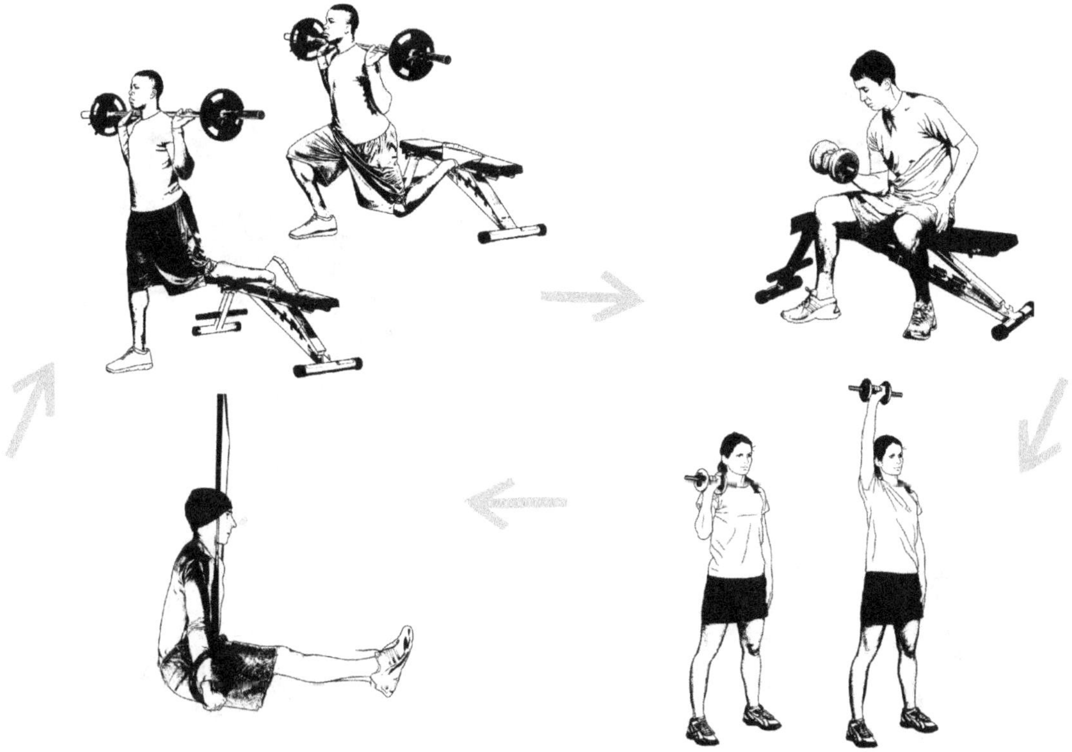

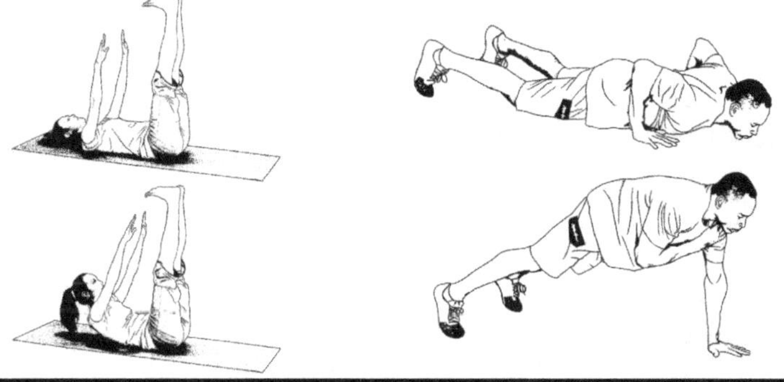

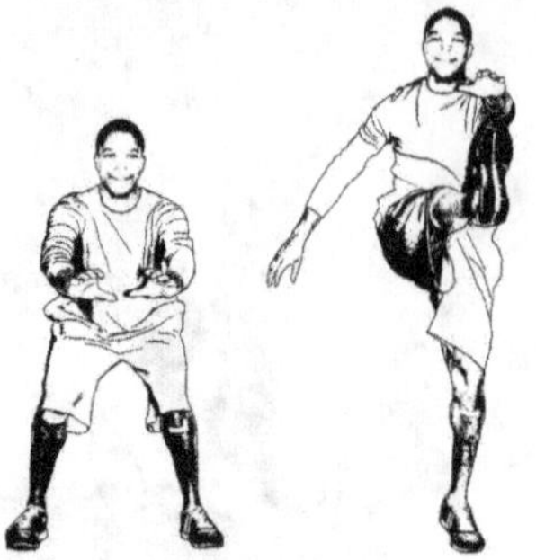

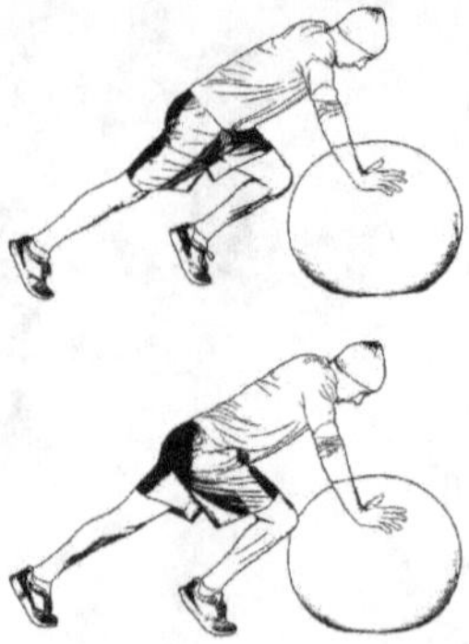

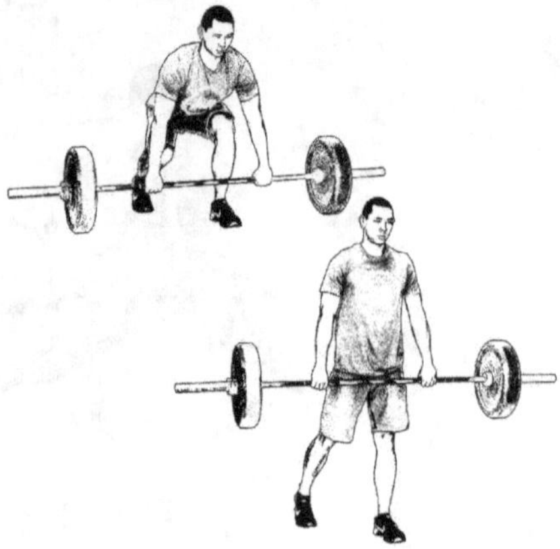

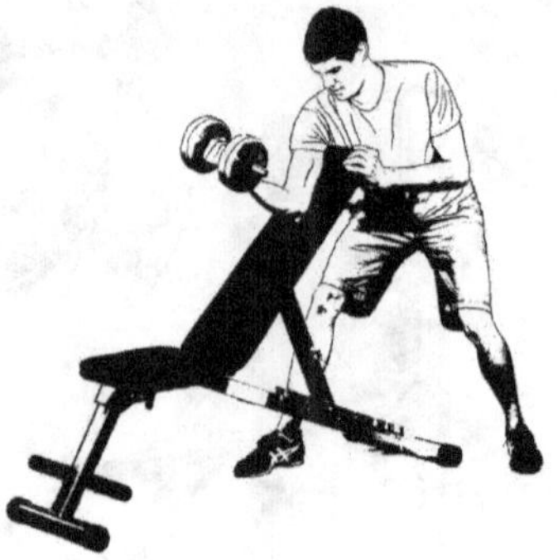

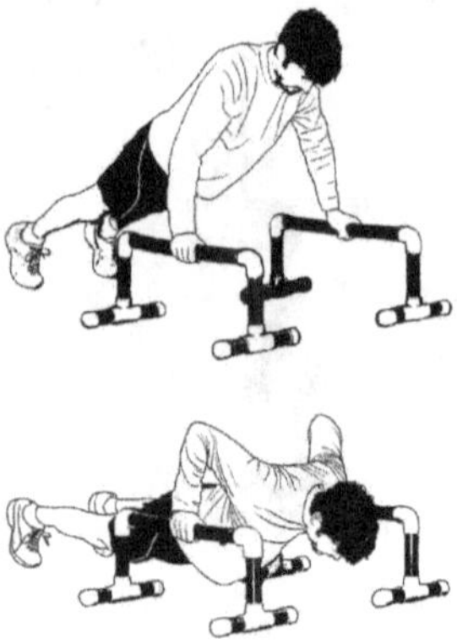

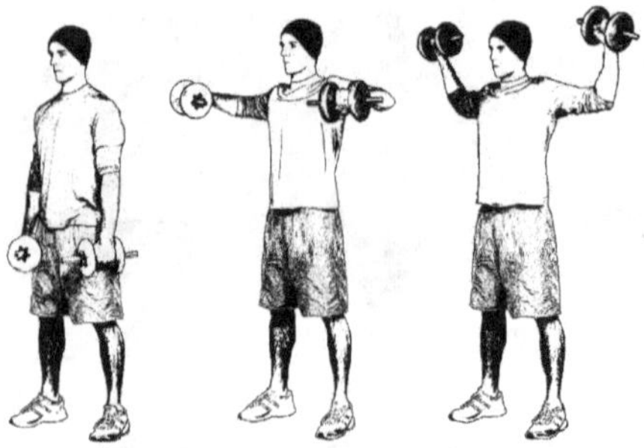

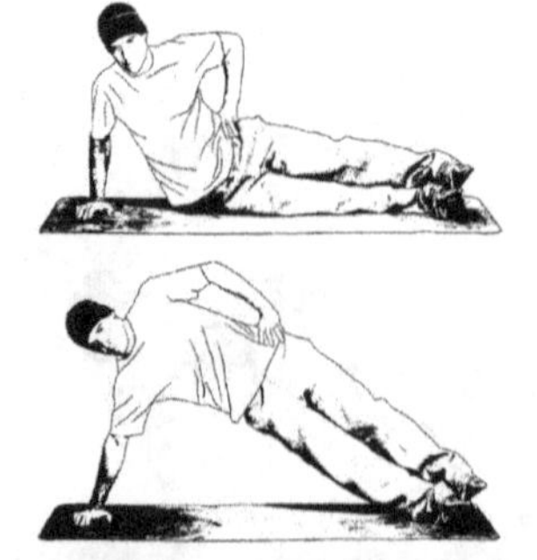
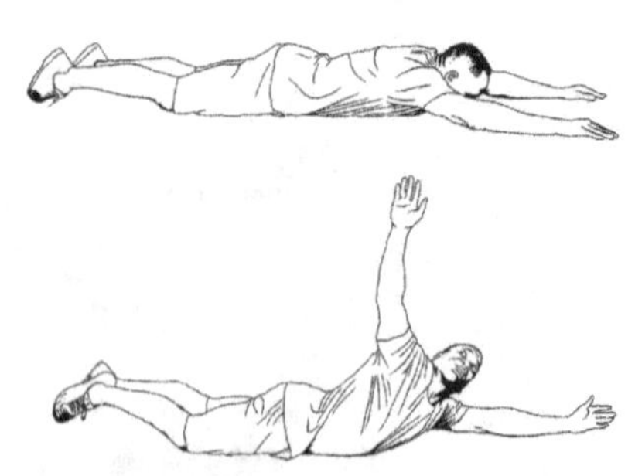

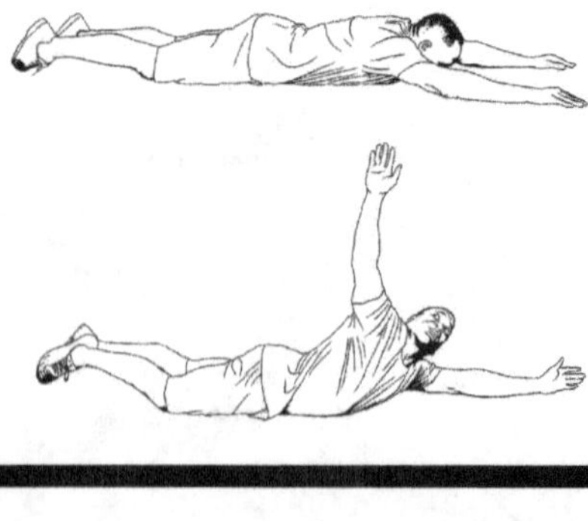

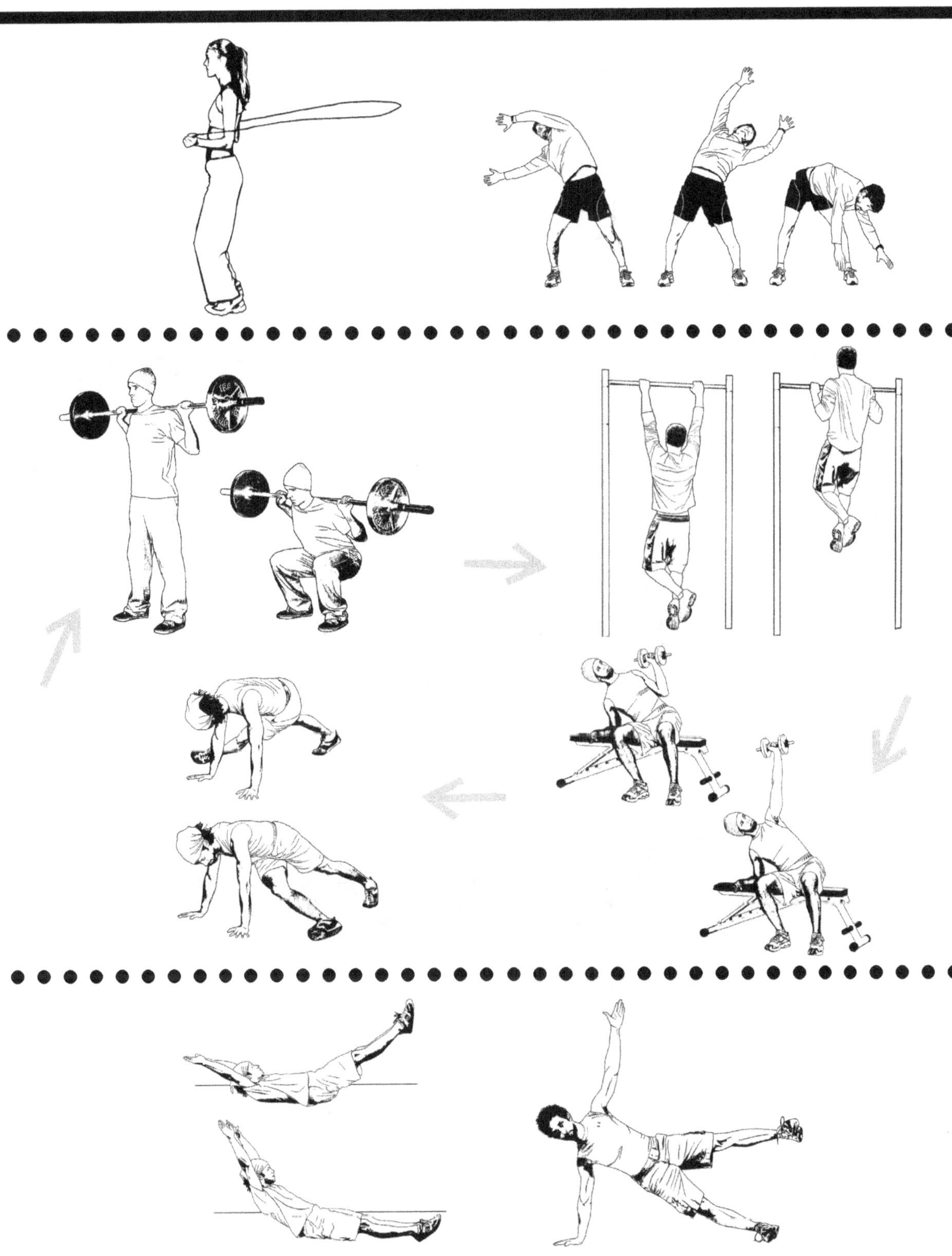

Hungry for more?

Stay to tuned for the next mixtape!

&

See more workouts at:

www.StrengthMob.com

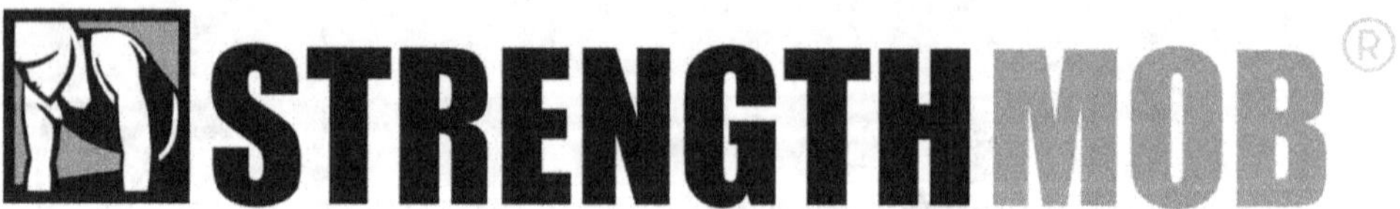

Appendix A
WORKOUT DESCRIPTIONS

LINER NOTES
Appendix A

KEY

KB = Kettlebell   SB = Stability Ball
DB = Dumbbell   BB = Barbell
WP = Weight Plate
"Hold" = the exercise is static, held for time
"Reps" = the exercise is dynamic, performed for repetitions
"Distance" = Do the exercise for a set distance across the floor

WORKOUTS

001.
Warm-up: Jump Rope & Trunk Twists
Circuit: BB Back Squats, DB Chest Presses, KB 3-point (aka Single Bent Over) Rows
Cool-down: Side Plank Reaches, Toe Touch Crunches

002.
Warm-up: High Stepping & Mountain Climbers
Circuit: BB Thrusters, Supported Single Arm Reverse Flyes, Ring Push-ups, Knees to Elbows
Cool-down: Dynamic Planks, Reverse Hypers
Note: Make the Ring Push-ups easier by starting in a more vertical position.

003.
Warm-up: Jumping Jacks & Reverse Lunge + Reaches
Circuit: BB Squat Pushes, Narrow Grip Chin-ups, Dive Bomber Push-ups, V-ups
Cool-down: Tuck Hollow Hold, Dynamic Side Planks

004.
Warm-up: KB Swings & Cossack Squats
Circuit: BB Hang Cleans, Parallette Push-ups, Ring Rows, DB Lateral Raise & External Rotation
Cool-down: L Hang (hold), Prone Leg Extension (hold)
Note: Make the Ring Rows easier by starting in a more vertical position.

005.
Warm-up: Split Jumps & Overhead Band Pull-aparts
Circuit: BB Deadlift, Toes to Bar, Ring Dips
Cool-down: Russian Twists, 3-point Plank on Elbows (hold)

LINER NOTES
Appendix A

006.
 Warm-up: Twisting Jumps & Split Squats
Circuit: Single Leg WP Deadlift, T Push-ups
Cool-down: Plank Splits, Arch Hold

007.
Warm-up: Butt Kicks & Air Squats
Circuit: BB Lunges, Burpees, DB Supported Single Arm Rows, KB Single Leg
Romanian Deadlift
Cool-down: Decline Push-ups, Tuck-ups

008.
Warm-up: Sumo Squat Jumping Jacks & Shoulder Dislocates
Circuit: Double KB Swings, Pull-ups, BB Bent Over Rows, Push-ups
Cool-down: Straddle V-ups, Arch Rocks

009.
Warm-up: Split Jacks, Squatting Knee Pushes
Circuit: BB Overhead Squats, KB Windmills, Squat Jumps, Inverted Rows
Cool-down: Med Ball Mountain Climbers, Parallette L-sit

010.
Warm-up: Squat Kicks & Plank Tucks
Circuit: BB Romanian Deadlift, Ring Push-ups, B Renegade Push-ups
Cool-down: Knees to Elbows, Box Donkey Kicks

011.
Warm-up: Single Leg Mountain Climbers & Bent Over Twists
Circuit: KB Belt Squats, DB Pull-overs, BB Shoulder Presses, Knees to Elbows
Cool-down: Shoulder Tap Push-ups, Side Plank Leg Raise (hold)

012.
Warm-up: Speed Skater Jumps & Knee Circles
Circuit: DB Step-ups, WP Halos, Ring Tuck Hold, Towel Pull-ups
Cool-down: 3-point Supine Plank, Feet on Wall Crunches

013.
Warm-up: Walking Toe Touches & Inchworms
Circuit: BB Sumo Deadlift High Pulls, KB Push Presses, Resisted Split Jumps,
DB Alternating Rows
Cool-down: Straddle (aka Leg Spread) Toe Touches, Bird Dog (hold)

LINER NOTES
Appendix A

014.
Warm-up: Commando Jacks & Burpees
Circuit: BB Hip Thrusts, DB Single Arm Thrusters, Chin-ups, DB Alternating Toe Touches
Cool-down: Hollow Hold, Prone Trunk Extension (hold)

015.
Warm-up: Run & Trunk Circles
Circuit: BB Thrusters, Box Jumps, DB Reverse Flyes
Cool-down: Horizontal Scissors, Parallette Push-ups

016.
Warm-up: Single Leg Toe Touches & Twisting Jumps
Circuit: BB Single Leg Romanian Deadlifts, Spiderman Pull-ups, DB Single Arm Overhead Squats, Fist Push-ups
Cool-down: V-sit (hold), Reverse Hyper Kick-outs

017.
Warm-up: KB Single Arm Swings & Side Step Squats
Circuit: BB Push Presses, KB Goblet Squats, KB 3-point Rows
Cool-down: Hollow Arch Rolls, Side Plank (hold)

018.
Warm-up: Jumping Jacks & Twisting Lunges
Circuit: BB Front Squats, KB Side Presses, Wood Chop Lunges, KB Bent Over Rows
Cool-down: Knees to Elbows, Diamond Push-ups

019.
Warm-up: Speed Skater Jumps & Arm Circles
Circuit: BB Bench Presses, DB Step-ups, Chin-ups, KB Single Arm Front Squats
Cool-down: Windshield Wipers, Leg Drops

020.
Warm-up: Split Jumps & Quadrupedal Movement
Circuit: BB Single Arm Squat Pushes, Parallette Push-ups, Ring Pull-ups
Cool-down: Quadruped Core Twists, Table Top Extensions

021.
Warm-up: Twisting Jumps & Indian Club Backstroke
Circuit: BB Clean & Presses, Wide Grip Pull-ups, Ring Dips, V-ups
Cool-down: Twisting Toe Touches, Prone Trunk Extension (hold)

022.
Warm-up: Jump Rope & Single Leg Good Mornings
Circuit: Toe Touch BB Deadlift, Single Arm DB Clean & Presses, Med Ball Slams
Cool-down: Mountain Climbers, Dynamic Side Planks

LINER NOTES
Appendix A

023.
Warm-up: DB Skier Raises & Trunk Twists with Bar
Circuit: BB Good Mornings, Jackknife Push-ups, Reverse Lunge & Chops, L Pull-ups
Cool-down: Cross-Over Stretch (hold), Cat Cows

024.
Warm-up: Prisoner Squats & Supine Scorpions
Circuit: BB Bulgarian Deadlifts, DB Seated Reverse Flyes, Burpees, Bench Dips
Cool-down: Side Plank Leg Swings, Roll-ups

025.
Warm-up: Carioca & Side Crawls
Circuit: BB Side Lunges, DB Diagonal Shoulder Presses, Plank KB Drags, Ring Rows
Cool-down: Hollow Holds, Uneven Push-ups (reps)

026.
Warm-up: Side to Side Lunges & German Arm Swings
Circuit: BB Split Squats, Ring Pull-ups, Pike Push-ups, KB Snatches
Cool-down: Reverse Crunches, Prone Alternating Arm & Leg Raises

027.
Warm-up: Jumping Jacks & Froggers (distance)
Circuit: BB Front Rack Lunges, Ring Push-ups, Wall Balls
Cool-down: Parallette L Sit, Reverse Hypers

028.
Warm-up: Ankle Hops & Overhead Squats
Circuit: BB Neider Presses, Med Ball Squat Cleans, Side-lying Reverse Flyes, Sit-ups
Cool-down: Butt Scoots (distance), Pull-ups

029.
Warm-up: Speed Skater Jumps & Crab Walk
Circuit: BB Sumo Deadlift, Push-ups, Narrow Grip Chin-up, DB Cuban Rotation & Presses
Cool-down: Quadruped Skiers, Dead Bugs

030.
Warm-up: Reverse Lunge + Reaches & Squatting Calf Raises
Circuit: WP Overhead Squats, Single Arm BB Long Bar Row, Elevated Feet Wall Push-ups, KB Low Windmill
Cool-down: Flutter Kicks, Side Plank & Knee Tuck (hold)

031.
Warm-up: Walking Toe Touches & Trunk Twists
Circuit: KB Waiter Carries, DB Squats, Inverted Rows, Parallette Push-ups
Cool-down: Tuck Hollow Holds, Box Donkey Kicks

LINER NOTES

Appendix A

032.
Warm-up: Toe Taps & Deep Lunge + Twists
Circuit: BB Z Presses, Spiderman Pull-ups, KB Front Squats
Cool-down: Quadruped Core Twists, Tuck-ups

033.
Warm-up: Jumping Jacks & Tiptoe Walking
Circuit: BB Lateral Split Lunges, DB Lateral Raises, Bench Jumps, DB Alternating Presses
Cool-down: Twisting Planks, Natural Hamstring Curls

034.
Warm-up: KB Alternating Swings & Forward Lunges
Circuit: BB Back Squats, KB Push Presses, DB Supported Single Rows
Cool-down: Hollow Rocks, Prone Leg Extension (hold)

035.
Warm-up: Med Ball Mountain Climbers & Bodyweight Good Mornings
Circuit: WP Thrusters, BB Bicep Curls, DB Single Arm Tricep Kickbacks, SB Pikes
Cool-down: T Push-ups, Resisted Sit-ups

036.
Warm-up: Commando Jacks & Lunge Kicks
Circuit: BB Front Squats, Inverted Rows, Single Leg Good Mornings, Ring Dips
Cool-down: Side to Side Push-ups, Rowing Crunches

037.
Warm-up: Split Jumps & Standing Crunches
Circuit: BB Single Leg Bulgarian Deadlifts, DB Alternating Forward Raises, Wood Chops, Parallette Push-ups
Cool-down: Straddle Hollow Holds, Dynamic Side Planks

038.
Warm-up: Hip Rotations & Arm Circles
Circuit: BB Overhead Squats, KB Turkish Get-ups, Pull-ups
Cool-down: Parallette Tuck Hold, Reverse Hyper Kick Outs

039.
Warm-up: High Stepping, Pelvis Circles
Circuit: BB Hang Cleans, KB Side Presses, Box Pistols, Burpees
Cool-down: Plank Splits, Split Leg Crunches

040.
Warm-up: Twisting Lunges & Inchworms
Circuit: BB Squat Pushes, Jackknife Push-ups, Ring Bicep Curls
Cool-down: V-ups, Arch Holds

LINER NOTES
Appendix A

041.
Warm-up: Walking Lunges, Twisting Jumps
Circuit: Resisted Side Lunges, KB Thrusters, DB Alternating Rows
Cool-down: Outrigger Push-ups, SB Skiers

042.
Warm-up: Walking Toe Touches & Dive Bomber Push-ups
Circuit: BB Deadlifts, Ring Push-ups, SB Jackknifes, DB Toe Touches
Cool-down: Airplane Pose (hold), Revolved Standing Forward Bend (hold)

043.
Warm-up: Jumping Jacks & Kangaroo Crawls
Circuit: Double KB Swings, Resisted Split Jumps, DB Alternating Rows
Cool-down: Knees to Elbows, Shoulder Tap Push-ups

044.
Warm-up: Jump Rope & Single Leg Mountain Climbers
Circuit: BB Zercher Lunges, Wrist Grip Chin-ups, KB Shoulder Presses, KB Russian Twists
Cool-down: 3-point Plank (hold), Tuck Hollow Hold

045.
Warm-up: Twisting Jumps & Diagonal Shoulder Swings
Circuit: BB Thrusters, DB Bent Over Rows, Toes to Bar, Plank Up Downs
Cool-down: KB Press Crunches, Camel Pose (hold)

046.
Warm-up: Lateral Leg Swings & Bent Over Twists
Circuit: BB Push Presses, Squat Jumps, DB Forward Lunges, V-ups
Cool-down: Cat Cow, Revolved Chair Pose (hold)

047.
Warm-up: Single Leg Toe Touches & Natural Leg Extensions
Circuit: KB Snatches, Dips, Uneven Pull-ups
Cool-down: Rowing V-sits, 3-point Plank on Elbows

048.
Warm-up: Crouched Walk & Lateral Bench Hops
Circuit: BB Stiff Leg Deadlifts, KB Bent Presses, DB Step-ups,
Supported Single Arm Reverse Flyes
Cool-down: Windshield Wipers, Push-up Arm Raises

049.
Warm-up: Split Jumps & Knee to Face
Circuit: BB Elevated Front Foot Split Squat, DB Alternating Curl, Ab Roller,
DB Single Arm Skull Crushers
Cool-down: SB Weight Rolls, Boat Pose (hold)

050.
Warm-up: Sumo Squat Jumping Jacks & Marching Bridges
Circuit: BB Shoulder Presses, KB Double Windmills, Broad Jumps, WP Shoulder Curls
Cool-down: Med Ball Push-ups (reps), Raised Knee Crunches

051.
Warm-up: Sumo Squats & Trunk Twists
Circuit: Sandbag Shoulder Cleans, BB Forward Raises, Ring Archer Pull-ups, Speed Skater Jumps
Cool-down: Plank Side Hops, Table Top Extensions

052.
Warm-up: Carioca & Plank Side Steps
Circuit: BB Drop Lunges, KB Twisting Crunches, KB Renegade Push-ups
Cool-down: Knees to Elbows, Reverse Hyper Kick Outs

053.
Warm-up: Jumping Jacks & Forearm Crawls
Circuit: WP Clean & Presses, Bodyweight Skull Crushers, KB Bird Dog Rows
Cool-down: Tuck-ups, Hanging Leg Scissors

054.
Warm-up: Indian Club Overhead Swings & Trunk Circles
Circuit: BB Half Moons, Parallette Push-ups, Commando Pull-ups, DB Single Arm Overhead Squats
Cool-down: Quadruped Skiers, Frog Leg Raises

055.
Warm-up: High Stepping & Kneeling Rocks
Circuit: BB Single Leg Hip Thrusts, DB Plank Rows, Tuck-ups, Push-ups
Cool-down: Fish Hook Crunches, Plank Arm Raises

056.
Warm-up: Prisoner Lunges & Bent Over Twists
Circuit: KB Swings, BB Long Bar Chest Presses, Inverted Rows, Squat Jumps
Cool-down: Backward Push-ups, Frog Leg Crunches

057.
Warm-up: Forward Leg Swings & Twisting Lunges
Circuit: BB Deficit Deadlifts, DB Clean & Presses, WP Rows, Cossack Squats
Cool-down: Bicycle Crunches, Dive Bomber Push-ups

LINER NOTES
Appendix A

058.
Warm-up: Jumping Jacks & Med Ball Mountain Climbers
Circuit: BB Back Squats, KB Push Presses, Supported Plank Rows
Cool-down: Dynamic Side Planks, Arch Swimmers

59.
Warm-up: Single Arm kb Swings & Tip Toe Squats
Circuit: Med Ball Squat Cleans, Mace 360s, Plyo Push-ups, Roll-ups
Cool-down: Plank Side Crunches, Prone Trunk Raise (hold)

060.
Warm-up: Split Jumps & Quadruped Core Twists
Circuit: Mace Barbarian Squats, Ring Dips, BB Bent Over Rows, Saxon Side Bends
Cool-down: Toe Touch Crunches, Hip Thrusts

061.
Warm-up: Marching Knee Tucks & Frogger (distance)
Circuit: DB Forward Lunges, Narrow Grip Chin-ups, BB Teeter Totter Presses
Cool-down: Scorpion Push-ups, Horizontal Scissors

062.
Warm-up: Narrow Squats & Inchworms
Circuit: Shrimp Squats, Bridge & WP Presses, SB Preacher Curls, KB Get-up Sit-up
Cool-down: Split Leg Crunches, Prone Leg Extension (hold)

063.
Warm-up: Commando Jacks & Split Squats
Circuit: BB Suitcase Deadlift, DB Calf Raises, T Push-ups, Mace Pivot Uppercut
Cool-down: Parallette Single Leg L-sit (hold), Single Arm Table Tops

064.
Warm-up: High Stepping & Prone Scorpions
Circuit: Med Ball Thrusters, Rotating Lunges, Renegade Push-ups, BB Kneeling Roll-outs
Cool-down: Teaser V-ups, Side Planks – Feet Elevated

065.
Warm-up: Air Squats & Bear Crawls (distance)
Circuit: BB Overhead Squats, Parallette Push-ups, Mixed-grip Pull-ups
Cool-down: Russian Twists – Feet Elevated, Twisting Supermans

066.
Warm-up: Lateral Leg Swings & Trunk Twists
Circuit: BB Front Rack Lunges, Ring Bicep Curls, Sandbag Cleans,
Twisting Shoulder Presses
Cool-down: Hollow Rocks, Incline Push-ups

067.
 Warm-up: Twisting Jumps & Single Leg Mountain Climbers
Circuit: Zercher Squats, DB Alternating Rows, KB Side Presses, SB Skiers
Cool-down: Narrow Grip Push-ups, Raised Knee Crunches

068.
Warm-up: Squat Kicks & Side Lunges,
Circuit: Mace Joust Lunges, DB Single Arm Thrusters, 3-point DB Rows, Box Jumps
Cool-down: 2-point Plank (hold), Alternating Sit-ups

069.
Warm-up: Side Step Squats, Reaching Backbends
Circuit: BB Push Presses, Resisted Split Jumps, Toes to Bar, WP Shoulder Curls
Cool-down: Supine Plank (hold), SB Pikes

070.
Warm-up: Forward Leg Swings, Backward Leg Drag (distance)
Circuit: DB Thrusters, Split Arm Pull-ups, KB Good Mornings, Push-up Arm Raises
Cool-down: Side Plank Leg Raise (hold), Pike Compressions

071.
Warm-up: KB Swings & Hip Cradles
Circuit: BB Squat Pushes, Inverted Rows, Mace Reverse Lunge & Uppercuts,
Pike Push-ups
Cool-down: Quadruped Skiers, DB Alternating Toe Touches

072.
Warm-up: Jump Rope & Quadrupedal Movement (distance)
Circuit: BB Single Leg Romanian Deadlifts, Pull-ups, Parallette Dips, Wood Chops
Cool-down: SB Back Extensions, Twisting Toe Touches

073.
Warm-up: Split Jacks & Trunk Twists with Bar
Circuit: DB Single Arm Overhead Squats, Pike Push-ups, Single Arm BB Long Bar
Rows
Cool-down: Hanging Knee Raises, DB Side Bends

074.
Warm-up: Walking Toe Touches &Trunk Circles
Circuit: BB Toe Touch Deadlifts, KB Figure Eights, DB Hammer Curls,
DB Single Arm Shoulder Presses
Cool-down: Single Leg Push-ups (reps), Prone Leg Extension (hold)

LINER NOTES
Appendix A

075.
Warm-up: Prisoner Lunges & Pelvis Circles
Circuit: BB Overhead Lunges, DB Supported Single Arm Rows, Single Leg
Corkscrews, Bench Dips with Ball
Cool-down: SB Hip Rolls, Pelvic Thrusts

076.
Warm-up: Butt Kicks & Crab Walk (distance)
Circuit: BB Split Good Mornings, Parallette Shoot Throughs, DB Cross Curls,
WP Thrusters
Cool-down: Crunches, Decline Push-ups (reps)

077.
Warm-up: Jumping jacks & Overhead Squats
Circuit: BB Thrusters, DB Lateral Raises, KB 3-point Rows, Pseudo Planche Push-ups
Cool-down: Reverse Hypers & Side Plank (hold)

078.
Warm-up: Prisoner Squats & Inchworms
Circuit: BB Rack Deadlifts, DB Supported Single Arm Rows, KB Side Presses
Cool-down: Shoulder Tap Push-ups, Leg Tosses (reps)

079.
Warm-up: Jump Rope & SB Mountain Climbers
Circuit: KB Goblet Squats, Ring Bicep Curls, Russian Twists, BB Javelin Presses
Cool-down: Leg Scissors, Prone Leg Extension (hold)

080.
Warm-up: Butt Kicks & Plank Tucks
Circuit: DB Front Squats, BB Supinated Bent Over Rows, Walking Overhead Lunges,
Ring Push-ups
Cool-down: Negative Sit-ups, Arch Swimmers

081.
Warm-up: Sumo Squat Jumping Jacks & Quadrupedal Movement (distance)
Circuit: BB Zercher Good Mornings, DB Alternating Rows, DB Single Arm Curl &
Presses, Side Plank Reaches
Cool-down: Knee Grab Sit-ups, Spiderman Push-ups

082.
Warm-up: Ginga & Prisoner Lunges
Circuit: Box Jumps, KB Push Presses, KB Single Leg Romanian Deadlifts, Twist
& Lateral Raises
Cool-down: Circular Toes to Bar, Arch Hold

083.
Warm-up: Split Jumps & Diagonal Shoulder Swings
Circuit: KB Head Cutters, Squat Jumps, Staggered Push-ups, Mace Bent Over Rows
Cool-down: Side Plank & Leg Lift (hold), Reverse Hypers

084.
Warm-up: High Stepping & Side to Side Lunges
Circuit: BB Front Squats, Ring Dips, Toes to Bar, WP Rows
Cool-down: Straddle V-ups, Plank Splits

085.
Warm-up: KB Alternating Swings & Bear Crawls (distance)
Circuit: BB Lunges, Chin-ups, KB Push Presses
Cool-down: Reverse Crunches, Single Leg Push-ups (reps)

086.
Warm-up: Marching Knee Tucks, Bent Over Twists
Circuit: BB Toe Touch Deadlifts, Bench Dips, WP Halos, DB Seated Reverse Flyes
Cool-down: Narrow Grip Push-ups, KB Renegade Push-ups

087.
Warm-up: Air Squats & Mountain Climbers
Circuit: KB Thrusters, Parallette Push-ups, Inverted Rows
Cool-down: Parallette L-sit (hold), Hanging Trunk Twists

088.
Warm-up: Split Jacks, Supine Scorpions
Circuit: BB Shoulder Presses, DB Alternating Bicep Curls, KB Single Arm Front Squats, Box Jumps
Cool-down: KB Press Crunches, Stacked Feet Push-ups

089.
Warm-up: Lateral Leg Swings & Indian Club Shoulder Rotations
Circuit: BB Hang Cleans, DB Step-ups, Ring Push-ups, Spiderman Pull-ups
Cool-down: V-ups, Dynamic Side Planks

090.
Warm-up: Speed Skater Jumps & DB Alternating Toe Touches
Circuit: BB Back Squats, Ring Pull-ups, Cartwheel Push-ups (reps)
Cool-down: Russian Twists – Feet Elevated, Box Donkey Kicks

LINER NOTES
Appendix A

091.
Warm-up: Butt Kicks & Trunk Twists
Circuit: Jackknife Push-ups, Wide Grip Pull-ups, KB Front Squats
Cool-down: Boat Pose (hold), Revolved Chair Pose (hold)

092.
Warm-up: Med Ball Mountain Climbers & Trunk Circles
Circuit: BB Single Arm Squat Pushes, T Push-ups, KB Halos, KB Upright Rows
Cool-down: Quadruped Core Twists, Arch Hold

093.
Warm-up: Jump Rope & Sprawl
Circuit: BB Single Leg Romanian Deadlifts, WP Curl & Raises, Side Plank Leg Swings, DB Single Arm Reverse Flyes
Cool-down: Plank Side Crunches, Single Leg Glute Bridge (hold)

094.
Warm-up: Run & Burpees
Circuit: Med Ball Squat Cleans, DB Twist & Lateral Raises, BB Hold Leg Raises, Reverse Lunge with Chops
Cool-down: Plank Press-ups, SB Oblique Crunches

095.
Warm-up: Jumping Jacks & Squatting Y Raises
Circuit: BB Overhead Squats, Dive Bomber Push-ups, Ring Rows
Cool-down: Knees to Elbows, Floor Trunk Twists

096.
Warm-up: Prisoner Lunges & Trunk Twists
Circuit: BB Sumo Deadlift High Pulls, WP Truck Drivers, Jackknife Push-ups, Rotating Lunges
Cool-down: Split Leg Crunches, Hip Adduction Side Planks

097.
Warm-up: Hip Rotations & Reverse Lunge + Reaches
Circuit: BB Bent Over Rows, DB Single Arm Squats, Corkscrews
Cool-down: Butterfly Sit-ups, Russian Push-ups

098.
Warm-up: Ankle Hops & Crab Walk (distance)
Circuit: BB Deadlifts, KB Push Presses, DB Reverse Flyes
Cool-down: Pull-ups, Incline Push-ups

099.
Warm-up: Toe Taps & Kangaroo Crawls
Circuit: DB Forward Lunges, DB Alternating Rows, BB Calf Raises, DB Single Arm Tricep Kickbacks
Cool-down: SB Roll-outs, Twisting Planks

100.
Warm-up: DB Swings, Butt Scoots
Circuit: DB Thrusters, WP Single Leg Deadlifts, BB High Pulls
Cool-down: Plank Rows, Ring Tuck Hold

101.
Warm-up: Jump Rope & Horse Stance Squats
Circuit: KB Alternating Swings, DB Supported Single Arm Reverse Flyes, Box Pistols, Ring Dips
Cool-down: Hollow Rocks, Reverse Hypers

102.
Warm-up: Split Jumps & Trunk Circles
Circuit: DB Single Arm Overhead Squats, Pull-ups, Renegade Push-ups
Cool-down: Parallette Tuck Hold, Plank Up Downs

103.
Warm-up: Split Jacks & Side Crawls (distance)
Circuit: KB Snatches, Knees to Elbows, Pike Push-ups, BB Long Bar Rows
Cool-down: V-sit (hold), Prone Leg Extension (hold)

104.
Warm-up: Jump Rope & Knee Circles
Circuit: BB Bench Presses, KB Low Windmills, KB Cleans, Ring Rows
Cool-down: Overhead Weighted Sit-ups, Push-up Plusses

105.
Warm-up: Swing Squats & Bear Crawls
Circuit: KB Goblet Squats, Resisted Split Jumps, KB Halos, DB Single Arm Skull Crushers
Cool-down: SB Oblique Crunches, 3-point Plank on Elbows

106.
Warm-up: Twisting Lunges & Squat Jumps
Circuit: BB Front Squats, Ring Dips, Parallette Straddle L-sit (hold), Commando Pull-ups
Cool-down: Uneven Push-ups (reps), Crunches

LINER NOTES
Appendix A

107.
Warm-up: Jumping Jacks & Trunk Twists
Circuit: BB Deadlifts, KB Side Presses, Chin-ups
Cool-down: Narrow Grip Push-ups, Dynamic Side V-sits

108. Warm-up: High Stepping & Med Ball Trunk Twists
Circuit: BB Single Leg Romanian Deadlifts, Inverted Rows, Burpees
Cool-down: Plank Side Crunches, V-ups

109.
Warm-up: Split Jumps & Squat Rotations
Circuit: BB Bulgarian Split Squats, DB Concentration Curls, DB Single Arm Shoulder Presses, Ring L-sit
Cool-down: Toe Touch Crunches, Shoulder Tap Push-ups

110.
Warm-up: Squat Kicks & SB Mountain Climbers
Circuit: BB Toe Touch Deadlifts, DB Single Arm Preacher Curls, Parallette Push-ups, DB Lateral Raise & External Rotations
Cool-down: Dynamic Side Planks, Twisting Supermans

111.
Warm-up: Jump Rope & Trunk Circles
Circuit: BB Back Squats, Pull-ups, DB Diagonal Shoulder Presses, Quadruped Core Twists
Cool-down: Hollow Rocks, Side Plank & Leg Lift (hold)

Appendix B
EXERCISE PROGRESSIONS

These progressions are suggestions only. Your baseline mobility or strength could make a more "advanced" movement seem easier than its predecessor. Proceed with an open mind.

Squat Progression

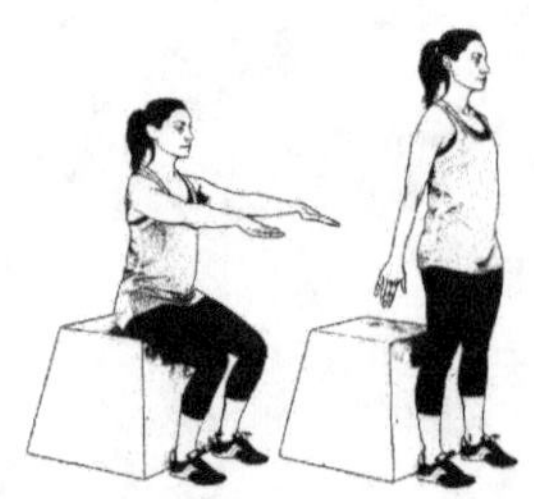

1.

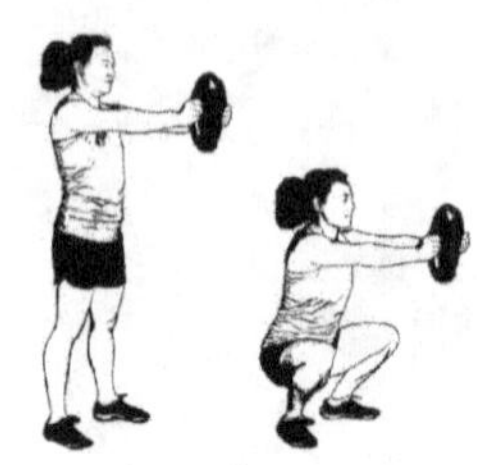

2.

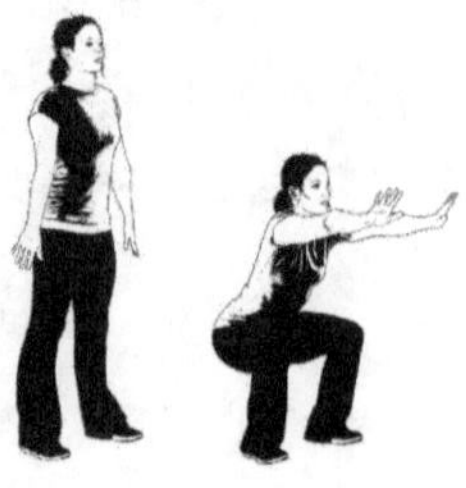

3.

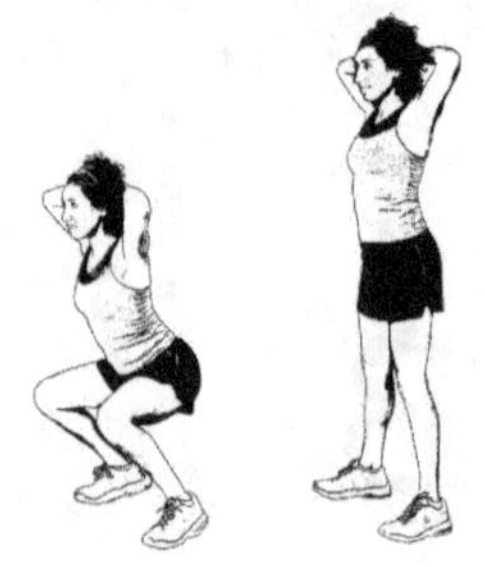

4.

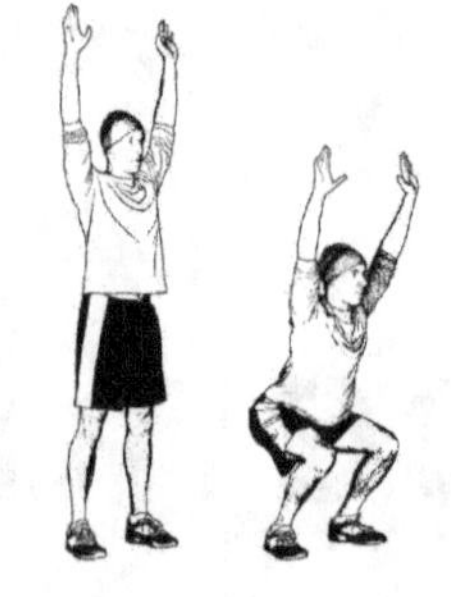

5.

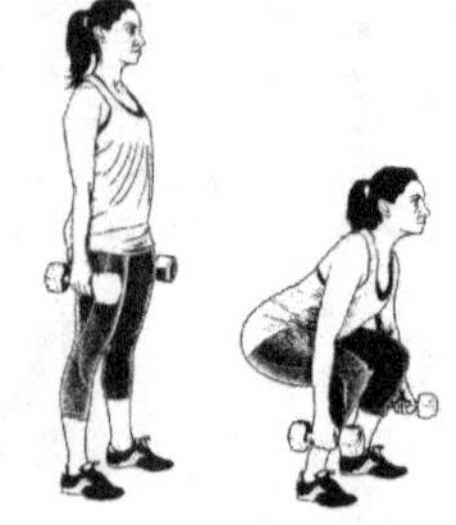

6.

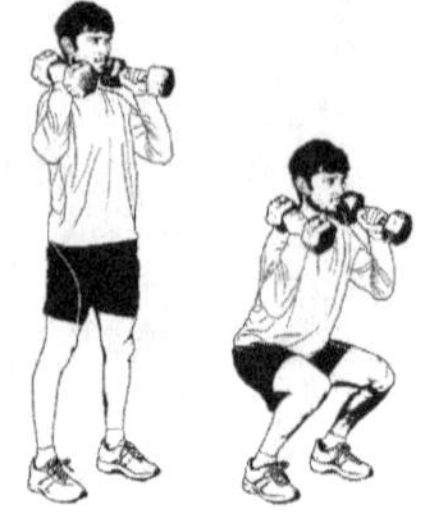

7.

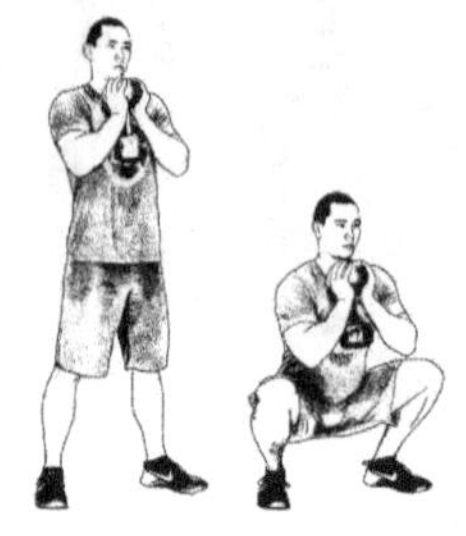

8.

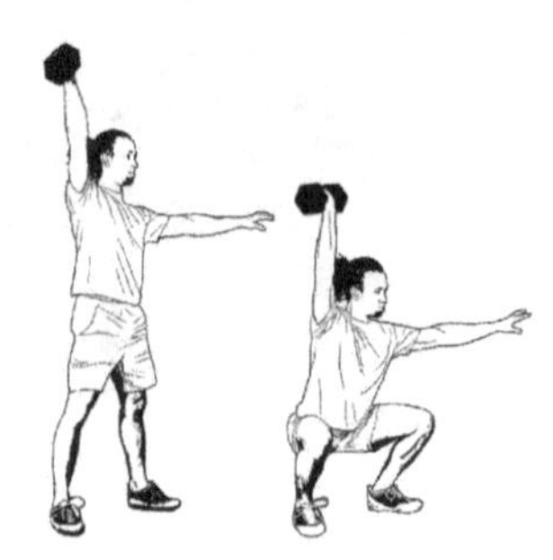

9.

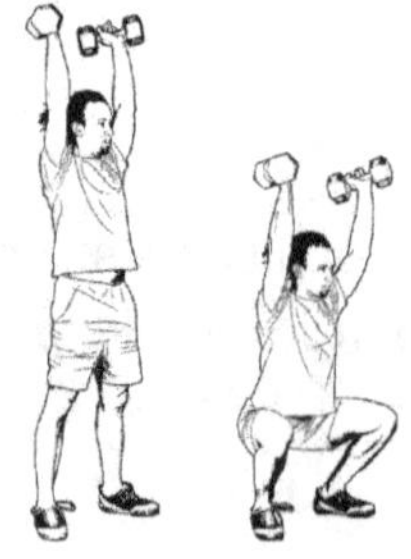

10.

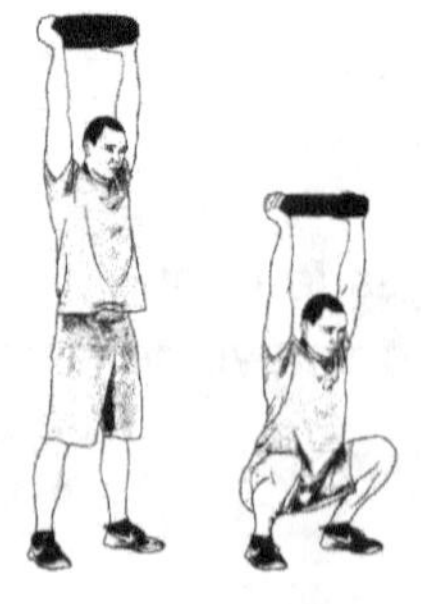

11.

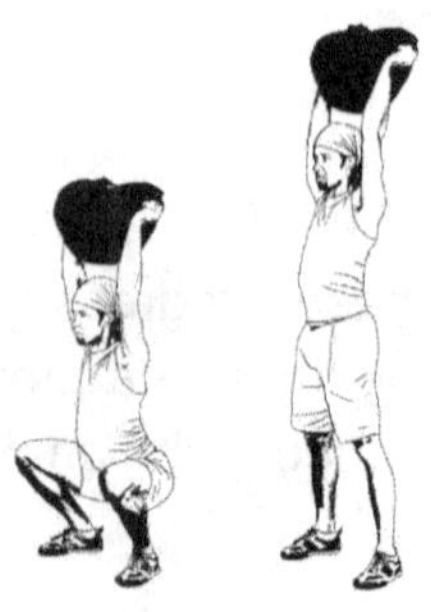

12.

Pistol Progression

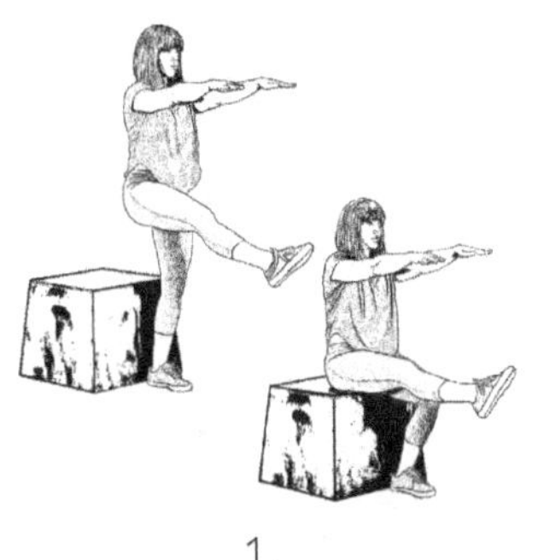

1.

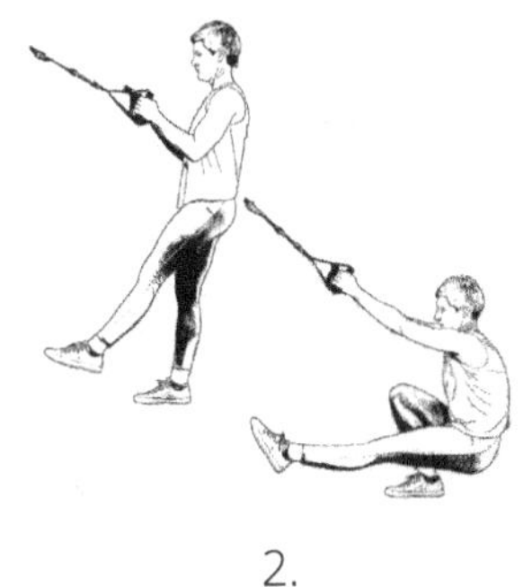

2.

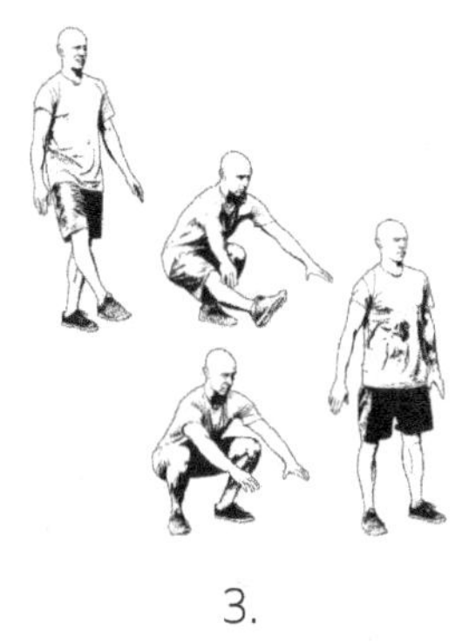

3.

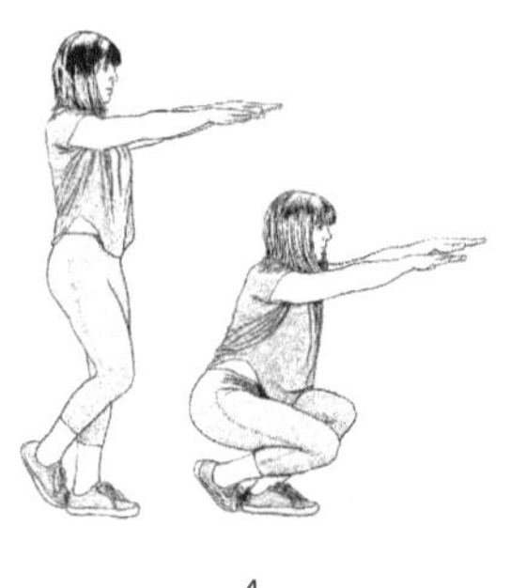

4.

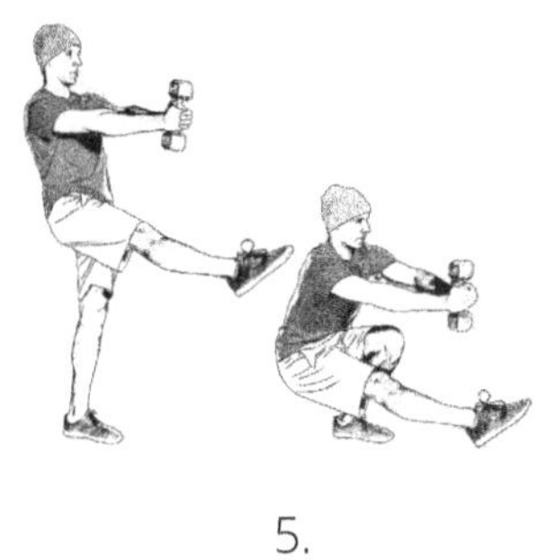

5.

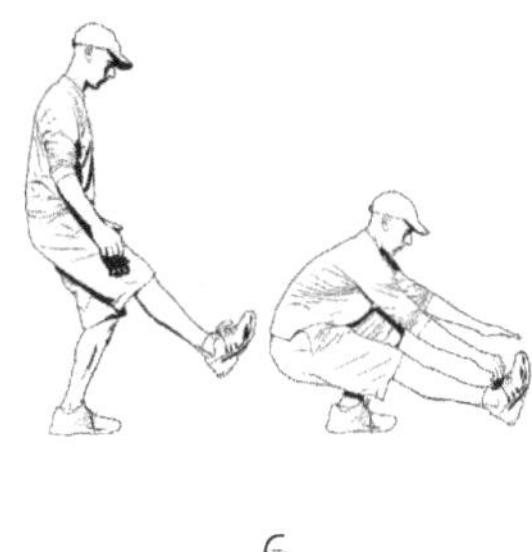

6.

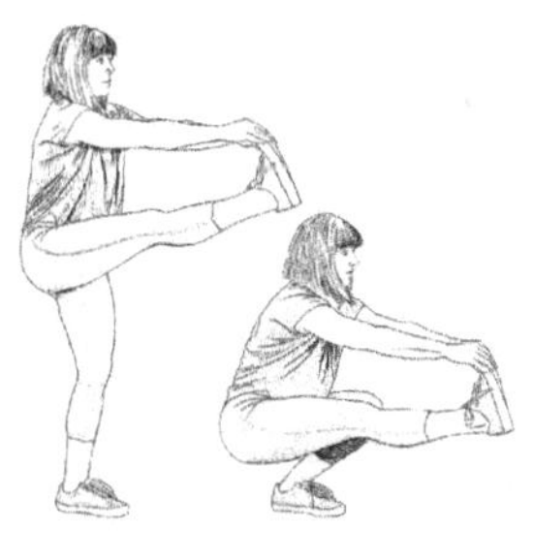

7.

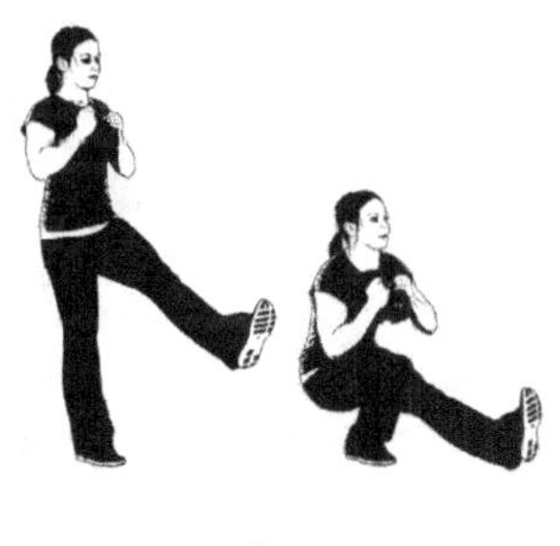

8.

Liner Notes
Appendix B

Push-up Progression

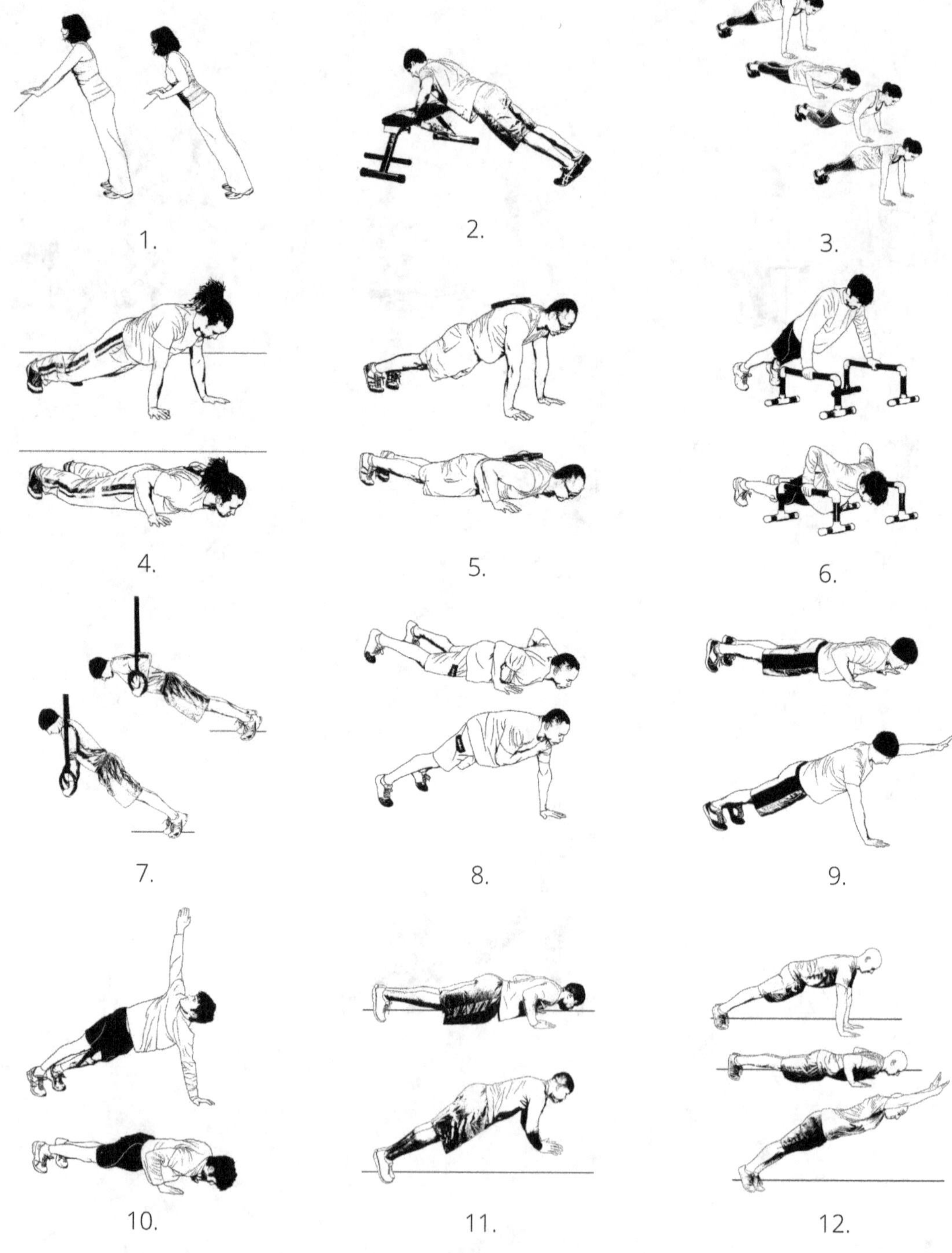

1.

2.

3.

4.

5.

6.

7.

8.

9.

10.

11.

12.

LINER NOTES
Appendix B

Pull-up Progression

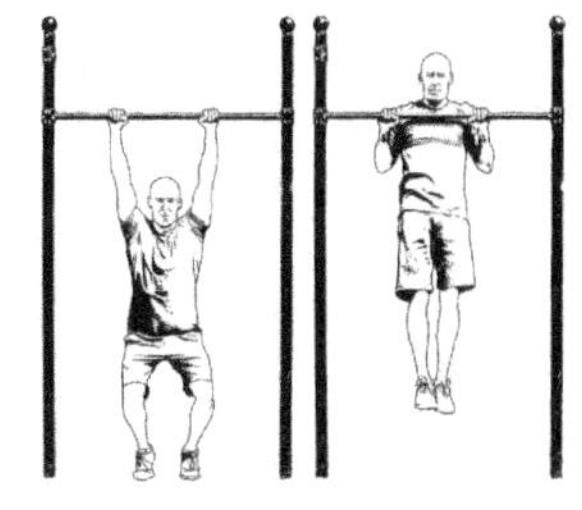

1.

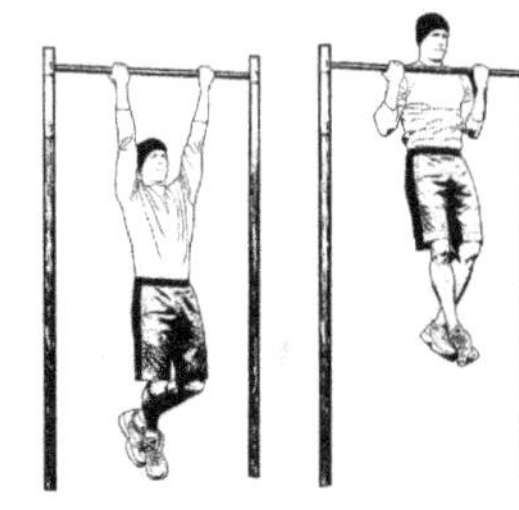

2.

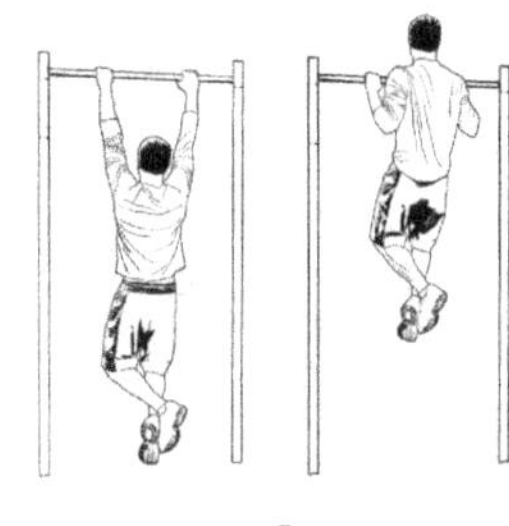

3.

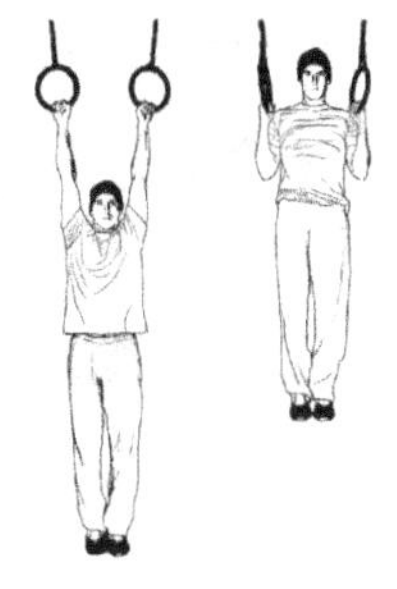

4.

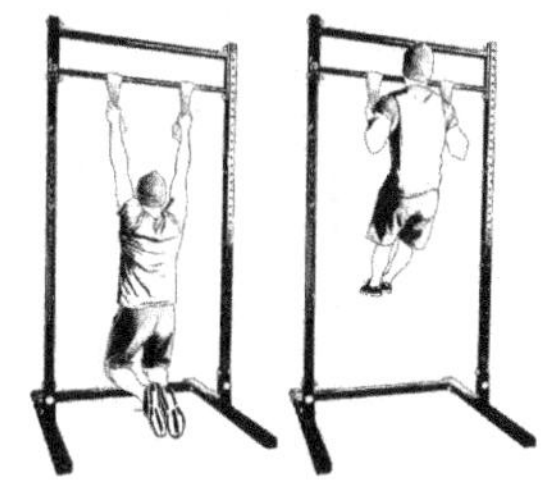

5.

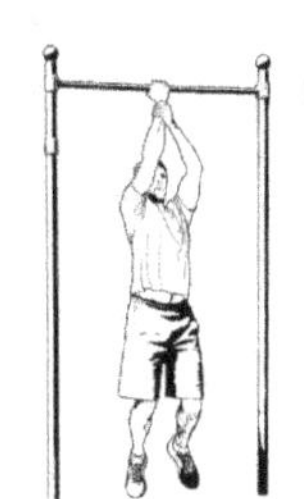

6.

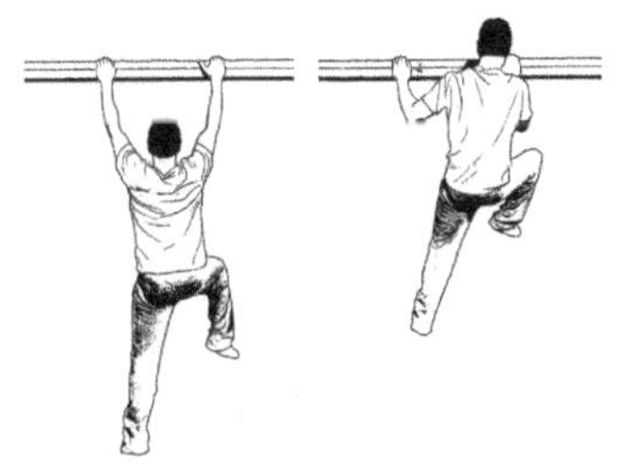

7.

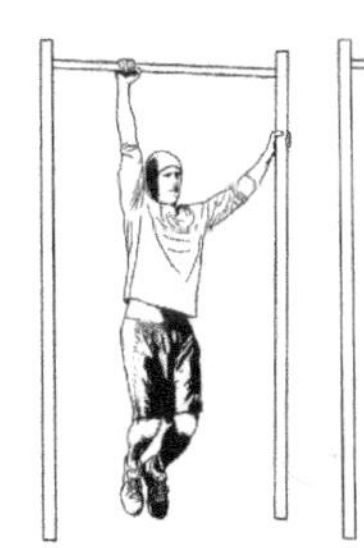

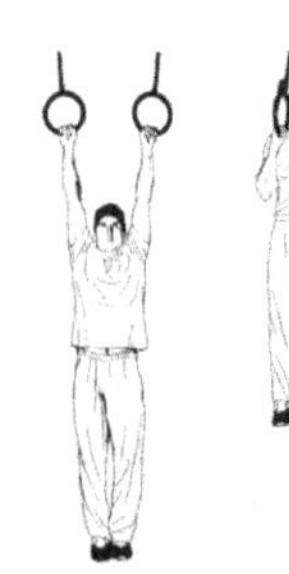

8.

9.

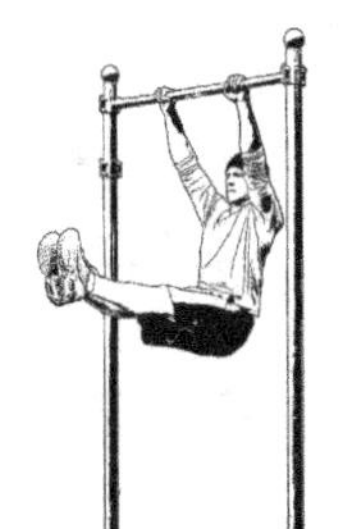
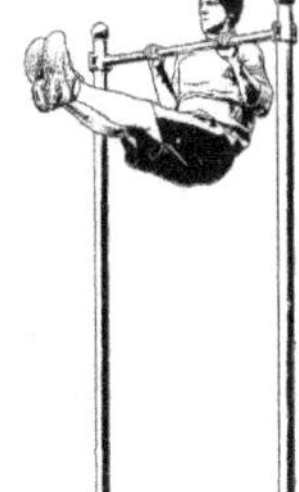

10.

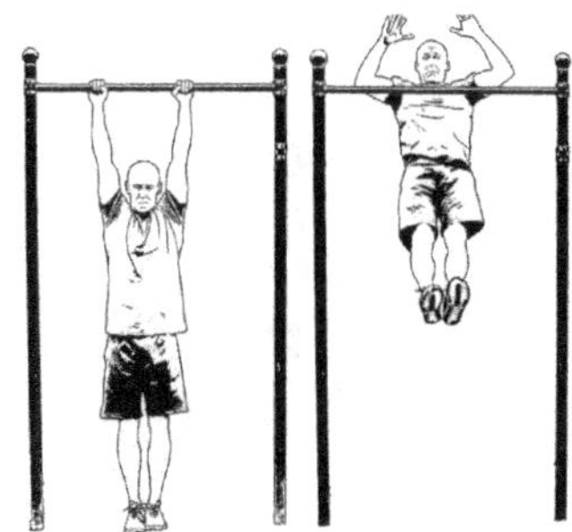

11.

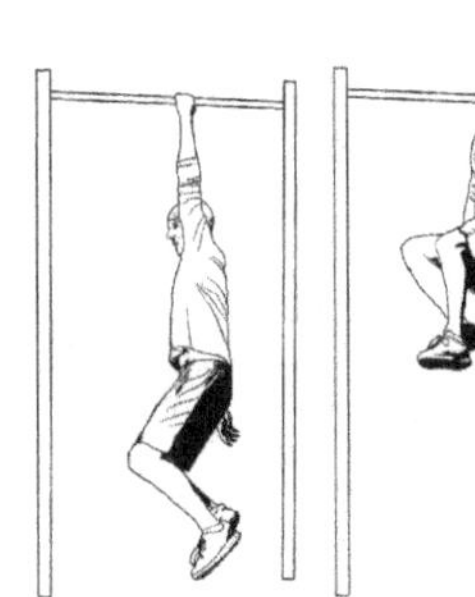

12.

LINER NOTES
Appendix B

Leg Raise Progression

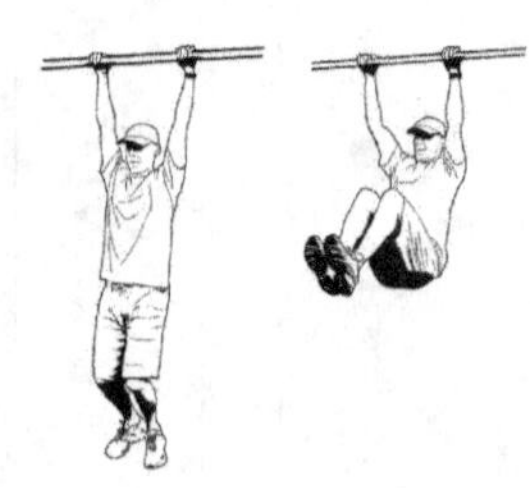

1.

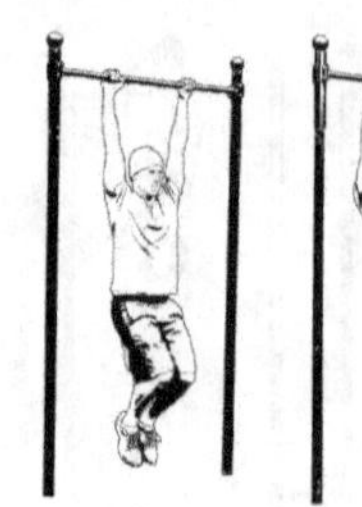

2.

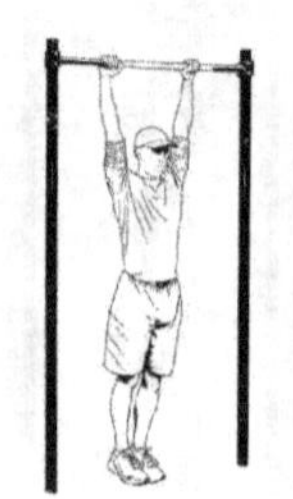

3.

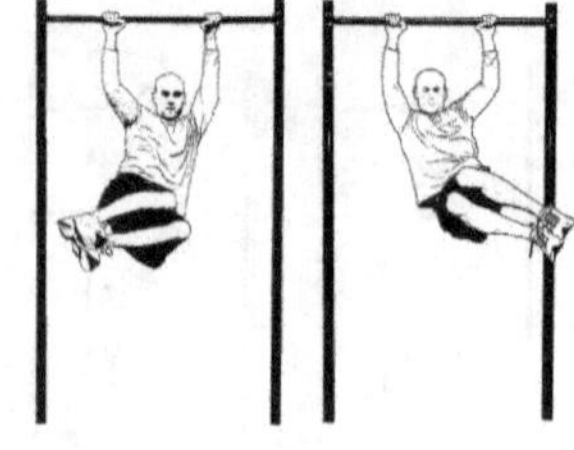

4.

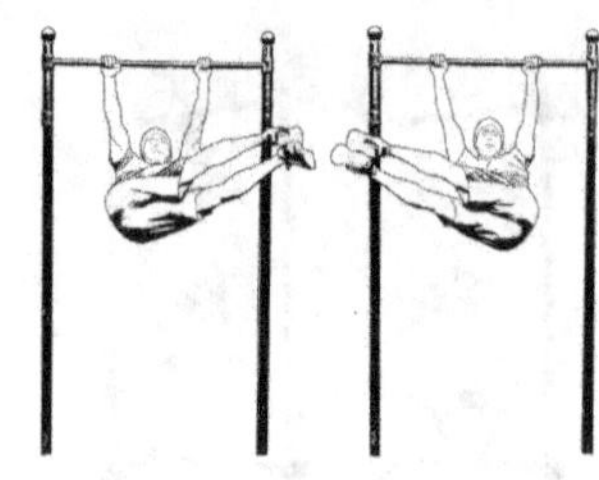

5.

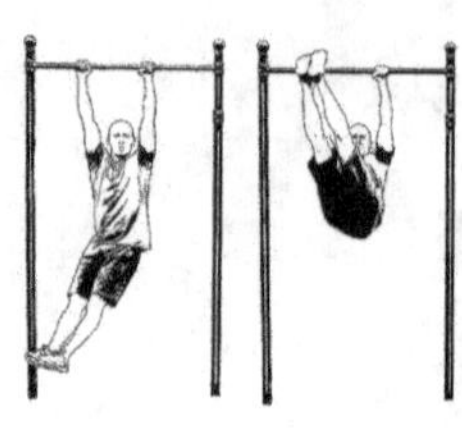

6.

V-sit Progression

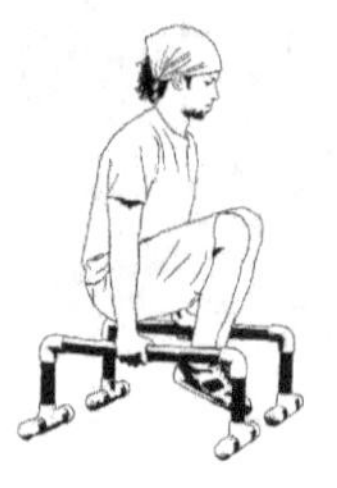

1.

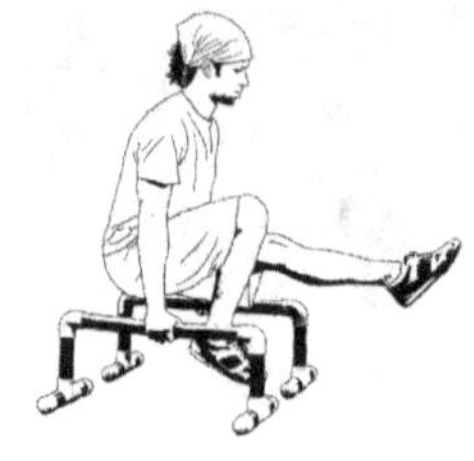

2.

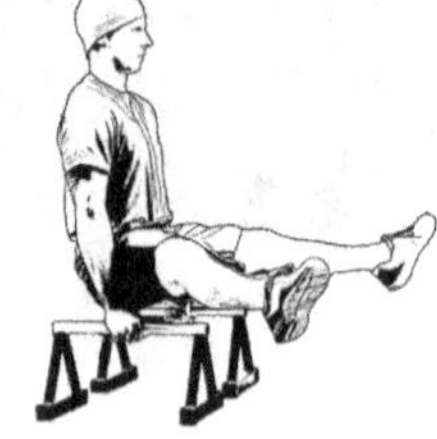

3.

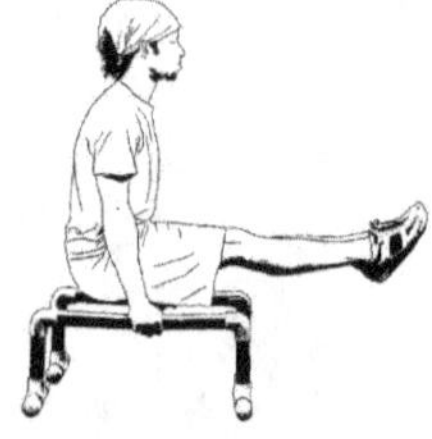

4.

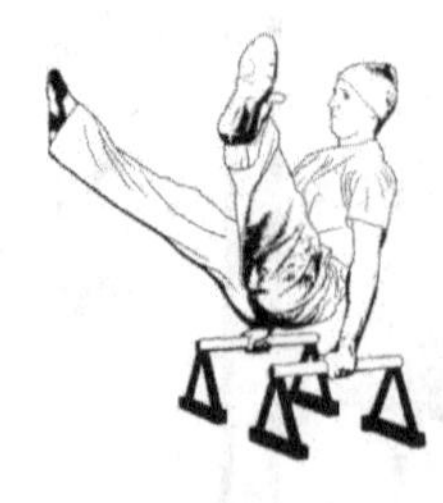

5.

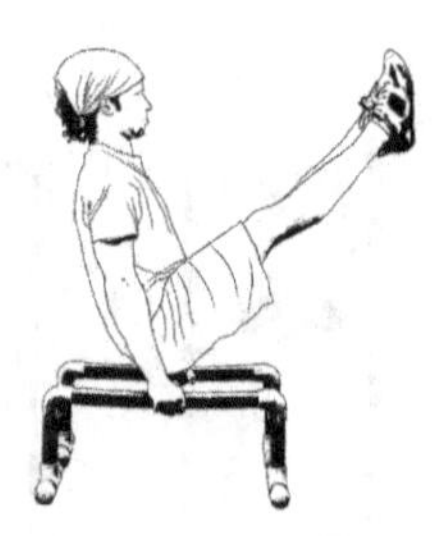

6.

LINER NOTES
Appendix B

Handstand Push-up Progression

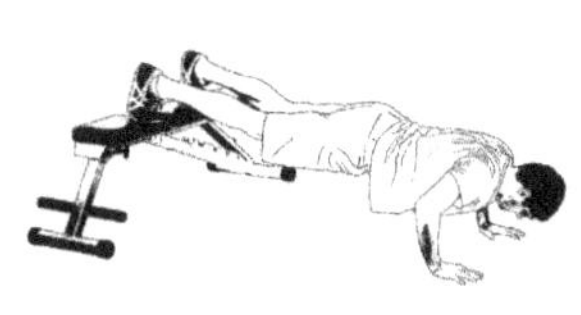

1.

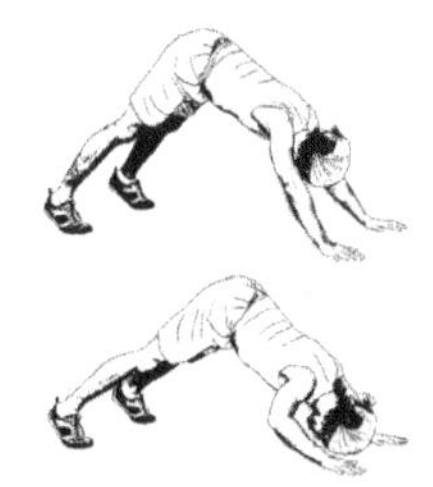

2.

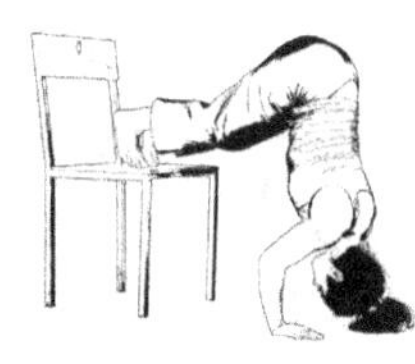

3.

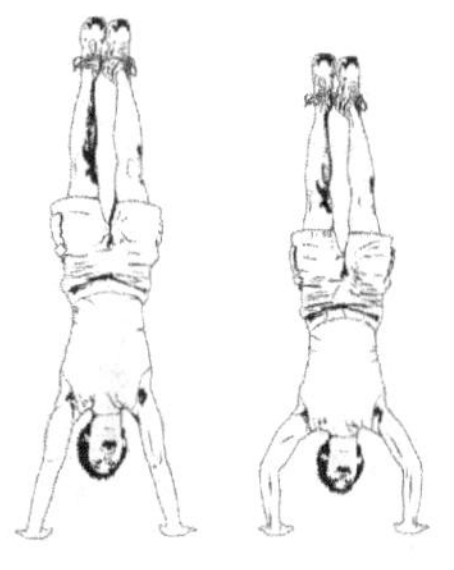

4.

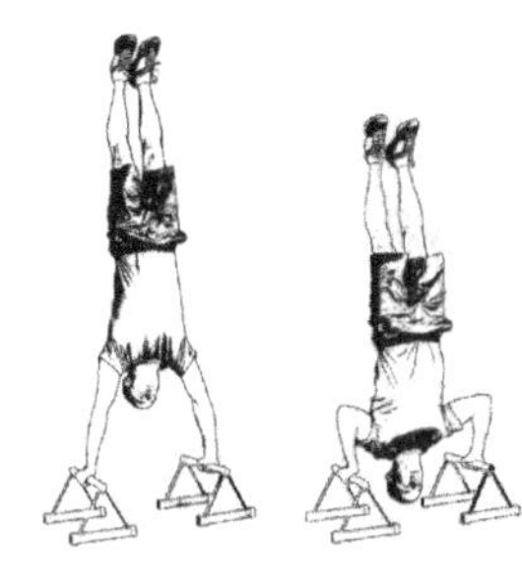

5.

Plank Progression

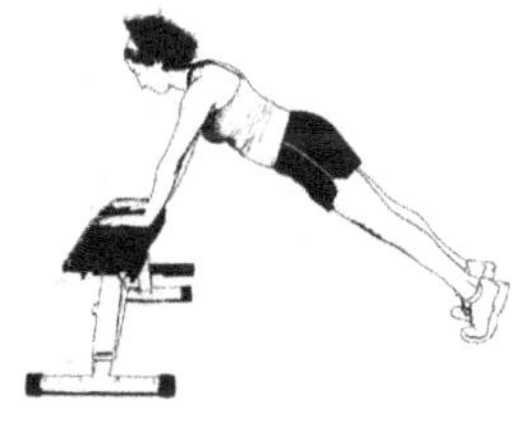

1.

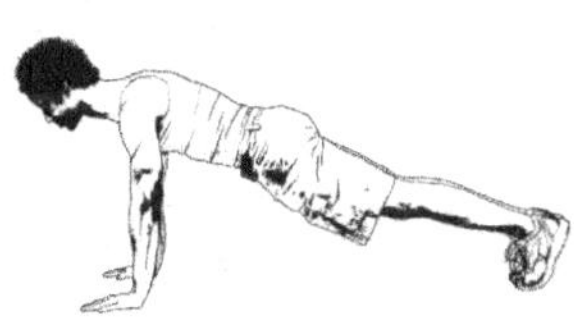

2.

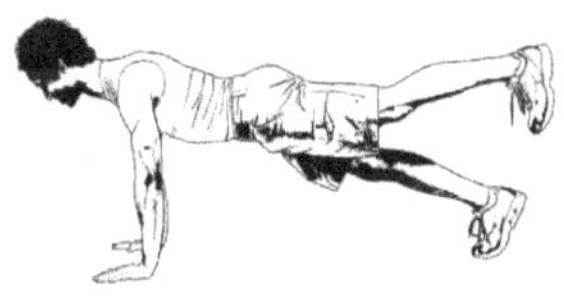

3.

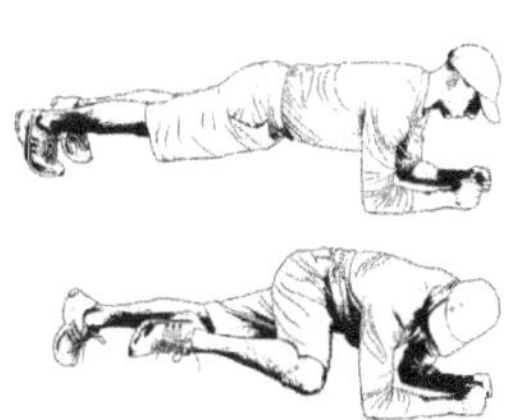

4.

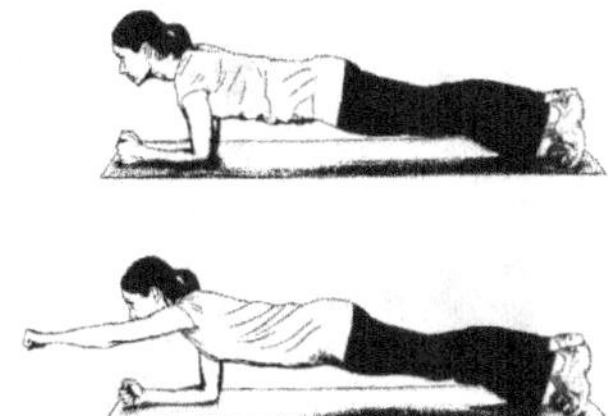

5.

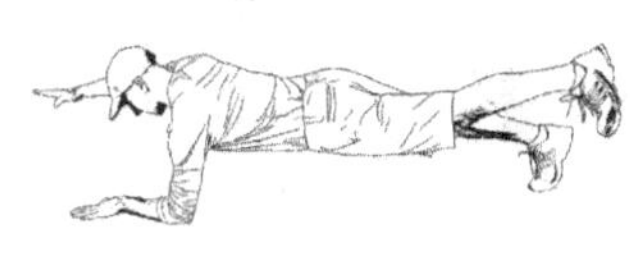

6.

LINER NOTES
Appendix B

Barbell Squat Progression

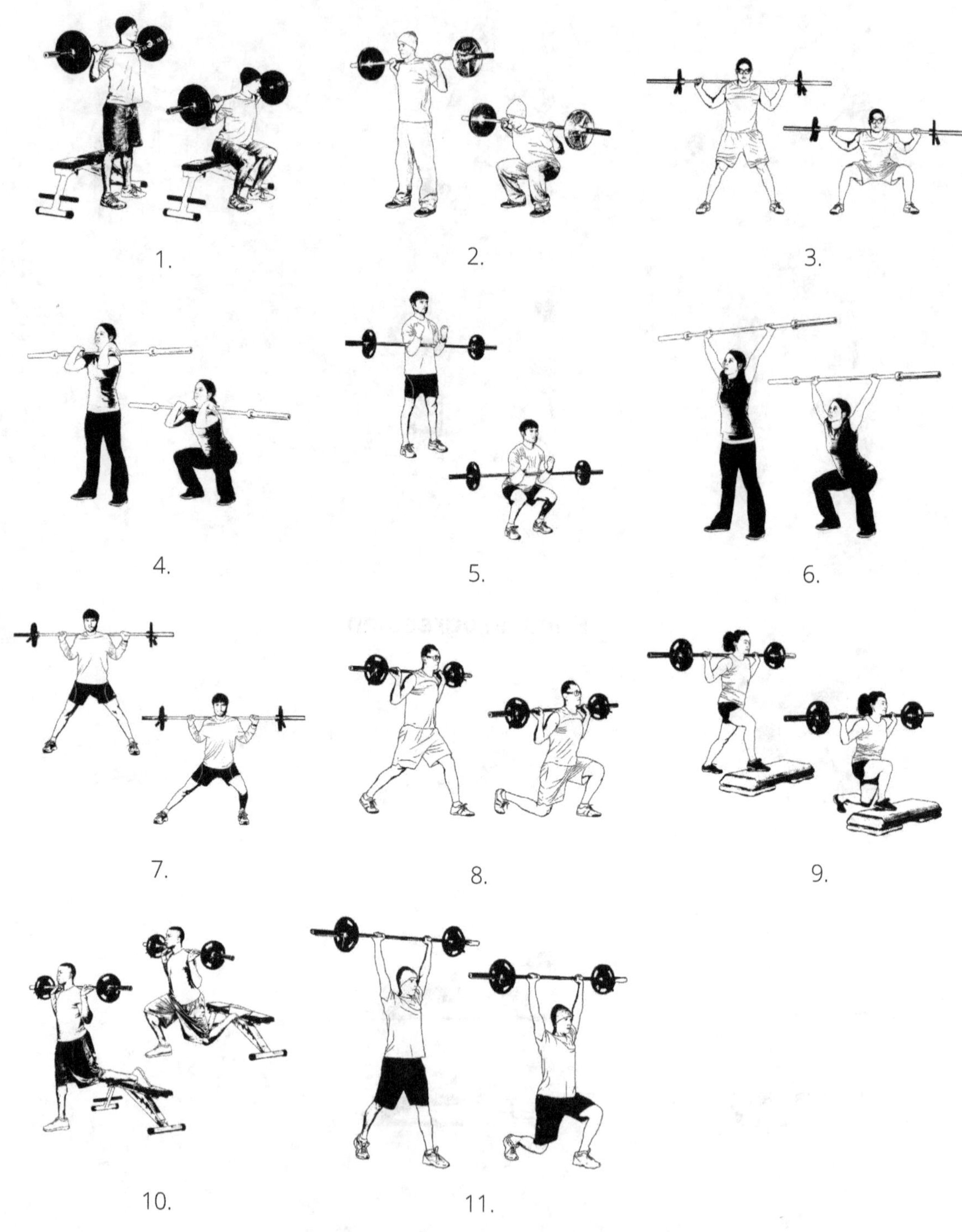

1.

2.

3.

4.

5.

6.

7.

8.

9.

10.

11.

AB-07

LINER NOTES
Appendix B

Deadlift Progression

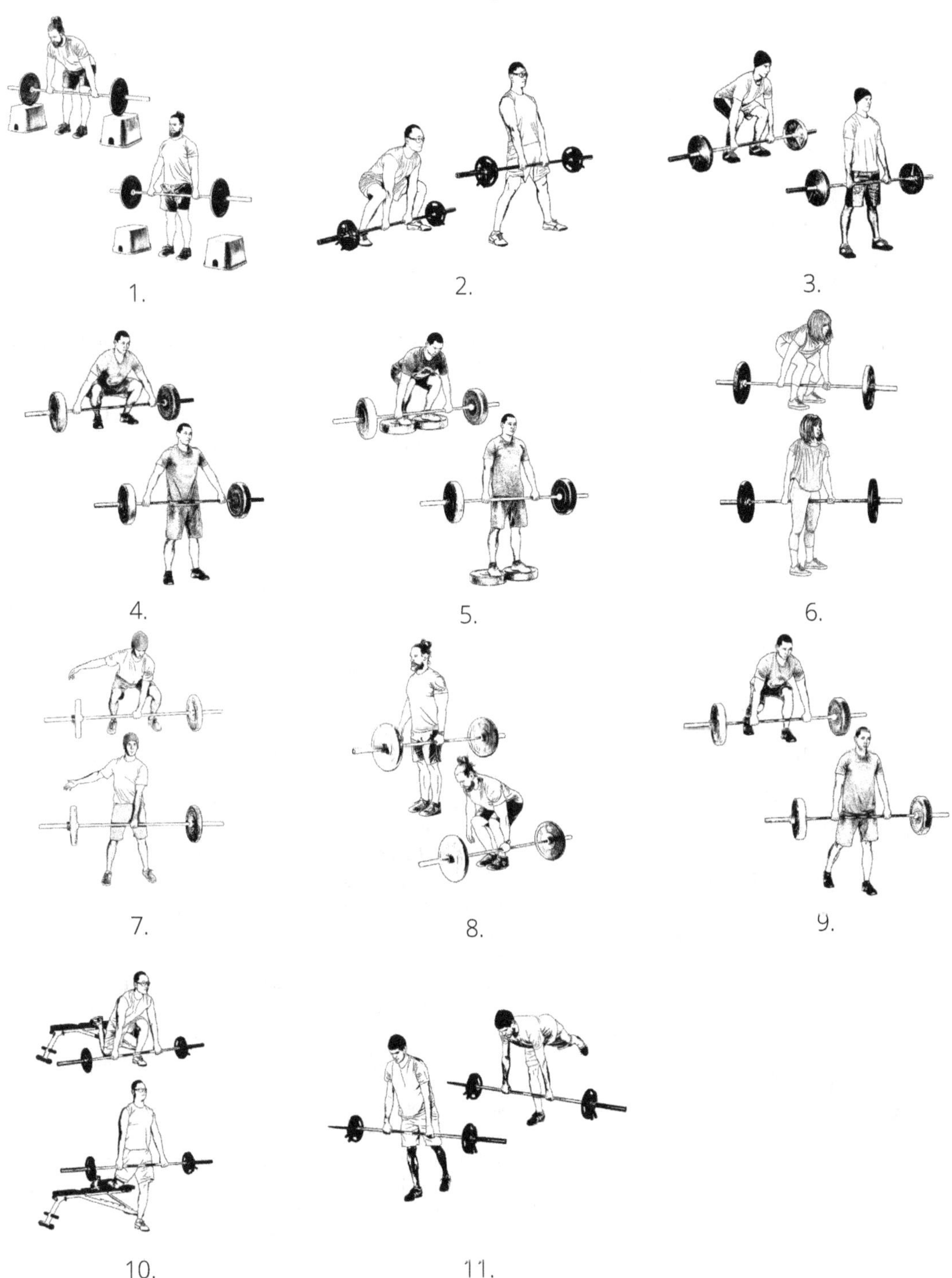

More books by this publisher

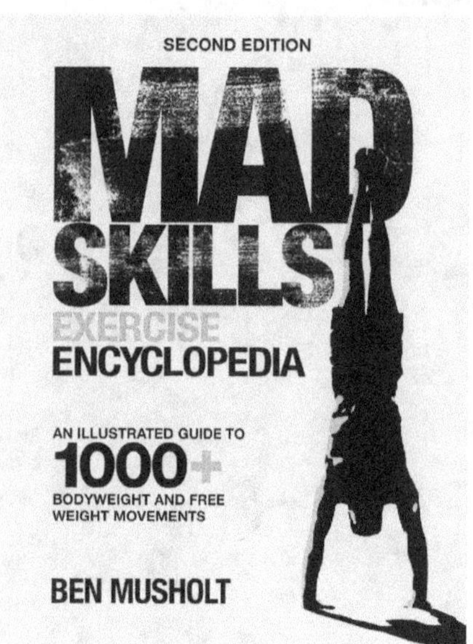

Are you hungry for more variety in your training?
Do you want to become a more well-rounded athlete?

Get ready because **Mad Skills** will help you:
- Warm-up before a training session
- Master bodyweight and calisthenics-type exercises
- Learn classic weight lifting techniques
- Build strength with barbell and kettlebell lifts
- Challenge yourself with whole body movements
- Incorporate single arm and double leg drills
- Fashion a rock-solid core for better athletic performance
- Improve your mobility with yoga postures and stretching variations.
- Have fun with partner-based skills
- Design killer at-home and garage gym workouts
- Never be boerd with fitness again!

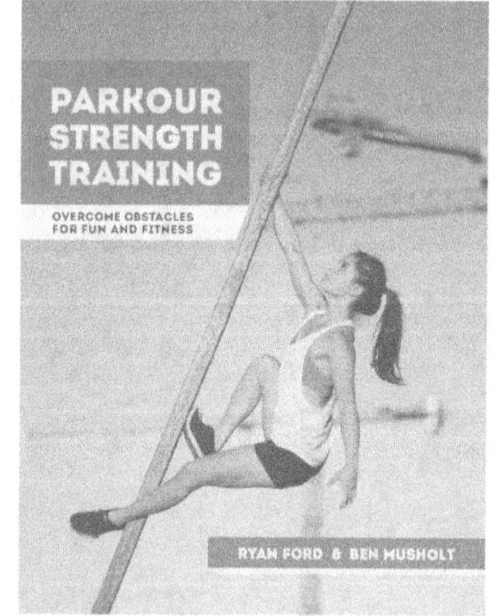

In **Parkour Strength Training,** you will learn how to:
• Accelerate your athletic development with three fundamental bodyweight exercises
• Promote the flexibility and mobility necessary for safe obstacle-based fitness
• Prepare and condition your joints to avoid injuries
• Train safely outdoors
• Remedy the common faults and errors that plague parkour newcomers
• Incorporate ground-based exercises, such as quadrupedal movement, bounding, and jumping into your workouts
• Use low obstacles such as benches, handrails, and walls for full-body strength training
• Fly over barriers using three basic vaults
• Mount, traverse, and overcome head-high walls and bar structures
• Master proper climb-up technique using many supplemental exercises
• Design an effective strength training program
• Combine skill-based drills and games to become a more well-rounded practitioner
• Dominate obstacle courses

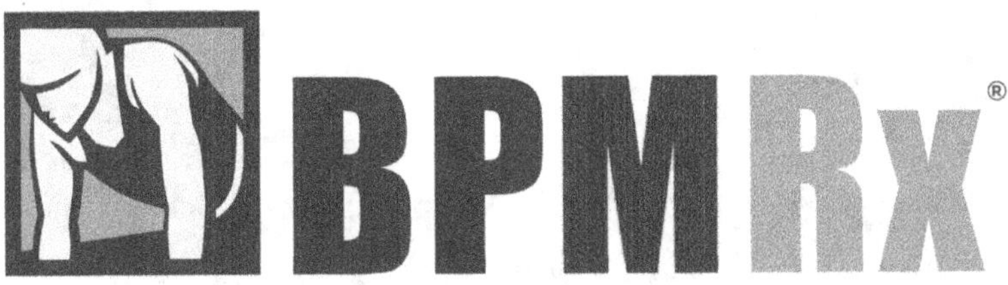

Do you prescribe exercise for a living?

Would you like to use the images in this book with your clientele?

Head over to:

www.BPMRx.com

Start giving your clients high-quality exercise handouts built from the BPM Rx image library!

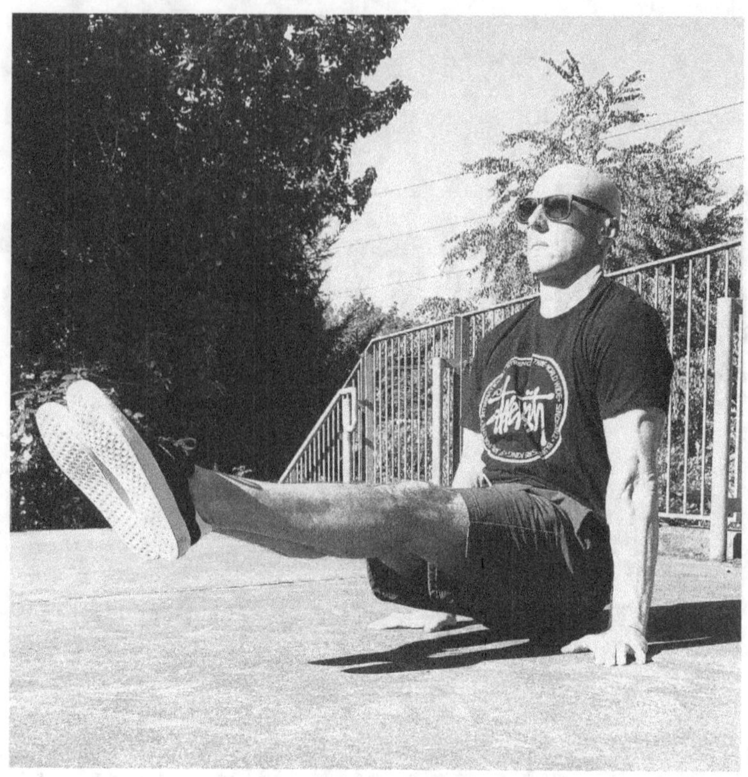

Ben Musholt is an athlete and physical therapist in Portland, Oregon. He co-authored Parkour Strength Training in 2016, and he first published the Mad Skills Exercise Encyclopedia in 2013. When not coaching or helping his clients move better, he can be found exploring the Pacific Northwest wonderland.

His goal is to do 3 fun physical activities per day.
Good luck keeping up!

www.BenMusholt.com

Instagram: @benmusholt
Facebook: madskillsbook